Response and Adaptation
to Hypoxia

CLINICAL PHYSIOLOGY SERIES

Response and Adaptation to Hypoxia
Organ to Organelle

EDITED BY Sukhamay Lahiri
Department of Physiology
University of Pennsylvania
School of Medicine
Philadelphia, Pennsylvania

Neil S. Cherniack
Department of Medicine
Case Western Reserve University
and University Hospitals of Cleveland
Cleveland, Ohio

Robert S. Fitzgerald
Departments of Environmental Health
  Sciences and of Physiology
The Johns Hopkins Medical Institutions
Baltimore, Maryland

New York   Oxford
Published for the American Physiological Society
by Oxford University Press
1991

Oxford University Press

Oxford   New York   Toronto
Delhi   Bombay   Calcutta   Madras   Karachi
Petaling Jaya   Singapore   Hong Kong   Tokyo
Nairobi   Dar es Salaam   Cape Town
Melbourne   Auckland

and associated companies in
Berlin   Ibadan

Copyright © 1991 by the American Physiological Society

Published for the American Physiological Society by
Oxford University Press, 200 Madison Avenue, New York, New York 10016

Oxford is a registered trademark of Oxford University Press

Library of Congress Cataloging-in-Publication Data
Response and adaptation to hypoxia : organ to organelle / edited by
Sukhamay Lahiri, Neil S. Cherniack, Robert S. Fitzgerald.
   p.   cm.   (The American Physiological Society series in clinical physiology)
Based on two meetings sponsored by the American Physiological
Society and the Federation of American Societies for Experimental
Biology.
Includes bibliographical references.   Includes index.   ISBN 0-19-506244-2
1. Anoxemia—Congresses.   2. Anoxemia—Molecular aspects— Congresses.
3. Oxygen—Physiological effect—Congresses.
4. Adaptation (Physiology)—Congresses.
5. Chemoreceptors— Physiological effect—Congresses.   I. Lahiri, Sukhamay.
II. Cherniack, Neil S.   III. Fitzgerald, Robert S., 1931–
IV. American Physiological Society (1887–   )
V. Federation of American Societies for Experimental Biology.   VI. Series.
[DNLM: 1. Adaptation, physiology.   2. Cell Hypoxia—congresses.
3. Chemoreceptors—physiology—congresses.
4. Erythropoietin— Physiology—congresses.
5. Mitochondria—physiology—congresses.
6. Oxygen—physiology—congresses.   QA 312 R434]
RB150.A67R47   1991   616.2—dc20
DNLM/DLC   for Library of Congress   90-14241

9 8 7 6 5 4 3 2 1

Printed in the United States of America
on acid-free paper

Preface

The underlying theme of this book is the biology of oxygen. The 22 chapters cover aspects of molecular, cellular, and integrative physiological functions. A fundamental evolutionary feature of the oxygen-consuming organism is that it developed a oxygen-sensing mechanism as a part of feedback control at the levels of molecules, organelles, organs, and systems. Oxygen sensing is particularly expressed in certain specific cells and tissues like peripheral chemoreceptors, erythroprotein-producing cells, and vascular smooth muscle. A part of the book is focused on the current issues of this basic question of chemosensing. Mitrochondria as the major site for cellular oxygen consumption is a natural candidate for cellular oxygen sensitivity and adaptation. A section deals with this question. A perennial question concerns chronic environmental oxygen and the organism's response and adaptation to it. This theme runs through several chapters. Because comparative physiology often provides insight into the mechanisms of environmental adaptation, a chapter on respiration of high altitude birds has been incorporated. Obviously this book gives only glimpses of the immense field of oxygen biology.

The book grew out of two meetings where these subjects were discussed. These meetings were sponsored by the American Physiological Society and the Federation of American Societies for Experimental Biology. We are grateful to the FASEB Program Committee and APS publication committee for their support. We owe much to Ms. Anne Miller for her editorial assistance.

Philadelphia   *S. L.*
Cleveland   *N. S .C.*
Baltimore   *R. S. F.*
January, 1990

Contents

IV. OXYGEN BIOLOGY OF ADAPTATION

Contributors

Allen, P. S.
*Department of Applied Physics
   in Medicine*
University of Alberta
Edmonton, Alberta
Canada

Anand, A.
*DST Centre for Visceral
   Mechanisms*
V. Patel Chest Institute
Delhi University
Delhi, India

Aw, T. Y.
*Department of Biochemistry and Winship
   Cancer Center*
Emory University School of Medicine
Atlanta, GA

Bai, C.
*Department of Biochemistry and Winship
   Cancer Center*
Emory University School of Medicine
Atlanta, GA

Bariety, J.
INSERM U 28
Hôpital Broussais
Paris, France

Beckman, B.
Department of Pharmacology
Tulane University
School of Medicine
New Orleans, LA

Bernstein, M. H.
Department of Biology
New Mexico State University
Las Cruces, NM

Bruneval, P.
INSERM U 28
Hôpital Broussais
Paris, France

Camilleri, J. P.
INSERM U 28
Hôpital Broussaids
Paris, France

Caro, J.
Department of Medicine
Thomas Jefferson University
Philadelphia, PA

Cerretelli, P.
Department of Physiology
University of Geneva School of Medicine
Geneva, Switzerland

Cherniack, N. S.
Department of Medicine
*Case Western Reserve University and
   University Hospital*
Cleveland, OH

Chesne, C.
INSERM U 49
Hôpital de Pontchaillou
Rennes, France

Da Silva, J. L.
INSERM U 28
Hôpital Broussais
Paris, France

Dehghani, G. A.
*Department of Environmental
   Health Sciences*
The Johns Hopkins Medical Institutions
Baltimore, MD

Edelman, N. H.
Department of Medicine
*University of Medicine and Dentistry of
   New Jersey*
Robert Wood Johnson Medical School
Piscataway, NJ

Farber, H. W.
School of Medicine Pulmonary Center
Boston University
Boston, MA

Fisher, J. W.
Department of Pharmacology
Tulane University
School of Medicine
New Orleans, LA

Fitzgerald, R. S.
Department of Environmental
    Health Sciences
The Johns Hopkins Medical Institutions
Baltimore, MD

Fraij, B.
Department of Medicine
Jefferson Medical College
Philadelphia, PA

Guillouzo, A.
INSERM U 49
Hopital de Fontchaillou
Rennes, France

Haxhiu, M. A.
Department of Medicine
Case Western Reserve University and
    University Hospital
Cleveland, OH

Hochachka, P. W.
Department of Zoology and Sports
    Medicine Division
University of British Columbia
Vancouver, British Columbia
Canada

Hoppeler, H.
Department of Anatomy
University of Berne
Berne, Switzerland

Jelkmann, W.
Department of Physiology
Medical University of Luebeck
Luebeck, Germany

Jones, D. P.
Department of Biochemistry and Winship
    Cancer Center
Emory University School of Medicine
Atlanta, GA

Jones, R.
Department of Medicine
University of Alberta
Edmonton, Alberta
Canada

Katz, D. M.
Department of Medicine and Center
    for Neuroscience
Case Western Reserve University School
    of Medicine
Cleveland, OH

Kayser, B.
Department of Physiology
University of Geneva School of Medicine
Geneva, Switzerland

Lacombe, C.
INSERM U 152
Hôpital Cochin
Paris, France

Lahiri, S.
Department of Physiology
University of Pennsylvania School
    of Medicine
Philadelphia, PA

Man, S. F. P.
Department of Medicine
University of Alberta
Edmonton, Alberta
Canada

Matheson, G. O.
Department of Zoology and Sports
    Medicine Division
University of British Columbia
Vancouver, British Columbia
Canada

Mathieu-Costello, O.
Department of Medicine
University of California
School of Medicine
San Diego, CA

McKenzie, D. C.
Department of Zoology and Sports
    Medicine Division
University of British Columbia
Vancouver, British Columbia
Canada

Melton, J. E.
Department of Medicine
University of Medicine and Dentistry of
    New Jersey
Robert Wood Johnson Medical School
Piscataway, NJ

Merkt, J.
Concord Field Station
Harvard University
Bradford, MA

Monge, C.
Department of Physiology
University of Peruana
Cayetano Heredia,
Lima, Peru

Nakashima, J.
Department of Pharmacology
Tulane University
School of Medicine
New Orleans, LA

Neubauer, J. A.
Department of Medicine
University of Medicine and Dentistry of
New Jersey
Robert Wood Johnson Medical School
Piscataway, NJ

Pagel, H.
Department of Physiology
Medical University of Luebeck
Luebeck, Germany

Paintal, A. S.
DST Centre for Visceral Mechanisms
V. Patel Chest Institute
Delhi University
Delhi, India

Parkhouse, W. S.
Department of Kinsiology
Simon Fraser University
Burnaby, British Columbia
Canada

Pette, D.
Department of Physiology
University of Geneva School of Medicine
Geneva, Switzerland

Prabhakar, N.
Department of Medicine
Case Western Reserve University and
University Hospital
Cleveland, OH

Raff, H.
Department of Medicine
Medical College of Wisconsin
Milwaukee, WI

Ramirez, S.
Department of Medicine
Jefferson Medical College
Philadelphia, PA

Rumsey, L.
Department of Biochemistry
and Biophysics
University of Pennsylvania
Medical School
Philadelphia, PA

Runold, M.
Department of Medicine
Case Western Reserve University and
University Hospital
Cleveland, OH

Schuster, S. J.
Department of Medicine
Thomas Jefferson University
Philadelphia, PA

Sham, J. S. K.
Department of Environmental
Health Sciences
The Johns Hopkins Medical Institutions
Baltimore, MD

Shirahata, M.
Department of Environmental
Health Sciences
The Johns Hopkins Medical Institutions
Baltimore, MD

Sillau, A.
Department of Physiology
University of Puerto Rico
School of Medicine
Puerto Rico

Stanley, C.
Department of Zoology and Sports
Medicine Division
University of British Columbia
Vancouver, British Columbia
Canada

Sumar-Kalinowski, J.
Veterinary Research Station
San Marcos University
La Raya, Peru

Tambourin, P.
INSERM U 152
Hôpital Cochin
Paris, France

Ueno, M.
Department of Pharmacology
Tulane University
School of Medicine
New Orleans, LA

I

MITOCHONDRIAL RESPONSE
AND ADAPTATION TO HYPOXIA

1

Respiratory System Adaptation to Hypoxia: Lung to Mitochondria

EWALD R. WEIBEL AND HANS HOPPELER

EWALD R. WEIBEL AND HANS HOPPELER

THE RESPIRATORY SYSTEM: A CONCEPT FOR
STRUCTURE–FUNCTION CORRELATION

The delivery of O_2 from the atmosphere to the mitochondria is determined by
an orderly sequence of functions that are associated with a sequence of structures, from the lung through the circulation of the blood to the mitochondria,
as in muscle cells. This constitutes an integral respiratory system, and one
may postulate that the structures and functions involved are set up in a balanced fashion, specifically that they are designed to serve the supply of O_2 and
the removal of CO_2 according to the energetic needs of the organism, taking
into account the prevailing boundary conditions. Among the latter, ambient
Po_2 plays a major role as the overall driving force for O_2 flow to the mitochondria. The question, therefore, arises how this system copes with a reduction in
this driving force as it occurs in hypoxia.

   Our own work has been based on the hypothesis that the structural design
of the respiratory system is not wasteful. We consider structural parameters
to be the primary candidates as potential limiting factors for physiological regulation, the reason being that regulating structures to functional demand is a
slow and costly process that requires morphogenesis. On the basis of these
arguments, we have formulated the hypothesis of symmorphosis, defining it
as the state of structural design commensurate to functional needs, resulting
from regulated morphogenesis (32). This hypothesis predicts that each part of
the system is matched to all others and to the limit of aerobic performance of
the entire system, considering the prevailing boundary conditions.

   If the boundary conditions, that is, the energetic needs or the prevailing
Po_2, are varied, then we would expect the system components at each level to
become adapted to the new conditions, and this could concern either structural
or functional parameters, or both (28). Symmorphosis would predict that these
changes should occur in a balanced fashion.

MODELS OF THE RESPIRATORY SYSTEM

The model of Fig. 1.1 shows an attempt to structure the respiratory system
into a sequence of steps of O_2 flow. On the one hand these steps are related to
the sequence of structures or compartments that connect the mitochondria to

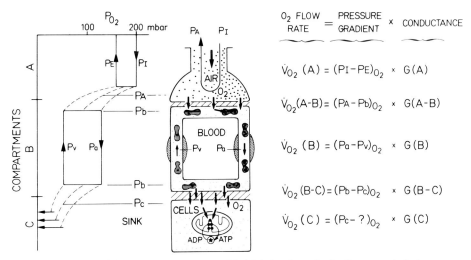

FIGURE 1.1. Model of the respiratory system. The driving force is the Po_2 cascade between ambient air and the O_2 sink in the mitochondria. At each level, the O_2 flow rate is the product of the pressure gradient and the conductance. (Modified after Taylor and Weibel, 1981.)

ambient air. On the other hand, they are related to the Po_2 cascade that establishes the overall driving force for O_2 flow from inspired air to the O_2 sink in the mitochondria. Under steady-state conditions, values for O_2 flow are the same for each step. What varies is the driving force across each step and the associated conductance, the product of the two being the oxygen flow, $\dot{V}o_2$.

As a further step in the analysis of the system, we can identify morphometric and physiological parameters that affect $\dot{V}o_2$, mostly through the conductance term (Fig. 1.2). Thus, the size of the O_2 sink in the cells is related to the total volume of mitochondria or their inner membrane area, which determines the number of respiratory chain complexes that perform oxidative phosphorylation (23, 33); or the pulmonary diffusing capacity is related to the alveolar and capillary surfaces and the barrier thickness (30). It is noteworthy that one morphometric parameter, the hematocrit or erythrocyte volume density, affects three steps in the cascade: O_2 uptake in the lung, O_2 transport by the heart and circulation, and O_2 delivery from the microcirculation. This marks the central importance of blood for the entire respiratory system.

TESTING SYMMORPHOSIS BY VARING $\dot{V}o_2$MAX

In our previous work we have tested the hypothesis of symmorphosis by varying the limit of aerobic metabolism, $\dot{V}o_2$max, under conditions of normoxia, that is, keeping the ambient Po_2 as a constant boundary condition. By exploiting experiments of nature we have used two strategies to vary $\dot{V}o_2$max: (1) allometric variation where mass-specific $\dot{V}o_2$max of small mammals, such as mice, is about six times higher than that of large mammals, such as cows (25, 32); and (2) adaptive variation, where "normal" animals are compared with

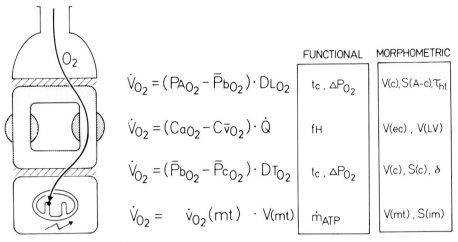

	FUNCTIONAL	MORPHOMETRIC
$\dot{V}_{O_2} = (P_{A_{O_2}} - \bar{P}_{b_{O_2}}) \cdot D_{L_{O_2}}$	$t_c, \Delta P_{O_2}$	$V(c), S(A-c), \tau_{ht}$
$\dot{V}_{O_2} = (C_{a_{O_2}} - C_{\bar{v}_{O_2}}) \cdot \dot{Q}$	f_H	$V(ec), V(LV)$
$\dot{V}_{O_2} = (\bar{P}_{b_{O_2}} - \bar{P}_{c_{O_2}}) \cdot D_{T_{O_2}}$	$t_c, \Delta P_{O_2}$	$V(c), S(c), \delta$
$\dot{V}_{O_2} = \dot{V}_{O_2}(mt) \cdot V(mt)$	$\dot{m}_{ATP}$	$V(mt), S(im)$

FIGURE 1.2. At each level of the respiratory system the flow of oxygen, $\dot{V}_{O_2}$, is given by the product of two terms, the first being determined mostly by functional and the second by morphometric factors. Some functional and morphometric parameters that enter into play are listed in the boxes. The morphometric symbols are volumes (V), surface areas (S), barrier thickness (τ), and diffusion distance (δ), related to capillaries (c), erythrocytes (ec), alveoli (A), left ventricle (LV), mitochondria (mt), and inner mitochondrial membrane (im).

"athletic" species of the same size, which achieve two to three times higher $\dot{V}_{O_2}$max (14, 27). In all these studies we have used an integrated approach, first extensively studying the physiology of the animals while they ran on a treadmill up to $\dot{V}_{O_2}$max; at the end of this part of the study the animals were sacrificed, and tissue samples were collected for the morphometric study of all organs involved. We, thus, obtained consistent data sets with functional and morphometric data determined on the same animals.

The results of these studies can be summarized as follows (28):

1. In locomotor muscles *mitochondria* are invariant building blocks. In both allometric and adaptive variation, the volume of mitochondria is strictly proportional to $\dot{V}_{O_2}$max. We have, therefore, concluded that mitochondria consume up to 4 to 5 ml of O_2/min/ml (12); accordingly, their amount determines the capacity for oxidative phosphorylation and thus O_2 demand by exercising muscle.

2. The length and volume of *capillaries* in muscle are about proportional to mitochondrial volume. In athletic species, however, we found hematocrit to be increased as well. The oxygen capacity of capillary blood is matched to the oxidative capacity of the muscle cells supplied, but in this case two structural components (capillaries and erythrocytes) may share the adaptive effort (7).

3. The convective *transport of O_2 by the circulation* is adapted in a different way in the two types of variation: by combining a change in cardiac output through stroke volume (ventricle size) with a change in O_2 capacity of the blood through hematocrit in adaptive variation; and by modulating cardiac output essentially through heart frequency in allometric variation.

4. The *pulmonary diffusing capacity* is only partially adapted to $\dot{V}o_2$max in adaptive variation; it maintains an excess capacity by about a factor of 2, which is partly exploited in athletic species (8, 15, 31). In allometric variation, the diffusing capacity of the lungs for oxygen (DLo_2) varies with body mass and is, thus, not related to $\dot{V}o_2$max, which changes with the 0.8 power of body mass (11).

On the whole, this study of allometric and adaptive variation of the aerobic capacity of mammals has revealed that symmorphosis does apply to a large extent in the respiratory system, but that there are some important variants to be noted (28). In the mitochondria of muscle cells, symmorphosis appears to hold in its simplest form: the volume of mitochondria varies directly in proportion to $\dot{V}o_2$max, regardless of how the energetic demand is varied. At the level of O_2 delivery from the microcirculation to the mitochondria, both structural and functional variables are involved. With respect to O_2 transport by the circulation, a match to varied maximal O_2 needs is achieved in adaptive variation purely by structural adaptation such as changing heart size and erythrocyte concentration. In allometric variation, it is mostly the functional variable, heart frequency, that is changed. It should be mentioned that these conclusions are valid for quadrupedal mammals, whereas the conditions may be somehow different in humans because of their bipedal locomotion.

The lung appears as the major exception in this scheme. In adaptive variation, we find that the pulmonary diffusing capacity, as determined by structural design, is only partly adapted to the higher $\dot{V}o_2$max in athletic species; in allometric variation, the diffusing capacity is not matched to $\dot{V}o_2$max. In an attempt to assess the process of O_2 uptake in the lung by Bohr integration (15), we found that only 40 to 80% of pulmonary capillary transit time is required to equilibrate capillary blood with alveolar air in the large animals. This suggests that the pulmonary gas exchanger has excess diffusing capacity when compared with the maximal needs for O_2 uptake. In other words, its design is redundant by about a factor of 2. In small athletic animals, such as foxes, however, we found that the pulmonary diffusing capacity is completely exploited and could well be the limiting factor for O_2 uptake (20).

REDUNDANCY: SURVIVAL STRATEGY AT THE INTERFACE TO
THE ENVIRONMENT

The finding that lung design establishes an excess capacity for O_2 uptake and thus deviates from the other parts of the respiratory system is intriguing. The simplest explanation would be that lung design is established early on during growth and that it is not greatly malleable because of the design properties. This is not very satisfactory, however, particularly because instances of quantitative malleability of diffusing capacity are known, such as, the compensatory growth of the pulmonary gas exchanger that occurs in the residual lung after pneumonectomy (4).

An hypothetical explanation can perhaps be found by noting that the lung establishes the interface of the respiratory system to the environment, and that this may impose redundancy on lung design if the organism is to cope with variations in environmental conditions. Indeed, taking a broader look, we note that genetically programmed redundancy may be one of the general survival strategies of living creatures and of plants in those instances where survival depends on an interaction with the environment. Perhaps the most striking examples are the excessive number of seeds strewn by plants onto the soil, or the large number of eggs deposited by lower animals into their breeding grounds, or even the large number of offspring delivered by small mammals. From these examples, it appears that the chances of survival determine the degree of redundancy with which animals and plants secure their successful procreation, the survival of the species. The environment has always been—not only in modern civilized times—hostile to survival of living creatures.

The lung is faced with a number of problems related to its position at the interface between internal milieu and environment, as well as to the requirement that the structure of the gas exchanger be kept extremely delicate over a large internal surface area. The dangers of dehydration, heat loss, or attack by inhaled matter are examples, as well as the difficulty in maintaining a well-matched distribution of perfusion and ventilation because of the effect of gravity. Redundancy may be necessary to cope with these difficulties.

HYPOXIC ENVIRONMENT MAY IMPOSE REDUNDANCY IN THE LUNGS

The O_2 flow from ambient air to the O_2 sink in the mitochondria is essentially driven by inspired Po_2. A problem is that the pressure head for this flow is primarily effective in the pulmonary gas exchanger. To maintain a certain redundancy in pulmonary diffusing capacity should, therefore, allow the respiratory system to tolerate a reduction in ambient Po_2 (hypoxia) as it occurs naturally at elevated altitudes, without loss in overall performance.

We have tested whether this is the case by determining the level of hypoxia tolerated by goats running on a treadmill at their predetermined $\dot{V}o_2$max. By measuring the relevant physiological variables we could then use the Bohr integration model to estimate the progression of O_2 uptake as blood flows through the capillaries (15). Figure 1.3 shows that progressively more lung is used for O_2 uptake as fraction of inspired oxygen (Fio_2) is decreased from 0.21 to 0.15, but $\dot{V}o_2$max remained unchanged. Down to an ambient Po_2 of about 110 mm Hg (equivalent to an altitude of about 3000 m), goats tolerate hypoxia well, without a loss in the overall aerobic performance of the respiratory system. It is likely that this is due, at least in part, to the redundancy built into their pulmonary gas exchanger. It is clear, however, that the reduction in O_2 concentration in the blood must also involve an increase in cardiac output if O_2 delivery to the tissues is to be maintained at $\dot{V}o_2$max, and this would reduce capillary transit time. The lung can, therefore, become the main limiting factor for $\dot{V}o_2$ in hypoxia. This conclusion is perhaps supported by the observation that similar experiments with gradual reduction of Fio_2 in dogs were unsuccessful, possibly because dogs need about 75% of their pulmonary diffusing capacity even in normoxia and, thus, have a much smaller redundancy.

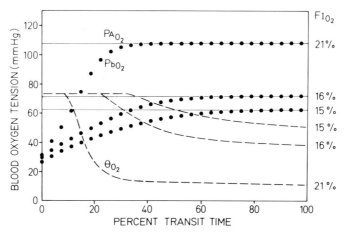

FIGURE 1.3. Hypoxia test of model for calculating O_2 transfer in the lung of the goat at $\dot{V}O_2$ max. The increase in PO_2 and decrease of ΘO_2 of the blood in the pulmonary capillaries is plotted as a function of transit time in the lung for inspired O_2 of 21%, 16%, and 15%. (From Karas et al., 1987.)

COPING WITH CHRONIC HYPOXIA: WHERE IS ADAPTATION USEFUL?

Hypoxia reduces the total driving force for O_2 flow to the mitochondria. But this reduction takes place primarily at the pressure head, the inspired partial pressure of oxygen (PiO_2) under conditions of environmental hypoxia. PiO_2 is reduced by about 60 mm Hg when barometric pressure drops from 760 to 450 mm Hg. Changes in PO_2 become more attenuated as the mitochondria are approached, with the PO_2 at that locus being only 10 mm Hg lower when barometric pressure is lowered from 760 to 450 mm Hg. The question we must now ask is where are adaptations of structural and functional parameters of the respiratory system useful in helping the system to maintain its aerobic capacity as near normal as possible. We shall then also look at the evidence available to see whether and to what extent the organism reacts to chronic hypoxia by adapting its system to cope with hypoxia.

Oxidative Phosphorylation in Mitochondria

The rate at which mitochondria perform oxidative phosphorylation appears to be rather independent of prevailing PO_2, as long as it does not fall below 0.5 mm Hg (10). Very little would be gained by modifying the mitochondrial volume in response to hypoxia. When studying muscle biopsies from mountaineers trained for extreme altitude climbing, Oelz and co-workers (21) found that the locomotor muscles contained a normal amount of mitochondria in relation to the state of physical fitness of these athletes. In guinea pigs raised under hypoxic conditions, no changes in the volume density or in the distribution of mitochondria were observed in myocardial cells (17).

Oxygen Delivery From the Microcirculation

Hypoxia causes a reduction in capillary P_{O_2}, the driving force for O_2 delivery. Using simple Krogh cylinder models, Stainsby et al. (24), as well as others, estimated that hypoxia may cause parts of the muscle cells located near the venous end of the capillary to become anoxic. This may, however, not be of functional consequence for two reasons: (1) the mitochondria are not homogeneously distributed throughout the muscle cell, but are rather concentrated in the region near the capillary (18) and (2) the muscle capillary network becomes denser as it approaches the venous end, causing the maximal diffusion distances to become shorter as the P_{O_2} in the capillary falls (33). These two design features combined may prevent *anoxic mitochondria* to occur in muscle cells, even in hypoxia (Fig. 1.4).

Studies in guinea pigs, exposed throughout 16 weeks to hypoxia and cold, have revealed some interesting adaptations in locomotor muscles: the capillary density was increased significantly, reducing the diffusion distances into the muscle cells (2).

Oxygen Transport by the Circulation of Blood

The O_2 transport in the blood is determined primarily by cardiac output and the O_2 capacity of the blood. It is well known that one of the first adaptations to chronic hypoxia is an increase in hematocrit and hemoglobin concentration;

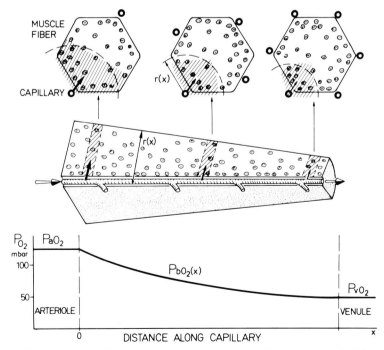

FIGURE 1.4. Because the capillary density increases toward the venular end of the capillary path, the Krogh tissue "cylinder" is tapering in the form of a cone. As the P_{O_2} falls, the diffusion distance is reduced. (From Weibel et al., 1981.)

this adaptive change seems, however, quite variable from species to species (1). In addition to increasing the amount of O_2 that can be contained in the unit volume of blood at low Po_2, the increase in hematocrit also improves O_2 delivery in the muscle by increasing O_2 concentration, and it improves O_2 uptake in the lung. As mentioned previously, hemoglobin concentration affects the three O_2 transport steps: uptake, delivery, and discharge.

It has been shown repeatedly that chronic hypoxia leads to right ventricular hypertrophy because of increased pulmonary vascular resistance (1). In spite of an increased cross-sectional area of myocardial fibers in the right ventricle, related to the hypertrophy, the diffusion distances are shorter because the length of capillaries increases, thus improving O_2 delivery (16).

Oxygen Uptake in the Lung

As outlined earlier, the redundancy in pulmonary diffusing capacity is a safeguard against hypoxia and allows O_2 uptake to be completed during transit time even in hypoxia. Wagner et al. (29) have shown that the pulmonary diffusing capacity of trained men becomes totally exploited when they perform heavy exercise in hypoxia equivalent to an altitude of 4500 m (P_B, 429 mm Hg). Under these conditions the lung may become the limiting factor for aerobic performance (Fig. 1.5), a result similar to that obtained on goats (see Fig. 1.3).

Does the lung adapt to chronic hypoxia by increasing its diffusing capacity? It has long been known that high altitude natives may have developed a greater efficiency for pulmonary gas exchange, and that their lungs may be larger (9, 13, 22). Two simultaneous, but independent, studies established that growing rats raised at high altitude developed a larger pulmonary gas exchange apparatus (3, 5). In our own study we raised young rats in the High Altitude Research Station on Jungfraujoch (3450 m) where an ambient Po_2 of 100 mm Hg prevailed; they were kept at room temperature. The matched controls were kept in Berne (ambient Po_2, 150 mm Hg), and a third group was

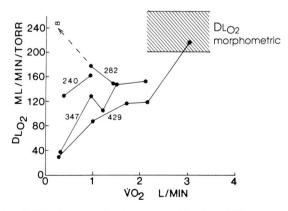

FIGURE 1.5. Calculated diffusing capacity for oxygen (DLo_2) at different exercise levels and at different altitudes (all data are average values for all subjects) as obtained by Wagner et al. (30). Numbers next to plotted points are values of barometric pressure. The *shaded area* in the upper right hand corner shows the range of morphometric estimates of DLo_2. (Modified after Wagner et al., 1987.)

exposed to mild hyperoxia (40% O_2, P_{O_2} 290 mm Hg). After 3 weeks, the high-altitude animals had developed a pulmonary diffusing capacity 20% larger than the lowland controls when expressed per unit body mass (5, 6); interestingly, the rats raised under hyperoxic conditions developed a significantly smaller diffusing capacity (about 15% less than lowland controls). This evidence, together with that of Bartlett and Remmers (3), suggested that the growing rat can adjust the growth of its lung to environmental levels of O_2 supply, presumably to the pressure head for O_2 flow through the respiratory system, at least within certain bounds. In a similar, but somewhat different, study on guinea pigs, Lechner et al. (19) arrived at the conclusion that exposure to hypoxia combined with cold caused lung growth to become accelerated, so that the alveolar surface area was larger after 2 to 10 weeks of exposure. But this difference from the controls was abolished when the animals reached the end of their growth period. Thus, it remains unclear whether the lung can, in a definite fashion, adapt its gas exchanger to variations in environmental O_2 supply.

CONCLUSIONS

When considering the respiratory system as a whole we find that its different levels respond in a different fashion to acute or chronic hypoxia. It appears that the size of the O_2 sink, determined by the amount of mitochondria, remains largely invariant. There may be some variable adaptations in the capillary network to improve the delivery of O_2 to the mitochondria, as well as in the O_2 capacity of blood. The diffusing capacity of the lung appears excessive by a factor of up to 2 under normoxic conditions when compared with the rate of O_2 uptake needed to sustain $\dot{V}_{O_2}$max. This can be seen as a redundancy required to allow high aerobic performance even under natural conditions of hypoxia, allowing $\dot{V}_{O_2}$max to be maintained up to altitudes of 3000 m, except in highly aerobic athletes such as dogs. It is possible that the pulmonary diffusing capacity is the ultimate limiting step for O_2 transport in the respiratory system when environmental O_2 becomes reduced. The redundancy built into the pulmonary gas exchanger could, therefore, be a survival strategy for animals living at variable altitude.

ACKNOWLEDGMENTS

This work was supported by Swiss National Science Foundation Grant No. 3.172.88. We thank Dr. Vilma Navarro and Elsbeth Hanger for their help in the preparation of this manuscript.

REFERENCES

1. BANCHERO, N. Cardiovascular responses to chronic hypoxia. *Ann. Rev. Physiol. 49*: 465–476, 1987.
2. BANCHERO, N., S. R. KAYAR, AND A. J. LECHNER. Increased capillarity in skeletal muscle of growing guinea pigs acclimated to cold and hypoxia. *Respir. Physiol. 62*:245–255, 1985.
3. BARTLETT, D., JR., AND J. E. REMMERS. Effects of high altitude exposure on the lungs of young rats. *Respir. Physiol. 13*:116–125, 1971.

4. BURRI, P. H., AND S. SEHOVIC. The adaptive response of the rat lung after bilobectomy. *Ann. Rev. Respir. Dis. 119*:769–777, 1979.

5. BURRI, P., AND E. R. WEIBEL. Morphometric estimation of pulmonary diffusion capacity. II. Effect of environmental Po_2 on the growing lung. *Respir. Physiol. 11*:247–264, 1971.

6. BURRI, P. H., AND E. R. WEIBEL. Morphometric evaluation of changes in lung structure due to high altitude. In: Ciba Foundation. *High Altitude Physiology: Cardiac and Respiratory Aspects,* ed. R. Porter and J. Knight. Edinburgh: Churchill Livingstone, 1971, pp. 15–30.

7. CONLEY, K. E., S. R. KAYAR, K. RÖSLER, H. HOPPELER, E. R. WEIBEL, AND C. R. TAYLOR. Adaptive variation in the mammalian respiratory system in relation to energetic demand. IV. Capillaries and their relationship to oxidative capacity. *Respir. Physiol. 69*: 47–64, 1987.

8. CONSTANTINOPOL, M., J. H. JONES, E. R. WEIBEL, C. R. TAYLOR, A. LINDHOLM, AND R. H. KARAS. Oxygen transport during exercise in large mammals. II. Oxygen uptake by the pulmonary gas exchanges. *J. Appl. Physiol. 67*:871–878, 1989.

9. DEMPSEY, J. A., W. G. REDDAN, M. L. BIRNBAUM, H. V. FORSTER, J. S. THODEN, R. F. GROVER, AND J. RANKLIN. Effects of acute through life-long hypoxic exposure on exercise pulmonary gas exchange. *Respir. Physiol. 13*:62–89, 1971.

10. GAYESKI, T. E. J., AND C. R. HONIG. Intracellular Po_2 in axis of individual fibers in working dog gracilis muscles. *Am. J. Physiol. 254*:H1179–H1186, 1988.

11. GEHR, P., D. K. MWANGI, A. AMMANN, G. M. O. MALOIY, C. R. TAYLOR, AND E. R. WEIBEL. Design of the mammalian respiratory system. V. Scaling morphometric pulmonary diffusing capacity to body mass: wild and domestic mammals. *Respir. Physiol. 44*: 61–86, 1981.

12. HOPPELER, H., AND S. L. LINDSTEDT. Malleability of skeletal muscle in overcoming limitations: structural elements. *J. Exp. Biol. 115*:355–364, 1985.

13. HURTADO, A. Respiratory adaptation in Indian natives of the Peruvian Andes. Studies at high altitude. *Ann. J. Phys. Anthropol. 17*:137–165, 1932.

14. JONES, J. H., K. E. LONGWORTH, A. LINDHOLM, K. E. CONLEY, R. H. KARAS, S. R. KAYAR, AND C. R. TAYLOR. Oxygen transport during exercise in large mammals: I. Adaptive variation in oxygen demand. *J. Appl. Physiol. 67*:862–870, 1989.

15. KARAS, R. H., C. R. TAYLOR, J. H. JONES, S. L. LINDSTEDT, R. B. REEVES, AND E. R. WEIBEL. Adaptive variation in the mammalian respiratory system in relation to energetic demand: VII. Flow of oxygen across the pulmonary gas exchanges. *Respir. Physiol. 69*:101–116, 1987.

16. KAYAR, S. R., AND N. BANCHERO. Myocardial capillarity in acclimation to hypoxia. *Pflügers Arch. 404*:319–325, 1985.

17. KAYAR, S. R., AND N. BANCHERO. Volume density and distribution of mitochondria in myocardial growth and hypertrophy. *Respir. Physiol. 70*:275–286, 1987.

18. KAYAR, S. R., H. HOPPELER, B. ESSEN-GUSTAVSSON, AND K. SCHWERZMANN. The similarity of mitochondrial distribution in equine skeletal muscles of differing oxidative capacity. *J. Exp. Biol. 137*:253–263, 1988.

19. LECHNER, A. J., M. S. GRIMES, L. AQUIN, AND N. BANCHERO. Adaptive lung growth during chronic cold plus hypoxia is age dependent. *J. Exp. Zool. 219*:285–291, 1982.

20. LONGWORTH, K. E., J. H. JONES, J. E. P. W. BICUDO, C. R. TAYLOR, AND E. R. WEIBEL. High rate of O_2 consumption in exercising foxes: large Po_2 difference drives diffusion across the lung. *Respir. Physiol. 77*:263–276, 1989.

21. OELZ, O., H. HOWALD, P. DIPRAMPERO, H. HOPPELER, H. CLAASEN, R. JENNI, A. BÜHLMANN, G. FERRETTI, J. -C. BRUECKNER, A. VEICSTEINAS, M. GUSSONI, AND P. CERRETELLI. Physiological profile of world class high altitude climbers. *J. Appl. Physiol. 60*:1734–1742, 1986.

22. REMMERS, J. E., AND J. C. MITHOEFER. The carbon monoxide diffusing capacity in permanent residents at high altitudes. *Respir. Physiol. 6*:233–244, 1969.

23. SCHWERZMANN, K., H. HOPPELER, S. R. KAYAR, AND E. R. WEIBEL. Oxidative capacity of muscle and mitochondria: correlation of physiological, biochemical and morphometric characteristics. *Proc. Natl. Acad. Sci. USA 86*:1583–1587, 1989.

24. STAINSBY, W. N., B. SNYDER, AND H. G. WELCH. A pictographic essay on blood and tissue oxygen transport. *Med. Sci. Sports Exerc. 20*:213–221, 1988.

25. TAYLOR, C. R., G. M. O. MALOIY, E. R. WEIBEL, V. A. LANGMAN, J. M. Z. KAMAN, H. J. SEEHERMANN, AND N. C. HEGLUND. Design of the mammalian respiratory system. III. Scaling maximum aerobic capacity to body mass: wild and domestic mammals. *Respir. Physiol. 44*:25–38, 1981.

26. TAYLOR, C. R., AND E. R. WEIBEL. Design of the mammalian respiratory system. I. Problem and strategy. *Respir. Physiol. 44*:1–10, 1981.

27. TAYLOR, C. R., AND E. R. WEIBEL. Adaptive variation in the mammalian respiratory system in relation to energetic demand I–VIII. *Respir. Physiol.* 69:1–127, 1987.
28. TAYLOR, C. R., E. R. WEIBEL, R. H. KARAS, AND H. HOPPELER. Matching structures and functions in the respiratory system. In: *Comparative Pulmonary Physiology*, ed. S. C. Wood. New York: Marcel Dekker, 1989, pp. 27–65.
29. WAGNER, P. D., J. R. SUTTON, J. T. REEVES, A. CYMERMANN, B. M. GROVES, AND M. K. MALCONIAN. Operation Everest II: Pulmonary gas exchange during a simulated ascent of Mt. Everest. *J. Appl. Physiol.* 63:2348–2359, 1987.
30. WEIBEL, E. R. *The Pathway for Oxygen. Structure and Function in the Mammalian Respiratory System*. Cambridge: Harvard University Press, 1984, 425 pp.
31. WEIBEL, E. R., L. B. MARQUES, M. CONSTANTINOPOL, F. DOFFEY, P. GEHR, AND C. R. TAYLOR. Adaptive variation in the mammalian respiratory system in relation to energetic demand. VI. The pulmonary gas exchanges. *Respir. Physiol.* 69:81–100, 1987.
32. WEIBEL, E. R., AND C. R. TAYLOR. Design of the mammalian respiratory system. I–IX. *Respir. Physiol.* 44:1–164, 1981.
33. WEIBEL, E. R., C. R. TAYLOR, P. GEHR, H. HOPPELER, O. MATTHIEU, AND G. M. O. MALOIY. Design of the mammalian respiratory system. IX. Functional and structural limits for oxygen flow. *Respir. Physiol.* 44:151–164, 1981.

2

Factors Affecting Adaptation of the Mitochondrial Enzyme Content to Cellular Needs

DAVID F. WILSON AND WILLIAM L. RUMSEY

Cells require a continuous supply of adenosine triphosphate (ATP) to carry out the synthesis of essential cellular components, to repair damage to these components, for various energy requiring transport and secretory functions, and to do mechanical work. The primary source of this ATP is mitochondrial oxidative phosphorylation. It is common knowledge that the cellular content of mitochondria varies widely among cell types and that the content of each cell type is, to a first approximation, matched to the cellular requirements for ATP from oxidative phosphorylation for that cell type. This is exemplified by the fact that cardiac myocytes, which have a high rate of ATP utilization and have a much higher content of mitochondrial enzymes than, for example, do cultured kidney cells, which have a lower rate of ATP utilization. This general observation suggests that cells have a mechanism(s) for changing their level of mitochondrial enzymes in response to the changing needs for ATP production resulting from chronic changes in cellular function. In this chapter we first examine our current understanding of the regulation of mitochondrial oxidative phosphorylation. The mitochondrial content of various cell types and of conditions that result in changes in their content of individual types of cells is evaluated. Last, we identify the possible mechanism(s) that serve to detect the need for alterations in the cellular level of mitochondria, thereby allowing cellular adaptation to occur in response to environmental needs.

MITOCHONDRIA IN CELLS: METABOLIC POWER SUPPLIES DEPEND ON BOTH THE INTRAMITOCHONDRIAL $[NAD^+]/[NADH]$ AND THE CELLULAR DEMAND FOR ADENOSINE TRIPHOSPHATE

Any system involved in regulating the amount of mitochondria in the cell must somehow "sense" the need for change, that is, a deficiency or excess of enzymatic capacity. The potential sensors for mitochondrial capacity are limited, because the mitochondria are surrounded by a double membrane, each membrane selectively permeable to cytoplasmic and mitochondrial components. Thus, the two compartments are effectively isolated from each other except for the flow of essential metabolites through specific transport systems in the membranes, a flow designed to maintain and regulate communication between the two compartments. In the complete system, the cytoplasm is responsible for supplying oxidizable substrates to the mitochondria, whereas the mitochondria are primarily responsible for supplying ATP to the cytoplasm. The regulation of mitochondrial oxidative phosphorylation may, therefore, be described as having "supply" and "demand" sides (9, 10, 24, 25).

The supply of oxidizable substrates for oxidative phosphorylation is concerned with both the chemical nature of the substrates (i.e., fatty acids vs. pyruvate), and the activity of the dehydrogenases by which the substrates are oxidized to provide reducing equivalents to the respiratory chain. This supply side of cellular energetics and mitochondrial oxidative phosphorylation is regulated at many levels by: (1) systemic hormonal systems by receptors on the plasma membrane and (2) the catabolic substrate(s) (fats, amino acids, or pyruvate) and other factors. Most of the dehydrogenases transfer the reducing equivalents to oxidized nicotinamide dinucleotide (NAD^+), producing reduced nicotinamide dinucleotide (NADH). The latter is then reoxidized by the respiratory chain, the reducing equivalents being used to reduce dioxygen to water. The intramitochondrial NAD^+ and NADH form a pool of reducing equivalents that, for most physiological conditions, defines the reducing power available for oxidative phosphorylation. This *reducing power* is most correctly expressed as the ratio of concentrations of unbound (free) NAD^+ to NADH in the intramitochondrial matrix ($[NAD^+]/[NADH]$).

The demand side of the regulation of oxidative phosphorylation is the rate of hydrolysis of ATP by the many energy-requiring reactions of the cell. As cellular ATP is continuously hydrolyzed by metabolic processes, it must, in the time average, be resynthesized at an equal rate or the cell will be unable to survive. Temporary inequalities, however, may occur in the rates of ATP hydrolysis and synthesis as part of cellular metabolic transitions, but these inequalities are an integral part of the control system. During rapid changes in the rate of ATP hydrolysis, for example, the rate of ATP hydrolysis may be less than or greater than the rate of ATP synthesis. As a result of this imbalance, the levels of ATP in the cell begin to rise or fall. Any change in the concentration of ATP results in even larger changes in the concentration of adenosine diphosphate (ADP) (the normal concentrations of ATP are from 10- to more than 100-fold greater above the concentrations of ADP and hydrolysis of 10% of the ATP increases ADP by 2- to 10-fold). Thus, an imbalance between the rate of ATP synthesis and hydrolysis is rapidly translated into a change in the cytoplasmic [ATP]/[ADP][Pi], a primary regulator of the rate of mitochondrial oxidative phosphorylation (9, 10, 13). When the [ATP]/[ADP][Pi] falls, the respiratory rate increases and when [ATP]/[ADP][Pi] increases, the respiratory rate decreases. The isolated, retrograde perfused rat heart responds to changes in perfusion pressure with changes in the rate of ATP utilization (16). Increases or decreases in perfusion pressure produced a parallel change in ATP consumption as reflected in the respiratory rate of the tissue. This may be considered an almost pure demand model because the respiratory rate correlated with the changes in cytoplasmic [ATP]/[ADP][Pi], whereas there were no measurable changes in the intramitochondrial [NAD^+]/[NADH].

Under physiological conditions both supply and demand mechanisms can operate simultaneously and independently. For any given rate of mitochondrial respiration, the factors regulating the supply side of mitochondrial oxidative phosphorylation can increase or decrease the intramitochondrial [NAD$^+$]/[NADH], independently of the rate of ATP hydrolysis. This occurs because in healthy cells the first two sites of mitochondrial oxidative phosphorylation are near equilibrium (11, 24, 25). The chemical equation for the first two sites of oxidative phosphorylation is:

$$\text{NADH} + 2c^{3+} + 2\text{ADP} + 2\text{Pi} \rightleftharpoons \text{NAD}^+ + 2c^{2+} + 2\text{ATP} \qquad (1)$$

where the NAD$^+$ and NADH are intramitochondrial, the ATP, ADP, and Pi are in the cytoplasm, and c^{2+} and c^{3+} are the reduced and oxidized forms of the mitochondrial cytochrome c, respectively. The equilibrium constant is expressed:

$$K_{eq} = [\text{NAD}^+]/[\text{NADH}] * ([c^{2+}]/[c^{3+}])^2 * ([\text{ATP}]/[\text{ADP}][\text{Pi}])^2 \qquad (2)$$

Any change in the [NAD$^+$]/[NADH] ratio can be compensated for by alterations in the [ATP]/[ADP][Pi] and/or the [c^{2+}]/[c^{3+}]. The respiratory rate increases with reduction of cytochrome c (increasing [c^{2+}]/[c^{3+}]) and with decreasing [ATP]/[ADP][Pi]. Under some metabolic conditions a decline in [NAD$^+$]/[NADH] (reduction of the mitochondrial pyridine nucleotide pool) is offset by an increase in [ATP]/[ADP][Pi] and in [c^{2+}]/[c^{3+}] sufficient to maintain a constant respiratory rate (19). On the other hand, a rise in the rate of ATP synthesis can occur with an increase, decrease, or no change in [ATP]/[ADP][Pi], depending on the direction of change in the intramitochondrial [NAD$^+$]/[NADH].

MITOCHONDRIAL ENZYME CONTENT IN CELLS WITH DIFFERENT RATES OF OXIDATIVE PHOSPHORYLATION

It is well known that the rates of cellular respiration are dependent on cell type, being much higher in some cells than in others. Table 2.1 summarizes the data taken from the literature on the energy metabolism and mitochondrial content of three different types of cells (10, 16). In each type of cell, the measured parameters included the content of mitochondrial cytochrome c, respiratory rate, intramitochondrial [NAD$^+$]/[NADH], and [ATP]/[ADP][Pi]. The respiration by the mitochondria in the cells are compared by calculating the turnover number for cytochrome c (the average number of times the cytochrome c was oxidized and reduced per second). This normalizes the respiration to the number of respiratory chains present in the cell. The rates of respiration per cytochrome c were similar in all of the cells, with values ranging from 3.6 to 14/sec. The respiratory rates for the hepatocytes and cultured kidney cells were measured at 23 to 25°C, whereas the respiration of the perfused heart was measured at 37°C, and correction for the temperature difference would make them essentially the same. The reported respiratory rate of he-

TABLE 2.1. Homeostasis in Cellular Energy Metabolism

Cell type	Cytochrome c (nmol/g wet wt)	Respiratory rate (μmol O₂/min/g)	Cytochrome c turnover (sec⁻¹)	[NAD⁺]/[NADH]	[ATP]/[ADP][Pi] (M⁻¹)
Hepatocytes	20	3.3	11	410	1,500
Kidney cells	16	3.9	16	180	2,000
Rat heart	56	8.2	10	1.3	60,000
Rat heart	51	10.3	14	2.4	31,000

Energy metabolism has been measured in three different types of cells. This included measurement of the levels of mitochondrial respiratory enzyme (cytochrome c), respiratory rate in μmol O₂/min/g wet weight (this was measured at room temperature for the cultured kidney cells and then the rate at 37°C assumed to be threefold higher, as observed for the hepatocytes), the intramitochondrial [NAD⁺]/[NADH] as indicated by a near equilibrium substrate couple (3-hydroxybutyrate dehydrogenase for hepatocytes and cultured kidney cells, glutamate dehydrogenase for heart). The total measured cellular concentrations of ATP, ADP, and Pi were used as indicators of the cytoplasmic [ATP]/[ADP] [Pi] for hepatocytes and cultured kidney cells, whereas the [creatine-phosphate]/[creatine] level was used to calculate the cytoplasmic [ATP]/[ADP] in heart assuming equilibrium of the creatine phosphokinase reaction. The inorganic phosphate in the heart was measured chemically in freeze-clamped tissue. The [ATP]/[ADP] [Pi] is in good agreement with that obtained using ³¹Pi (see Ref. 9 for discussion). Data were taken from Erecinska et al. (10) and Nishiki et al. (16).

patocytes at 37°C, (15) gives a turnover number for cytochrome c of approximately 11/sec. The values of the intramitochondrial [NAD$^+$]/[NADH] ratio range from 410 to 1.3, whereas the corresponding values for [ATP]/[ADP][Pi] are between 1.5×10^3 to 60×10^3/M. That the mitochondria of hepatocytes, with an [ATP]/[ADP][Pi] of 1,500/M should have a turnover number essentially the same as that of cardiac myocytes with an [ATP]/[ADP][Pi] of 60,000/M is seemingly in contrast to observations made using suspensions of isolated mitochondria. Mitochondria isolated from liver and heart, for example, and provided with the same experimental conditions (such as oxidizable substrate, i.e., glutamate and malate), have a very similar relationship of the respiratory rate to extramitochondrial [ATP]/[ADP][Pi]. In cells, in contrast to isolated mitochondria, the intramitochondrial [NAD$^+$]/[NADH] is under full metabolic control by the cell. Each cell can, by the regulation of the activity of the dehydrogenases of the citric acid cycle and fatty acid oxidation, set this value to that necessary for its metabolic function. The [NAD$^+$]/[NADH] is much more reducing in cardiac myocytes than in hepatocytes or cultured kidney cells (1.3 and 2.4 vs. 410 and 160), directly reflecting the differing needs of the cells. As discussed previously (see also Refs. 9, 18, 21, 24, 25), for any given respiratory rate a more reduced intramitochondrial pyridine nucleotide pool will result in an increased value of [ATP]/[ADP][Pi]. It is clear, however, that the content of mitochondrial enzymes is closely correlated with the metabolic activity of cells. Cells with a higher oxidative capacity have a higher content of mitochondrial enzymes. The higher concentration of mitochondria is required to allow the increased rate to occur without a decline in the [ATP]/[ADP][Pi] or an increase in intramitochondrial [NAD$^+$]/[NADH] that would otherwise be needed to attain the same increase in respiratory rate.

THE EFFECT OF ENDURANCE TRAINING ON THE CONTENT OF MITOCHONDRIAL ENZYMES IN SKELETAL MUSCLE

When untrained skeletal muscles are subjected regularly to heavy exercise for extended periods (endurance training), there are changes in the content of the mitochondrial enzymes (for review see Ref. 14). Several groups have confirmed and extended these observations (4, 5, 12), but the data in Table 2.2 were taken from Davies et al. (5) because the measurements of the mitochondrial enzymes were more extensive in a single paper. In this study, rats were subjected to extensive training on a treadmill each day for a period of 10 weeks. Both the maximal rate of whole body oxygen consumption and the time to exhaustion (a measure of endurance capacity) were measured at the beginning and end of the training period. In addition, the maximal activities of several enzymes in skeletal muscle were determined before training (control) and in separate animals after training. As a result of training, maximal whole body oxygen consumption (76.6 vs. 87.7 ml/kg per minute) and maximal endurance (36.3 vs. 182 minutes) were increased.

The maximal activities of mitochondrial enzymes in the skeletal muscles of the endurance trained animals were greater than that of the controls by approximately 100% or a twofold increase in the muscles of the trained ani-

TABLE 2.2. The Effect of Endurance Training on the Content of Mitochondrial Enzymes in the Skeletal Muscle of Rats

Enzyme	Normal	Endurance Trained	% Increase
Succinate dehydrogenase	11.9 μmol/min/g	24.9 μmol/min/g	209
NADH dehydrogenase.	71.8 μmol/min/g	122.8 μmol/min/g	171
Choline dehydrogenase.	0.31 μmol/min/g	0.83 μmol/min/g	268
Cytochrome a	6.4 nmol/g	13.3 nmol/g	208
Cytochrome $c + c_1$	13.5 nmol/g	28.7 nmol/g	211

Female Wistar rats were divided into two groups and endurance trained by exercising them 5 days a week for 10 weeks by running at 26.8 m/min and a grade of 8.5 degrees. From the beginning of week 5 through the end of the 10th week, the rats ran for 120 min/day. At the end of the training period the muscles were excised and used for assay of enzyme activity. The activities of the dehydrogenases are expressed as μmol acceptor reduced/min/g muscle weight and the contents of cytochromes are expressed as nmol/g muscle weight. Data taken from Davies et al. (5).

mals. This was true for several enzymes characteristic of mitochondria and a few of these enzymes are listed in Table 2.2. The increase in each enzyme activity or content was similar in all cases, approximately twofold, indicating that the entire enzyme complement of the mitochondria was induced as a whole. Thus, the capacity of the cells to carry out all aspects of oxidative phosphorylation was increased by about twofold. On the other hand, the ability of the animals to perform endurance exercise rose by fourfold, indicating that this capacity for exercise at a defined level of work was not entirely due to the rise in enzymatic activity. Other factors, such as improved O_2 delivery to the tissue, are likely also important in determining the time to exhaustion.

THE EFFECT OF THE TRANSITION FROM HYPOTHYROID TO
HYPERTHYROID ON THE RESPIRATORY ENZYMES OF RAT HEART

The heart is an unusual muscle because it is continuously active, even when the skeletal musculature is at rest. Thus, it is generally observed that the exercise training protocols that modify the enzyme contents of skeletal muscle have no effect on cardiac muscle (for review see Ref. 1). Thyroid hormone, however, changes the basal metabolic rate of the body, the metabolic rate increasing with increasing concentrations of the hormone. As a result, the heart is subjected to metabolic loads that are imposed for the full 24 hours of the day. Comparison of the mitochondrial enzyme content of the hearts of hypothyroid, euthyroid, and hyperthyroid rats allows an examination of the effects of such sustained changes in metabolic rate on the content of mitochondrial enzymes of heart muscle.

Nishiki and co-workers (17) studied heart metabolism and function, including the mitochondrial content of the heart muscle, using groups of rats that had been made hypothyroid by surgically removing the thyroid gland or made hyperthyroid by intraperitoneal injection of 35 μg of thyroid hormone/100 g body weight each day for 10 to 15 days. The heart muscle from each of these groups of animals was compared with that from healthy (euthyroid) an-

TABLE 2.3. Comparison of the Mitochondrial Respiratory Capacity of Hearts From Euthyroid, Hypothyroid, and Hyperthyroid Rats

Animal Condition	Cytochrome Content		Mitochondrial protein (mg/g)	O_2 Consumption (μmol/min/g)
	$c + c_1$ (nmol/g)	$a + a_3$ (nmol/g)		
Hypothyroid	39	23	66	5.5
Euthyroid	56	32	70	8.2
Hyperthyroid	69	42	80	11.3

Hearts were isolated from rats that were normal (euthyroid), had been made hypothyroid for 10 to 20 days by surgically removing the thyroid gland (hypothyroid), or had been given intraperitoneal injections of 35 μg thyroxine/100 g body weight per day (hyperthyroid). The hearts were perfused retrogradely at a perfusion pressure of 80 cm H_2O. The content of cytochromes is expressed as nmol/g wet weight of tissue and the respiratory rate as μmol O_2/min/g wet weight. Data from Nishiki et al. (17).

imals. Some of the results are reproduced in Tables 2.3 and 2.4. The tissue content of mitochondrial enzymes was higher in animals with higher thyroid hormone levels, with the hyperthyroid animals having an enzyme content 80% greater than that of the hypothyroid animals. The amount of respiratory enzymes per milligram of mitochondrial protein rose, indicating the fraction of mitochondrial protein contributed by the respiratory chain increased.

Hearts were isolated from animals of each group and retrogradely perfused. The hearts were maintained under comparable perfusion conditions until a steady state was attained (20 minutes) and then freeze clamped. The concentrations of ATP, ADP, Pi, creatine phosphate, and creatine were measured in extracts of the frozen tissue. The calculated [creatine phosphate]/[creatine], [ATP]/[ADP][Pi], and intramitochondrial [NAD$^+$]/[NADH] ratios were remarkably independent of the level of thyroid hormone. Thus, although each gram of heart muscle from hyperthyroid animals consumed almost twice as much oxygen each minute than did the hearts from hypothyroid animals, the correspondingly higher content of respiratory enzymes resulted in the respiratory chain operating at essentially the same rate per respiratory chain unit. As a result the cardiac cells were respiring at the same intramitochondrial [NAD$^+$]/[NADH] and [ATP]/[ADP][Pi] in the hearts of both hypothyroid and hyperthyroid animals.

TABLE 2.4. Comparison of Cardiac Energy Metabolism in Hearts From Hypothyroid, Euthyroid, and Hyperthyroid Rats

Animal Condition	[NAD$^+$]/[NADH]	[Cr-P]/[Cr]	[Pi] (μmol/g)	[ATP]/[ADP][Pi]
Hypothyroid	1.32	1.98	2.6	40.3×10^3/M
Euthyroid	2.23	2.31	3.1	64.8×10^3/M
Hyperthyroid	1.61	1.39	4.3	22.4×10^3/M

The hearts were taken from rats treated as described in the footnote of Table 2.3. The intramitochondrial [NAD$^+$]/[NADH] was calculated from the glutamate dehydrogenase equilibrium, the ratio of the concentration of creatine phosphate to that of creatine ([Cr-P]/[Cr]) was calculated from the measured concentrations of these compounds, and the cytoplasmic energy state ([ATP]/[ADP][Pi]) was calculated from the equilibrium constant for creatine phosphokinase at pH 7.0 and 1 mM Mg^{+2} and the measured concentration of inorganic phosphate.

THE EFFECT OF RESTRICTED OXYGEN DELIVERY AND EXERCISE ON THE
MITOCHONDRIAL CONTENT OF SKELETAL MUSCLE

The results presented suggest that the metabolic products of mitochondrial metabolism are part of the sensory mechanism for modulation of the cellular content of mitochondrial enzymes. If this is the case, there is a possibility that chronic hypoxia would enhance the effects of exercise. In chronic hypoxia, the oxygen pressure in the cells decreases below normal, particularly when the tissue is subject to conditions of increased ATP demand. The capacity of mitochondria in situ to synthesize ATP is dependent on the oxygen pressure at values less than about 30 mm Hg (21–23), and in this range below normal oxygen pressure would be expected to mimic a reduction in mitochondrial enzyme content. There have been several reports of effects of restricted oxygen delivery (vascular occlusion) on the mitochondrial content of skeletal muscle (2, 3, for review see Ref. 20), notably by Bylund-Fellenius and collaborators. The initial reports were for patients with peripheral vascular disease that reduced the blood flow to the lower extremities. When the affected legs of these patients were exercised, there was an increase in the levels of mitochondrial enzymes in muscles. The increase in enzyme content was similar to that induced by endurance exercise but occurred at much lower levels of exercise than required for normal endurance training.

This observation was confirmed and developed further using animal models (7, 8). Experiments were carried out in which one of the common iliac arteries of rats was ligated for 6 days. The enzymatic activities in both the soleus and extensor digitorum longus (EDL) muscle were measured and are presented in Table 2.5. The leg muscles of the rats were either used as controls or (the ligated leg) exercised by stimulating the sciatic nerve for 10 to 20 minutes, three to four times per day for 6 days. The measured activity of a key glycolytic enzyme, phosphofructokinase, was essentially unchanged by the exercise regimen, whereas the activities of the mitochondrial enzymes increased by more than 20%. The changes in mitochondrial enzyme content were similar for both the soleus and EDL muscles. Interestingly, the content of glycogen was also about 60% higher in both muscles after the exercise regimen. Such

TABLE 2.5. Effect of Exercise on the Oxidative Enzyme Content of Ischemic Skeletal Muscle in Rat

Enzyme	Control Leg (μmol/min/g)	Ligated Leg (μmol/min/g)
Soleus muscle		
Phosphofructokinase	331	353
Citrate synthetase	184	229
Cytochrome *c* oxidase	70	89
EDL muscle		
Phosphofructokinase	1262	1306
Citrate synthetase	184	222
Cytochrome *c* oxidase	55	68

One of the common iliac arteries of each rat was ligated and electrical stimulation of the sciatic nerves to both hindlimbs stimulated 10 to 20 minutes, three to four times a day for 6 days. The soleus and extensor digitorum longus (EDL) muscles were excised and then the enzyme activity measured and expressed per gram wet weight. Data taken from Elander et al. (8).

an increase in glycogen content is also observed to occur as a result of endurance training. When the muscles were perfused in situ to eliminate differences in oxygen delivery, the increased mitochondrial enzyme content of the exercised muscles of the ligated legs resulted in their [ATP]/[ADP][Pi] falling less at each level of exercise of the muscles than was the case for controls (8). This is consistent with the observations for endurance-trained muscle (4, 6).

DISCUSSION

When the data are considered as a whole, it is apparent that the signal for modulation of the cellular content of mitochondrial enzymes is related to the products of mitochondrial metabolism. The level of mitochondrial enzymes in tissue is clearly coupled to the metabolic need of that tissue for the synthesis of ATP. The sensor activity derives from long-term changes in the levels of the metabolic products of mitochondrial metabolism as evidenced by the necessity for long (days to weeks) periods of altered metabolic demand to alter the mitochondrial enzyme levels. In each case, the metabolic stress was submaximal and sustained for considerable periods. When muscles with enhanced content of mitochondrial enzymes and controls were subjected to similar intensities of exercise (4, 6, 7, 17), the changes in high energy phosphates (creatine phosphate, ATP) were substantially smaller in the muscles with greater enzyme content. The increase in mitochondrial content, therefore, alleviates the metabolic difficiency that is the signal for the increase.

The effect of thyroid hormone on heart muscle is also illuminating as the rates of respiration are increased only about twofold. This increase, however, was sustained throughout the 24-hour period. Thus the sensor is not detecting the intensity of the displacement of mitochondrial metabolism from the resting value per se, but rather to the integral of the stimulus over substantial periods (days). The sensor activity, therefore, involves a slow, progressive response to the modification of cellular energy state. This response is progressive, resulting in an effect that is cumulative, reflecting both the time and intensity of the metabolic modification. The involvement of metabolic products other than the [ATP]/[ADP][Pi], such as intracellular pH or of stress on the muscle fiber in sensing the mitochondrial enzyme content is unlikely. The intracellular pH was unlikely to be modified in the hearts of hyperthyroid versus hypothyroid animals, as minimal change in respiratory rate was involved. Stress on the muscle fibers is clearly less in exercise of ischemic muscle than in normal muscle. Likewise, the sensor does not appear to respond to the intramitochondrial [NAD$^+$]/[NADH], except indirectly, as the [NAD$^+$]/[NADH] is under independent control by many levels of metabolic regulators. Moreover, similar induction of mitochondrial enzymes was observed with endurance exercise and moderate exercise in ischemic muscle. The latter would be expected to be accompanied by a much greater increase in the reduction of the pyridine nucleotides than the former, due to the development of a relative hypoxia.

The *metabolic sensor* for regulation of the mitochondrial enzyme content has the following characteristics: (1) it operates over relatively long time intervals, responding only to those increases or decreases in ATP utilization that continue for extended periods and (2) it has the ability to operate selectively for different types of cells, that is, cells that normally operate at very different cytoplasmic [ATP]/[ADP][Pi] values. Thus, the sensor does not detect deviations of cytoplasmic [ATP]/[ADP][Pi] from a single value but rather it detects deviation from the value specific for the cell type in question.

CONCLUSION

The sensor responsible for regulating the cellular content of mitochondrial enzymes appears to be, by current evidence, the cytoplasmic phosphorylation potential ([ATP]/[ADP][Pi]). The cytoplasmic [ATP]/[ADP][Pi] is itself subject to modification according to the needs of cellular differentiation, as it is an important determinant of the metabolic capacity of the cell. The cytoplasmic phosphorylation potential is set by the mechanisms responsible for differentiation, and the mechanisms that determine the mitochondrial enzyme content are designed to provide sufficient enzyme to attain that value.

REFERENCES

1. BLOMQVIST, C. G., AND B. SALTIN. Cardiovascular adaptations to physical training. *Annu. Rev. Physiol.* 45:169–189, 1983.
2. BYLUND, A.-C., J. HAMMARSTEN, J. HOLM, AND T. SCHERSTEN. Enzyme activities in skeletal muscle from patients with peripheral arterial insufficiency. *Eur. J. Clin. Invest.* 6:425–429, 1976.
3. BYLUND-FELLENIUS, A. -C., P. M. WALKER, A. ELANDER, S. HOLM, J. HOLM, AND T. SCHERSTEN. Energy metabolism in relation to oxygen partial pressure in human skeletal muscle during exercise. *Biochem. J.* 200:247–255, 1981.
4. CONSTABLE, S. H., R. J. FAVIER, J. A. McLANE, R. D. FELL, M. CHEN, AND J. O. HOLLOSZY. Energy metabolism in contracting rat skeletal muscle: adaptation to training. *Am. J. Physiol.* 253:C316–C322, 1987.
5. DAVIES, K. J. A., L. PACKER, AND G. BROOKS. Biochemical adaptation of mitochondria, muscle, and whole-animal respiration to endurance training. *Arch. Biochem. Biophys.* 209:539–554, 1981.
6. DUDLEY, G. A., P. C. TULLSON, AND R. I. TERJUNG. Influence of mitochondrial content on the sensitivity of respiratory control. *J. Biol. Chem.* 262:9109–9114, 1987.
7. ELANDER, A., J. -P. IDSTROM, S. HOLM, T. SCHERSTEN, AND A. -C. BYLUND-FELLENIUS. Metabolic adaptation to reduced muscle blood flow. II. Mechanisms and beneficial effects. *Am. J. Physiol.* 249:E70–E76, 1985.
8. ELANDER, A., J. -P. IDSTROM, T. SCHERSTEN, AND A. -C. BYLUND-FELLENIUS. Metabolic adaptation to reduced muscle blood flow. I. Enzyme and metabolite alterations. *Am. J. Physiol.* 249:E63–E69, 1985.
9. ERECINSKA, M., AND D. F. WILSON. Regulation of cellular energy metabolism. *J. Memb. Biol.* 70:1–14, 1982.
10. ERECINSKA, M., D. F. WILSON, AND K. NISHIKI. Homeostatic regulation of energy metabolism: experimental characterization in vivo and fit to a model. *Am. J. Physiol.* 234:C82–C89, 1978.
11. FORMAN, N. G., AND D. F. WILSON. Energetics and stoichiometry of oxidative phosphorylation from NADH to cytochrome c in isolated rat liver mitochondria. *J. Biol. Chem.* 257:12908–12915, 1982.
12. HENDRIKSSON, J. Training induced adaptations of skeletal muscle and metabolism during submaximal exercise. *J. Physiol. (London)* 38:661–675, 1977.
13. HOLIAN, A., C. S. OWEN, AND D. F. WILSON. Control of respiration in isolated mitochondria: quantitative evaluation of the dependence of respiratory rates on [ATP], [ADP], and [Pi]. *Arch. Biochem. Biophys.* 181:164–171, 1977.
14. HOLLOSZY, J. O., AND F. W. BOOTH. Biochemical adaptation to endurance exercise in muscle. *Annu. Rev. Physiol.* 38:273–291, 1976.

15. KASHIWAGURA, T., D. F. WILSON, AND M. ERECINSKA. Oxygen dependence of cellular metabolism: the effect of O_2 tension on gluconeogenesis and urea synthesis in isolated rat hepatocytes. *J. Cellular Physiol.* *120*:13–18, 1984.
16. NISHIKI, N., M. ERECINSKA, AND D. F. WILSON. Energy relationships between cytosolic metabolism and mitochondrial respiration. *Am. J. Physiol.* *234*:C73–C81, 1978.
17. NISHIKI, N., M. ERECINSKA, D. F. WILSON, AND S. COOPER. Evaluation of oxidative phosphorylation in hearts from euthyroid, hypothyroid, and hyperthyroid rats. *Am. J. Physiol.* *235*(5):C212–C219, 1978.
18. NUUTINEN, E. M., J. K. HILTUNEN, AND I. E. HASSINEN. The glutamate dehydrogenase system and the redox state of mitochondrial free nicotinamide adenine dinucleotide in myocardium. *FEBS Letters* *128*:356–360, 1981.
19. STARNES, J. W., D. F. WILSON, AND M. ERECINSKA. Substrate dependence of metabolic state and coronary flow in perfused rat heart. *Am. J. Physiol.* *249*:H799–H806, 1985.
20. TERJUNG, R. L., G. M. MATHIEN, T. P. ERNEY, AND R. W. OGILIE. Peripheral adaptations to low blood flow in muscle during exercise. *Am. J. Cardiol.* *62*:15E–19E, 1988.
21. WILSON, D. F., AND M. ERECINSKA. Effect of oxygen concentration on cellular metabolism. *Chest* *88S*:229S–232S, 1985.
22. WILSON, D. F., M. ERECINSKA, C. DROWN, AND I. A. SILVER. The oxygen dependence of cellular energy metabolism. *Arch. Biochem. Biophys.* *195*:485–493, 1979.
23. WILSON, D. F., C. S. OWEN, AND M. ERECINSKA. Quantitative dependence of mitochondrial oxidative phosphorylation on oxygen concentration: a mathematical model. *Arch. Biochem. Biophys.* *195*:494–504, 1979.
24. WILSON, D. F., M. STUBBS, N. OSHINO, AND M. ERECINSKA. Thermodynamic relationships between the mitochondrial oxidation-reduction reactions and cellular ATP levels in ascites tumor cells and perfused rat liver. *Biochemistry* *13*:5305–5311, 1974.
25. WILSON, D. F., M. STUBBS, R. L. VEECH, M. ERECINSKA, AND H. A. KREBS. Equilibrium relations between the oxidation–reduction reactions and the adenosine triphosphate synthesis in suspensions of isolated liver cells. *Biochem. J.* *140*:57–64, 1974.

3

Regulation of Mitochondrial Distribution: An Adaptive Response to Changes in Oxygen Supply

DEAN P. JONES, TAK YEE AW,
CHANGLI BAI, AND A. H. SILLAU

Our recent research has focused on the functional and structural changes of cells in response to changes in O_2 supply. This research has been based on earlier studies that provide a working model for defining cellular O_2 dependence. This model was derived from experimental data that have been presented previously in detail (3, 18, 23, 24) and analyzed and reviewed elsewhere (19–21, 24, 25). In this discussion of mitochondrial distribution in response to changes in O_2 supply, we begin with a brief description of this model and a review of the factors that can affect the cellular O_2 dependence. Subsequent sections consider potential mechanisms for changing cellular O_2 dependence, experimental data on factors affecting the cellular O_2 dependence, and potential mechanisms for changing the geometry of mitochondrial distribution.

MITOCHONDRIAL CLUSTERING AS A DETERMINANT OF CELLULAR OXYGEN DEPENDENCE

A concentration gradient (ΔC) of O_2 will occur in any unmixed solution where there is a spatial separation of elements for O_2 supply and removal. In general, the magnitude of the gradient over a defined geometry is described by the equation

$$\Delta C = \frac{K}{D} \times G \tag{1}$$

where K is the O_2 consumption rate, D is the diffusion coefficient for O_2 in the medium, and G is a term or function appropriate for the geometry. For diffusion into an isolated sphere of radius b, $G = b^2/3$ (5) so that the equation for diffusion into mitochondria or mitochondrial aggregates in cells is:

$$\Delta C = \frac{Kb^2}{3D} \tag{2}$$

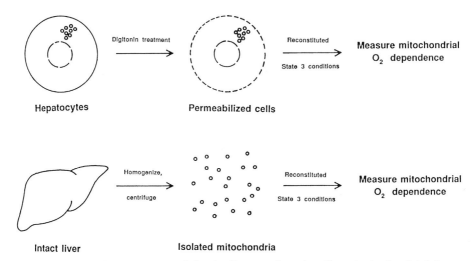

FIGURE 3.1. Use of digitonin-permeabilized cells to analyze the effect of mitochondrial clustering on cellular O_2 dependence.

For isolated cells, we can obtain information on the contribution of the spatial distribution of mitochondria to the cellular O_2 dependence by comparing the O_2 dependences of isolated liver mitochondria and mitochondria retained in the cytoskeleton of permeabilized hepatocytes (Fig. 3.1). By selecting a suitable concentration of digitonin, one can selectively disrupt the plasma membrane without detectable damage to the mitochondria and without substantial redistribution of mitochondria (12). When isolated mitochondria and digitonin-treated cells were suspended under identical conditions (same buffer, pH, and concentrations of cytochromes, ADP, and metabolic substrates), the O_2 concentration required for half-maximal oxidation of cytochrome $c + c_1$ (P_{50} value) was significantly lower for the isolated mitochondria (18). This difference was also present for mitochondria and digitonin-treated cells in the presence of an uncoupler, indicating that differences in respiratory control cannot account for the differences between mitochondria and permeabilized cells (18). Therefore, the difference in oxygen half-saturation pressure (P_{50}) values appears to be due to the difference in spatial distribution of mitochondria, that is, single in suspension or retained in clusters within the cytoskeleton.

Using the difference in P_{50} values as an estimate of the average O_2 concentration gradient into the mitochondria in the permeabilized cells, one can analyze the spatial distribution of the mitochondria for different geometries. We have used radial diffusion into O_2-consuming spheres as a first approximation, but other geometries could also be considered. Because of the cushioning effect of the mitochondrial chain (7), the O_2 consumption rate at the P_{50} value for cytochromes $c + c_1$ is very near the maximal O_2 consumption value; therefore, the latter can be used for analysis (23). With replacement of the aqueous cytoplasm by the suspending medium, the value for D can be safely assumed to be that of O_2 in a normal salt solution. With these considerations, the results show that the O_2 dependence of mitochondria in permeabilized cells responds as though the mitochondria are in clusters with an average radius of about 2 μm (18).

This analysis of permeabilized cells also provides an approach to estimate the intracellular diffusion coefficient for O_2 (D_c). This can be done with Equation 2 applied to the comparison of P_{50} values for intact cells and digitonin-permeabilized cells, and using the value for the average cluster radius determined from the above analysis (18). The value obtained from this approach ranges from about 2×10^{-6} to 4.5×10^{-6} cm^2/s, depending on the correction that is made for an extracellular unstirred layer (18). For cells and digitonin-treated cells (or mitochondria) treated with carbonylcyanide-p-trifluoromethoxyphenylhydrazone (FCCP) to eliminate respiratory control, the results for estimates of b and D were nearly identical, indicating that respiratory control characteristics have minimal effects on cellular O_2 dependence under these conditions.

POTENTIAL MECHANISMS FOR CHANGING CELLULAR OXYGEN DEPENDENCE

From these considerations, it is clear that there are several possible ways in which cells could adapt to hypoxia and function maximally at a lower O_2 concentration. The potential contributions of changes in respiration rate, distribution of mitochondria, and D_c can be compared by calculating ΔC from Equation 2 as a function of each of these parameters. This analysis (Fig. 3.2) shows that the magnitude of the gradient is directly proportional to the respiration rate and inversely proportional to D_c; in contrast, the magnitude is proportional to the square of the average radius of mitochondrial clusters. Thus, although changes in any of the three factors will affect the gradient, a change in the extent of clustering would appear to be most effective in changing the cellular O_2 dependence.

Compared to these changes that could occur within the cell, a reduction in the cell size alone is relatively ineffective in changing the cellular O_2 dependence (6). This occurs for two reasons. First, the diffusion coefficient in the cell is only 15% to 20% of the value in aqueous salts solutions (19). This means

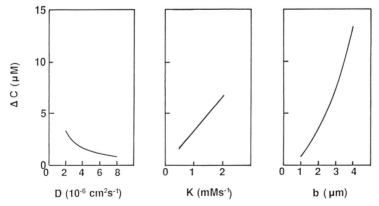

FIGURE 3.2. Effect of changes in diffusion coefficient (D_c), O_2 consumption rate (K) and radius of mitochondrial cluster on the magnitude of the O_2 gradient to mitochondria (ΔC).

that the contribution due to an unstirred layer outside the cell is always relatively small compared with the gradient inside the cell. Second, the transcellular diffusion gradient created by radial diffusion into cells is normally small relative to that created by radial diffusion into a cluster (A. H. Sillau, T. Y. Aw, and D. P. Jones, manuscript submitted). Because few cells with high O_2 consumption rate/volume ratios have a large radius (cardiac myocytes are the only cells that we have found where this is significant; 29), it is unlikely that a change in cell size provides a common mechanism to adjust the cellular O_2 dependence in response to hypoxia.

A potential mechanism to regulate cellular O_2 dependence by modulating the apparent affinity of the cytochrome oxidase has been considered in detail by Wilson and co-workers (43). They and others (9, 30, 35, 43) have found that a high adenosine triphosphate to adenosine diphosphate (ATP/ADP) ratio can inhibit mitochondrial respiration and increase the apparent K_{mO2}. This condition, however, may not be directly applicable to intracellular conditions because the ATP/ADP ratio falls during hypoxia. Thus, even though the apparent K_{mO2} is relatively high in isolated mitochondria incubated with high ATP/ADP, this does not mean that when one lowers $[O_2]$ in the cell that the apparent K_{mO2} will be high. In fact, because under these conditions the ATP/ADP falls, the apparent K_{mO2} in the cells should be a lower value as obtained with isolated mitochondria when ATP/ADP is low. This interpretation is supported by experiments in which mitochondria were treated with a protonophore to eliminate respiratory control in both isolated mitochondria and intact cells (18). Addition of FCCP, which results in elimination of coupling of oxidation to phosphorylation, resulted in an increase in the P_{50} in both mitochondria and cells but did not eliminate the difference between P_{50} values for the two preparations (18). Thus, changes in the K_{mO2} for mitochondrial oxidation due to changes in ATP/ADP are not the major contributor to the cellular O_2 dependence under usual conditions in cells with clustered mitochondria such as adult rat hepatocytes (18), cardiac myocytes (29), and proximal tubule cells (3). Because of this, a change in the respiratory control is not likely to have a great impact on the cellular O_2 dependence. On the other hand, in cells where mitochondria are not extensively clustered, a change in respiratory control characteristics could have a major effect on the cellular O_2 dependence. For instance, this could occur if an initial response of the cells is to inhibit ATP utilization such that ATP/ADP does not fall as $[O_2]$ falls.

EXPERIMENTAL DATA ON FACTORS AFFECTING THE
CELLULAR OXYGEN DEPENDENCE

The respiration rate of cells can vary considerably in different tissues depending on the demand for energy-requiring functions. As described previously, the magnitude of O_2 gradients into cells should be proportional to the O_2 consumption rate of the cells. This prediction has been confirmed in experiments with freshly isolated hepatocytes, cardiac myocytes, and proximal tubule cells (3, 23, 26). The results are most dramatic in the cardiac myocytes because these cells are noncontractile upon isolation and have an O_2 consumption rate similar to that in the arrested heart (29). As freshly isolated, these cells have an O_2 consumption rate of 66 nmol/10^6 cells/minute and a half-maximal oxidation of cytochrome $a + a_3$ at 5.8 µM. Electrical stimulation of these cells to contract results in stimulation of O_2 consumption to 121 nmol/10^6 cells/minute and an increase in P_{50} value to 11.6 µM (26). Similar changes in P_{50} value in response to changes in O_2 consumption rate occur in kidney cells, where the ATP demand can be differentially affected by inhibiting the Na^+, K^+-ATPase with ouabain or stimulating the activity by adding the Na^+ ionophore, nystatin (3). Thus, a twofold change in respiration roughly gives a twofold change in O_2 dependence of the cells. This indicates that an adaptation to hypoxia that would make cells less sensitive to O_2 deficiency would be to decrease cellular respiratory activity. The disadvantageous aspect of this mechanism of adaptation is that it would also result in a loss of functional capacity. Moreover, our studies of hepatocytes from chronically hypoxic rats have shown that respiration rate does not decrease significantly in the hypoxic cells. Thus, it appears that this mechanism may be involved under some conditions, but does not provide a highly effective or common mechanism of adaptation.

In contrast, redistribution of mitochondria from large clusters to give smaller clusters and more uniform distribution can have a much larger effect on the cellular O_2 dependence. Costa et al. (8) found that mitochondria in livers of rats that were maintained under hypobaric hypoxia for 6 months had relatively uniformly distributed mitochondria, whereas those from animals maintained at normoxia were extensively clustered. They found no difference in the characteristics of the mitochondria; we have examined the O_2 dependence of isolated mitochondria from control and chronically hypoxic cells and also found no difference in their P_{50} values (39). When we examined the O_2 dependence of hepatocytes from normoxic and chronically hypoxic (Pio_2, 70 mm Hg for 8 to 10 days) rats, however, we found that the P_{50} values for hypoxic cells are significantly lower than those of normoxic cells (39). This difference is also preserved in digitonin-treated cells that were reconstituted under state 3 conditions and also in the presence of FCCP. Thus, in the in vivo chronic hypoxia model, it appears that at least part of the acclimation to hypoxia is at the cellular level and due to a redistribution of mitochondria.

We have found a marked change in cellular O_2 dependence in association with differentiation of fetal hepatocytes as they mature to adult hepatocytes. Electron micrographs indicate that there is a lower density of mitochondria in hepatocytes from fetal and neonatal cells compared with adult cells (16, 27). Measurement of the O_2 dependence of respiratory function in hepatocytes from newborn and adult rats showed that the cells from the newborns required a substantially lower O_2 concentration for maximal function than did the cells from the adults (2). There was no difference in the O_2 dependence of the isolated mitochondria. Thus, the results indicate that major determinants of the cellular O_2 requirement in isolated hepatocytes are the density and extent of clustering of mitochondria; the cells from the newborn function maximally at relatively low O_2 concentrations but have a relatively low total functional capacity. During the first few weeks of life, the O_2 dependence of the hepatocytes shifts from the characteristics of the isolated mitochondria to that of the adult hepatocytes. This means that larger changes in cellular O_2 dependence are possible than those that we observed during 8 to 10 days adaptation to in vivo hypoxia.

A dramatic change in cellular O_2 dependence occurs when freshly isolated hepatocytes are placed in primary culture (22). Cultured cells frequently undergo a phenotypic change due to the loss of normal substratum for growth and due to the abnormal content of hormones and growth factors in the media. This change includes a loss of cytochromes and has characteristics similar to the dedifferentiation that occurs upon transformation of normal cells to malignant cells. The change in O_2 dependence of adult hepatocytes occurs rapidly; within 48 hours in culture, the O_2 dependence that is characteristic of adult cells is shifted to that of isolated mitochondria or fetal cells. Thus, one of the changes of dedifferentiated cells is that they have undergone a change that adapts them to better tolerate hypoxia.

These examples illustrate how mitochondrial changes that occur during development, exposure to hypoxia, and dedifferentiation (as occurs in carcinogenic transformation), result in adaptations of the cells with regard to O_2 dependence. This indicates that the distribution of mitochondria is a dynamic process; cells have the ability to adapt with new distributions according to O_2 supply and energy needs. This property is important to normal physiology because adaptation to dynamic changes in the microvasculature could be an ongoing process in cells. Several years ago, Quistorff (36) found that enzyme activities rapidly change in hepatocytes that are attached in a column and perfused with an O_2-containing medium such that the cells were exposed to a gradient of O_2 concentrations. In vivo, cells at the arterial end of a capillary are exposed to a higher O_2 concentration than cells at the venular end. In the liver, this results in a marked zonation of metabolism with gluconeogenesis being most active at the centrilobular end. Mitochondria are also distributed heterogeneously within the liver lobule. Loud (32) found that the mitochondria were larger and more densely packed in the periportal cells than in the centrilobular cells. We recently used a selective disruption technique (31) to isolate and study the O_2 dependences of periportal and centrilobular hepatocytes. The results of these studies showed that the P_{50} value for the periportal cells (6.0 μM) was higher than that for the centrilobular cells (4.9 μM; Fig. 3.3). Thus, the centrilobular cells are adapted to function maximally at a lower concentration of O_2 than the periportal cells.

MECHANISMS FOR CHANGE IN GEOMETRY OF
MITOCHONDRIAL DISTRIBUTION

The recognition that mitochondria have cell-specific distribution patterns in adult mammalian cells (10) and that they undergo redistribution in adaptation to physiological changes indicates that mechanisms must exist to move mitochondria and to anchor them in specific sites. Although considerable information is now available concerning molecular motors that function to move organelles in cells, the molecular details of the components responsible for moving mitochondria and anchoring them in specific sites remains fragmentary.

In nerve axons, mitochondria have been observed to be associated with

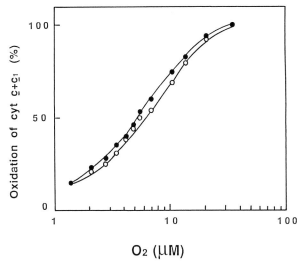

FIGURE 3.3. Oxygen dependence of cytochrome $c + c_1$ oxidation in periportal ($\bigcirc$) and centrilobular ($\bullet$) hepatocytes. Data are averages from five different cell preparations for each. Standard error was typically less than the size of the points in this figure, and P_{50} values were significantly different at $P < 0.01$.

microtubules and to be moved along the microtubule tracts. Deep-etch studies of Hirokawa (17) show that two types of cross-linking components are present that link mitochondria to microtubules and neurofilaments in the nerve axon. Microtubular transport, however, appears to be a system with a common function to move organelles; this alone cannot account for directional movement and accumulation of mitochondria in specific sites.

Studies of the localization of components that bind antitubulin and antimitochondrial antibodies show that mitochondria are associated with microtubules in cultured cells (15). Mitochondria also associate with intermediate filaments, and in some cells, with other cytoskeletal structures (41). For instance, Summerhayes et al. (40) showed an association of mitochondria with intermediate filaments by co-localization of antibodies to vimentin- and rhodamine-stained mitochondria. In addition, studies with immunofluorescence techniques have shown that antibodies raised from a component of intermediate filaments subpopulation reacts specifically with mitochondria of different cell types (33). Furthermore, Hirokawa (17) found cross-linking elements between mitochondria and neurofilaments in axons. Thus, there is reasonable evidence that mitochondria can associate with different cytoskeletal network elements.

In several cell types, there is an apparent association of mitochondria with the plasma membrane. This is clearly seen in transport epithelia, such as in distal convoluted tubule cells of the kidney (10). In some cases, specific junctional complexes have been found and microfilaments might be involved in these associations (13, 38). In cardiac muscle, two populations of mitochondria have been separated experimentally (34). One is located beneath the sarcolemma, and the other is between the myofibrils. Studies of biochemical and transport properties show that these populations are functionally different. In cultured cardiomyocytes and fibroblasts, mitochondrial clusters are connected by gap junctions to maintain a continuous proton gradient, and constitute a supernetwork for production of energy (1). Associations of mitochondria with other subcellular structures, such as endoplasmic reticulum, has also been demonstrated (14, 28). In injured cells and freshly plated cultured cells, there is frequently a high density of mitochondria in the perinuclear zone (21), and in both skeletal and heart muscle, there is typically a cluster of mitochondria adjacent to each cell nucleus (21). Thus, there are many different yet seemingly specific associations of mitochondria within cells.

The association of mitochondria with microtubules has been suggested to occur by microtubule-associated proteins (MAPs) (37). Because this group of proteins are widely distributed and in many cases are tissue- and species-specific (42), MAPs could be involved in the regulation of mitochondria distribution. It is currently unclear, however, whether they are the critical proteins that link mitochondria to microtubules and allow their controlled redistribution within cells.

At present it is unknown whether there are common or specific mechanisms for moving the mitochondria in different cells or whether there are common or specific "anchors" in different cell types and at different sites within cells. Perhaps the clearest example of the specificity of movement and anchoring mitochondria is in the development of avian sperm tail (11). During spermatogenesis, microtubules are initially laid down in a spiral manner around the contractile axoneme. Subsequently, the mitochondria that previously aligned along the axoneme were oriented surrounding the axoneme in association with the microtubules. Finally, the microtubules are removed and the mitochondria are retained with a spiral distribution. Thus, the process of distributing mitochondria to specific sites in the avian sperm tail includes a sequence of reactions involving establishment of a scaffold with a molecular motor to move mitochondria into position followed by an anchoring of mitochondria in place and removal of the scaffold. It is not clear whether this is a general sequence for distributing mitochondria, and additional studies in mammalian tissues will be needed to understand this process.

In an initial attempt to isolate proteins involved in binding mitochondria to other mitochondria and to other organelles, we have developed a filtration assay to measure mitochondrial aggregation and release from cytoskeletal components (4). This approach uses polycarbonate filters with uniform-sized cylindrical pores that allow only single mitochondria (or very small aggregates) to penetrate (Fig. 3.4). Thus, one can readily measure the release of mitochondria from the cytoskeleton to determine the factors that are critical to retain the association and also to measure the extent of aggregation caused by specific in vitro metabolic conditions. With this approach, we are hopeful to isolate and characterize the molecular components involved in the adaptation of cellular O_2 requirements that occurs through redistribution of mitochondria.

SUMMARY AND CONCLUSIONS

1. Studies with freshly isolated cells from adult rat show that the O_2 concentration requirement for mitochondrial function is about an order of magnitude higher than that of isolated mitochondria. Analysis of data from digi-

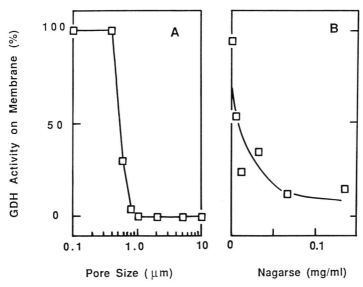

FIGURE 3.4. Use of membrane filtration to measure release of single mitochondria from clusters in hepatocytes. (**A**) Isolated single mitochondria penetrate polycarbonate pores greater than 1 μm. (**B**) Single mitochondria are not released from digitonin-permeabilized hepatocytes unless treated with the protease nagarse. GDH = glutamate dehydrogenase. Data redrawn from Ref. 4.

tonin-permeabilized cells and isolated mitochondria, each reconstituted in state 3 conditions, shows that spatial distribution of mitochondria within the cytoskeleton is an important determinant of the cellular O_2 dependence. Comparison of the magnitude of effects on O_2 gradients due to changes in diffusion coefficient, respiratory rate, and extent of clustering shows that regulation of cluster size provides a relatively more sensitive control of mitochondrial O_2 dependence.

2. Studies with several physiological conditions indicate that the cellular O_2 dependence is altered by changes in mitochondrial distribution. Chronic hypoxia results in decreased clustering of mitochondria and a decrease in the O_2 concentration required for mitochondrial function. The O_2 dependence of mitochondrial function in neonatal hepatocytes increases during postnatal development in association with increases in mitochondrial density and cluster size. Conversely, primary cultures of adult rat hepatocytes undergo a large decrease in cellular O_2 dependence within 48 hours of plating in association with a loss of mitochondrial density and a decrease in the extent of mitochondrial clustering. The results of O_2 dependence studies in periportal and pericentral cells also show that the periportal cells, which are normally exposed to a higher O_2 concentration and have a larger mitochondrial clustering, also require a higher O_2 concentration for maximal function. Thus, several examples indicate that regulation of mitochondrial distribution is an important adaptive response to O_2 supply.

3. Current knowledge is limited concerning the molecular mechanisms that determine mitochondrial distribution patterns in different cells. Mitochondria are known to associate with and to be moved along microtubular tracts. In addition, mitochondria are found to be associated with a variety of

other cellular elements. Thus, movement along microtubules may provide a general means to redistribute mitochondria, and specificity of distribution may be provided by selective interaction with other cellular components.

ACKNOWLEDGMENT

The research upon which this manuscript was based was provided by the National Institutes of Health grant GM 36538.

REFERENCES

1. Amchenkova, A. A., L. E. Bakeeva, Y. S. Chentsov, and V. P. Skulachev. Coupling membranes as energy-transmitting cables. I. Filamentous mitochondria in fibroblasts and mitochondrial clusters in cardiomyocytes. *J. Cell Biol. 107*:481–495, 1988.
2. Aw, T. Y., and D. P. Jones. Respiratory characteristics of neonatal rat hepatocytes. *Pediatr. Res. 21*:492–496, 1987.
3. Aw, T. Y., E. Wilson, T. M. Hagen, and D. P. Jones. Determinants of mitochondrial O_2 dependence in kidney. *Am. J. Physiol. 253*:F440–F447, 1987.
4. Bai, C., C. S. Slife, T. Y. Aw, and D. P. Jones. Fractionation and analysis of mitochondria with polycarbonate membrane filters. *Anal. Biochem. 179*:114–119, 1989.
5. Boag, J. W. Oxygen diffusion and oxygen depletion problems in radiobiology. *Curr. Top. Radiat. Res. 5*:141–195, 1969.
6. Boag, J. W. Cellular respiration as a function of oxygen tension. *Int. J. Radiat. Biol. 18*:475–477, 1970.
7. Chance, B. Cellular oxygen requirements. *Fed. Proc. 16*:671–680, 1957.
8. Costa, L. E., A. Boveris, O. R. Koch, and A. C. Taquini. Liver and heart mitochondria in rats submitted to chronic hypobaric hypoxia. *Am. J. Physiol. 255*:C123–C129, 1988.
9. Davis, E. J., and W. I. A. Davis-van Thienen. Control of mitochondrial metabolism by the ATP/ADP ratio. *Biochem. Biophys. Res. Communic. 83*:1260–1266, 1978.
10. Fawcett, D. W. The cell. In: *Mitochondria,* 2nd ed. Philadelphia: W. B. Saunders, 1981, pp. 410–485.
11. Fawcett, D. W., W. A. Anderson, and D. M. Phillips. Morphogenetic factors influencing the shape of the sperm head. *Dev. Biol. 26*:220–251, 1971.
12. Fiskum, G., S. W. Craig, G. L. Decker, and A. L. Lehninger. The cytoskeleton of digitonin-treated rat hepatocytes. *Proc. Natl. Acad. Sci. (USA) 77*:3430–3434, 1980.
13. Freddo, T. F. Mitochondria attached to desmosomes in the ciliary epithelia of human, monkey, and rabbit eyes. *Cell Tissue Res. 251*:671–675, 1988.
14. Gronblad, M., and K. E. O. Akerman. Electron-dense endoplasmic reticulum-like profiles closely associated with mitochondria in glomus cells of the carotid body after fixation with oxalate. *Expt. Cell Res. 152*:161–168, 1984.
15. Heggeness, M. H., M. Simon, and S. J. Singer. Association of mitochondria with microtubules in cultured cells. *Proc. Natl. Acad. Sci. (USA) 75*:3863–3866, 1978.
16. Herzfeld, A., M. Federman, and O. Greengard. Subcellular morphometric and biochemical analyses of developing rat hepatocytes. *J. Cell Biol. 57*:475–483, 1973.
17. Hirokawa, N. Cross-linker system between neurofilaments, microtubules, and membranous organelles in frog axons revealed by the quick-freeze, deep-etching method. *J. Cell Biol. 94*:129–142, 1982.
18. Jones, D. P. Effect of mitochondrial clustering on O_2 supply in hepatocytes. *Am. J. Physiol. 247*:C83–C89, 1984.
19. Jones, D. P. Intracellular diffusion gradients of O_2 and ATP. *Am. J. Physiol. 250*:C663-C675, 1986.
20. Jones, D. P. New concepts of the molecular pathogenesis arising from hypoxia. In: *Oxidases and Related Redox Systems,* eds. T. E. King, H. S. Mason and M. Morrison. New York: Alan R. Liss, 1988, pp. 127–144.
21. Jones, D. P., and T. Y. Aw. Mitochondrial distribution and O_2 gradients in mammalian cells. In: *Microcompartmentation,* ed. D. P. Jones. Boca Raton, Florida: CRC Press, 1988, pp. 37–53.
22. Jones, D. P., T. Y. Aw, B. C. Lincoln, and H. L. Bonkovsky. Oxygen concentration requirement for mitochondrial function in rat hepatocytes decreases dramatically during 2 days in primary culture. *The Physiologist 30*:123, 1987.

23. JONES, D. P., AND F. G. KENNEDY. Intracellular oxygen supply during hypoxia. *Am. J. Physiol. 243*:C247–C253, 1982.

24. JONES, D. P., AND F. G. KENNEDY. Analysis of intracellular oxygenation of isolated adult cardiac myocytes. *Am. J. Physiol. 250*:C384–C390, 1986.

25. JONES, D. P., F. G. KENNEDY, B. S. ANDERSSON, T. Y. AW, AND E. WILSON. When is a mammalian cell hypoxic? Insights from studies of cells versus mitochondria. *Mol. Physiol. 8*:473–482, 1985.

26. JONES, D. P., F. G. KENNEDY, AND T. Y. AW. Intracellular O_2 gradients and the distribution of mitochondria. In: *Hypoxia: The Tolerable Limits,* eds. J. R. Sutton, C. S. Houston and G. Coates. Carmel, Ind.: Benchmark Press, 1988, pp. 59–69.

27. KANAMURA, S., K. KANAI, M. OKA, Y. SHUGYO, AND J. WATANABE. Quantitative analysis of development of mitochondrial ultrastructure in differentiating mouse hepatocytes during postnatal period. *J. Ultrastruct. Res. 93*:195–204, 1985.

28. KATZ, J., P. A. WALS, S. GOLDEN, AND L. RAIJMAN. Mitochondrial–reticular cytostructure in liver cells. *Biochem. J. 214*:795–813, 1983.

29. KENNEDY, F. G., AND D. P. JONES. Oxygen dependence of mitochondrial function in isolated rat cardiac myocytes. *Am. J. Physiol. 250*:C374–C383, 1986.

30. KUSTER, U., R. BOHNENSACK, AND W. KUNZ. Control of oxidative phosphorylation by the extramitochondrial ATP/ADP ratio. *Biochem. Biophys. Acta 440*:391–402, 1976.

31. LINDROS, K. O., AND K. E. PENTILLA. Digitonin–collagenase perfusion for efficient separation of periportal or perivenous hepatocytes. *Biochem. J. 228*:757–760, 1985.

32. LOUD, A. V. A quantitative stereological description of the ultrastructure of normal rat liver parenchymal cells. *J. Cell Biol. 37*:27–46, 1968.

33. MOSE-LARSEN, P., R. BRAVO, S. J. FEY, J. V. SMALL, AND J. E. CELIS. Putative association of mitochondria with a subpopulation of intermediate-sized filaments in cultured human skin fibroblasts. *Cell 31*:681–692, 1982.

34. PALMER, J. W., B. TANDLER, AND C. L. HOPPEL. Biochemical properties of subsarcolemmal and interfibrillar mitochondria isolated from rat cardiac muscle. *J. Biol. Chem. 252*:8731–8736, 1977.

35. PETERSEN, L. C., P. NICHOLLS, AND H. DEGN. The effect of energization on the apparent Michaelis-Menten constant for oxygen in mitochondrial respiration. *Biochem. J. 142*:247–252,, 1974.

36. QUISTORFF, B. The use of a hepatocyte column in the study of metabolic zonation in the liver. In: *Isolation, Characterization and Use of Hepatocytes,* ed. R. A. Harris and N. W. Cornell. New York: Elsevier Biomedical, 1983, pp. 131–137.

37. RENDON, A., D. FILLIOL, AND V. JANCSIK. Microtubule associated proteins bind to 30 KD and 60 KD proteins of rat brain mitochondria: visualization by ligand blotting. *Biochem. Biophys. Res. Commun. 149*:776–783, 1987.

38. SANTANDER, R. G., G. M. CUADRADO, AND M. R. SAEZ. High-energy adhering junctional complexes or with mitochondrial coupling. *Histol. Histopath. 2*:153–161, 1987.

39. SILLAU, A. H., T. Y. AW, AND D. P. JONES. O_2 dependence of cytochrome *c* oxidation in hepatocytes from hypoxic rats. *The Physiologist 34*:A146, 1988.

40. SUMMERHAYES, I. C., D. WONG, AND L. B. CHEN. Effect of microtubules and intermediate filaments on mitochondrial distribution. *J. Cell Sci. 61*:87–105, 1983.

41. TRAUB, P. *Intermediate filaments, a review.* Berlin: Springer-Verlag, 1985, pp. 58–60.

42. VALLEE, R. B., G. S. BLOOM, AND F. C. LUCA. Differential cellular and subcellular distribution of microtubule associated proteins. In: *Molecular Biology of the Cytoskeleton,* ed. Borisy, G. G., Cleveland, D., Murphy, D. B. New York: Cold Spring Harbor, 1984, pp. 111–130.

43. WILSON, D. F., M. ERECINSKA, C. DROWN, AND I. A. SILVER. The oxygen dependence of cellular metabolism. *Arch. Biochem. Biophys. 195*:485–493, 1979.

II
CELL AND MOLECULAR BIOLOGY
OF ERYTHROPOIETIN

4

Control of the Production of Erythropoietin by a Renal Oxygen-Sensor?

WOLFGANG JELKMANN, HORST PAGEL,
AND CHRISTOPH WEISS

The glycoprotein hormone erythropoietin (Epo) is an obligatory growth and differentiation factor for the erythrocytic progenitors. The plasma level of Epo in the human is about 5 to 25 mU/ml under normoxic conditions. Tissue hypoxia is a major stimulus for erythropoiesis. The plasma level of Epo may increase to 1000 mU/ml or more after the induction of anemia or hypoxic hypoxia (12, 20, 31).

Jacobson et al. (29) first proposed that blood-borne Epo is mainly of renal origin, as the plasma level of the hormone did not rise in bilaterally nephrectomized rats after stimulation with hypoxia or cobalt. Subsequently, Naets (45) found that erythropoiesis subsides in nephrectomized dogs but can be restored by the application of Epo. Indeed, recombinant human Epo has been used lately in the treatment of the anemia of renal insufficiency (10, 63). In 1961, Kuratowska et al. (38) and Fisher and Birdwell (13) demonstrated Epo in the effluent of isolated blood-perfused kidneys. This finding was confirmed in kidneys perfused with serum-free medium (6). Erythropoietin was demonstrated in kidney extracts from hypoxic rats. Extracts were more active from the cortex of the kidney than from the medulla (21, 32). Erythropoietin messenger RNA (mRNA) was found to rise in the kidney 1 to 2 hours after the induction of anemia (1, 2) or hypoxemia (59). In situ hybridization has also been used to identify the type of cell that produces Epo in murine kidneys (37, 40). The cells positive for Epo mRNA were neither tubular nor glomerular. It is most likely that peritubular capillary endothelial cells or a subset of interstitial cells in the kidney cortex are the site of the synthesis of Epo in the kidney (37, 40).

Although the capacity of the kidney to produce Epo has been fairly well documented, its role in the mechanism of O_2 sensing is still not completely understood. Herein, the evidence is reviewed that suggests that the O_2 tension in the kidney tissue is the primary parameter in the control of the synthesis of Epo. The questions raised are (1) whether the production of Epo increases when the O_2 supply to the kidney alone is lowered and (2) whether this Epo response is quantitatively similar to the one seen after a reduction of the whole body O_2?

IN VIVO STUDIES

The plasma level of Epo increases in humans and in experimental animals when the O_2 content of the arterial blood is reduced. A reduction can be accomplished by lowering either the arterial Po_2 or the O_2 carrying capacity of the blood. Very few studies have been performed in which the O_2 content of the arterial blood was diminished in the renal artery but not in the general circulation. Of note are earlier clinical observations in patients with erythrocytosis due to a patent ductus arteriosus Botalli with a reversed shunt. Because the hypoxemia was confined to the lower part of the body, O_2-sensitive tissue below the diaphragm was apparently involved in the stimulation of erythropoiesis (57, 60). Attempts were partially successful to trigger the production of Epo in anesthetized dogs by creating a shunt so that venous blood from the right atrium perfused the renal artery (52). Plasma from 4 of 8 dogs displayed some erythropoietic activity when the perfusion was carried out for at least 5 hours. In control experiments, plasma Epo was elevated in 1 of 5 dogs after shunting of arterial blood from the femoral artery into the kidney. This finding together with the reported Epo increase in only 2 of 6 dogs ventilated with 10% O_2 (52) renders a more quantitative analysis of the data difficult.

Penington (53) had earlier pointed out that "if the determining factor in erythropoietin secretion is the oxygen tension in the peritubular capillary network, it might be expected to be governed by the balance of oxygen supply and oxygen tension." In addition to the O_2 content of the blood, Penington regarded the rate of blood flow and the O_2 consumption by the tubule as important variables (53). Reduction in the flow due to stenosis of the renal artery very rarely leads to erythrocytosis (3, 28, 62). Nevertheless, there appears to be a slight increase in plasma Epo in patients with renal artery stenosis (3, 25). The clipping of the renal arteries in experimental animals was found to be a stimulus for the production of Epo by several investigators (17, 18, 24, 44, 61), with few exceptions (5). It has been reported that the inhibition of prostaglandin synthesis by indomethacin prevents the increase in plasma Epo in dogs after renal artery constriction (24, 44).

The O_2 tension in most of the tissue of the kidney is little affected by fluctuations of renal blood flow. The rate of the renal O_2 consumption falls in proportion with the blood flow, because the energy-consuming tubular sodium chloride reabsorption decreases pari passu with the glomerular filtration (see Ref. 36). Note that plasma Epo levels are relatively low in hypoxic animals with kidney tubule lesions (14, 35, 41, 56).

We have recently investigated the relationship between renal blood flow, O_2 tension in the renal venous blood, and production of Epo. Details of the experimental procedures are described in the papers by Pagel et al. (49, 50). In brief, renal blood flow was acutely lowered in rats by applying silver clips to both renal arteries. A controlled reduction of the renal blood flow was achieved by using clips of different inner diameters. As shown in Fig. 4.1, glomerular filtration decreased in proportion with renal blood flow. When the flow was reduced below 60% of normal, the O_2 tension in the renal vein clearly fell. It reached values below 10 mm Hg, when renal blood flow was 10% of normal. Under these conditions the concentration of Epo in the plasma in-

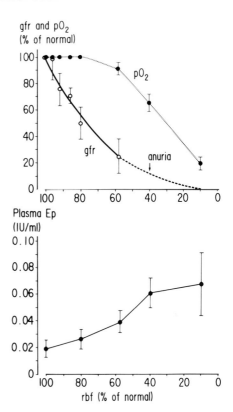

FIGURE 4.1. Effects of lowering renal blood flow (rbf) on glomerular filtration rate (gfr; mean ± SEM, $n = 5$) and renal venous O_2 tension (Po_2; $n = 10$; upper panel), and on plasma erythropoietin (Epo) bioactivity ($n = 3$ to 5; 18 to 20 hours after bilateral constriction of the renal arteries; lower panel) in male Sprague-Dawley rats. Based on studies by Pagel et al. (49, 50).

creased from a mean value of 20 to 69 mU/ml during the experimental period of 18 to 20 hours. This increase in Epo must be considered very moderate when compared with the response seen after a reduction of whole body O_2 content. For example, we have shown that the plasma Epo level in rats rises from 20 to 6000 mU/ml in severe anemia with blood hemoglobin values of 40 g/L blood (49) or to 4000 mU/ml when rats are exposed to simulated high altitude of 7000 m in a low-pressure chamber for 18 hours (30). Extrarenal sources clearly do not account for these high Epo levels, as extrarenal sites contribute only 10 to 25% to blood-borne Epo in anemic (8) or hypoxemic (35) rats.

In conclusion, our studies of the effects of reduced renal blood flow support the view that the production of Epo is stimulated, to some extent, when the O_2 supply to the kidney alone is reduced. The moderate increase in plasma Epo seen in association with very low renal venous O_2 tensions, however, leaves some doubt as to the exclusiveness of the renal O_2-sensitive mechanism controlling the production of Epo.

STUDIES IN ISOLATED PERFUSED KIDNEYS

Kuratowska et al. (38) first observed an increase in Epo activity in the blood perfusate of isolated rabbit kidneys after 3 hours of hypoxemic perfusion in a recirculation system. Some investigators confirmed these findings in rabbit

(55) and dog (15, 16, 64) kidneys perfused with blood at low O_2 tension. Other studies were negative (9). Erslev et al. (9) noted that the methods for the assay of Epo were quite crude in these early studies, and pH and blood gases were not quantified. Reissmann and Nomura (55) reported that several of their rabbit kidneys, including the technically best preparations, failed to produce Epo during hypoxemic perfusion. In addition, no Epo was generated when the kidneys were perfused with blood at low hemoglobin concentrations (55). We shall return to this interesting subject.

Because of the meager production of Epo in kidneys isolated from healthy animals, Malgor and Fisher (42) and Erslev (6) developed the model of the "programmed" kidneys, which were obtained from animals after previous exposure to hypobaric hypoxia. The release of Epo from programmed isolated perfused kidneys is enhanced, probably because the synthesis of the hormone is initiated in vivo. In addition, Erslev (6) showed that programmed isolated rabbit kidneys produce Epo when they are perfused with serum-free medium. Using serum-free perfused rat kidneys, Paul et al. (51) recently showed that the enzyme adenosine deaminase which breaks down adenosine, inhibits the formation of Epo. It had been reported earlier that the inhibition of prostaglandin synthesis prevents the elaboration of Epo in the programmed isolated perfused dog kidney (33). Renal arterial infusions of prostaglandin E or arachidonoic acid, on the other hand, stimulate the release of Epo from such kidneys (19). Thus, tissue hormones appear to play a regulatory role in the production of Epo by the kidney.

Using an optimized perfusion technique and a sensitive radioimmunoassay for Epo, we have reinvestigated the effects of reduced O_2 delivery on the production of Epo in isolated perfused rat kidneys. The kidneys were obtained from adult male Sprague-Dawley rats without prior "programming." As described by Schurek and Alt (58), the kidneys were perfused at constant pressure (100 mm Hg) in a recirculating system filled with 200 ml of substrate-enriched Krebs-Henseleit buffer supplemented with bovine serum albumin (60 g/L) and freshly drawn human erythrocytes. To ensure a high stability of the preparation, the perfusion medium was regenerated by dialysis as described in (58). The perfusion medium was equilibrated with 5% CO_2 (final pH 7.4) and various O_2 concentrations. In addition, different concentrations of erythrocytes were adjusted. Erythropoietin in the perfusate was measured by radioimmunoassay in fivefold-concentrated samples collected after a 3-hour perfusion period.

The radioimmunoassay was carried out using rat plasma Epo as the standard, ^{125}I-labeled recombinant human Epo (r-huEpo) as the tracer, and rabbit antiserum versus r-huEpo. The results shown in Table 4.1 indicate that the production of immunoreactive Epo increased when the O_2 tension of the perfusion medium was lowered. On the other hand, changes in the hematocrit—and thus, in the O_2-carrying capacity of the perfusate—had no major influence on the level of Epo. When the perfusion medium was equilibrated with air and the hematocrit was 0.05 ("anemic perfusion"), no Epo was produced in significant amounts. These findings would seem to indicate that the synthesis of Epo in isolated perfused rat kidneys depends on the O_2 tension rather than on the O_2-carrying capacity of the perfusion medium.

TABLE 4.1. Effects of Low O_2 Concentration and Hematocrit on the Production of
Immunoreactive Erythropoietin in Isolated Perfused Rat Kidneys

% O_2	Hematocrit	n	Erythropoietin (mU/g kidney)
95	0.05	10	156 ± 57
20	0.05	5	87 ± 54
3	0.00	4	661 ± 47[a]
3	0.05	5	882 ± 137[a]
3	0.20	5	618 ± 126[a]
3	0.40	4	528 ± 86[a]

Values are means ± SE. Isolated rat kidneys were perfused at 37°C for 3 hours in a recirculation system
with 200 ml substrate-enriched Krebs-Henseleit buffer supplemented with 60 g/L bovine serum albumin and
human erythrocytes. Erythropoietin was assayed in fivefold concentrated samples using rat erythropoietin
standard, ^{125}I-labeled recombinant human erythropoietin (r-huEpo), and antiserum from a rabbit immunized
with r-huEpo.
[a]Indicates significant difference from the value at 95% O_2 (P < 0.05, Dunnett's test).

RENAL CELL CULTURES

There have been several reports on the formation of erythropoiesis-stimulating
activity in cell cultures derived from healthy kidney tissue or from kidney tu-
mors (see Ref. 34). In co-cultures of newborn rabbit kidney cells with bone
marrow cells, Ozawa (48) observed increased heme synthesis by the bone marrow cells when the O_2 concentration in the incubator was reduced from 21% to
3%. McDonald et al. (43) reported Epo production by bovine kidney cells grown
at 5% O_2, but not in air. In addition, kidney cultures from rabbits previously
subjected to "programming" by phlebotomy or exposure to hypobaric hypoxia
were found to release into the culture medium an erythropoiesis-stimulating
activity (47). The observation of Epo production by cultures of the established
porcine kidney tubule cell line LLCPK$_1$ at low O_2 tension (4) was not confirmed
by other investigators (23, 35). Rat kidney glomerular mesangial cells incubated at low O_2 tensions release into the culture medium an erythropoiesis-
stimulating activity, which was originally considered to be Epo (39). The recent
localization, by in situ hybridization, of Epo mRNA selectively in peritubular
capillaries of the kidney cortex (37, 40), however, has cast doubt as to the correct interpretation of the cell culture studies previously reported. Frankly, a
renal cell culture system has not been clearly established that synthesizes Epo
dependency on O_2 supply. Presumably erythropoietic factors distinct from Epo
were produced in some of the renal cell culture systems. The use of immu-
noassays for Epo may be more satisfactory than the classic bioassays. In this
context, it should be noted that two human hepatoma cell lines, HepG2 and
Hep3B, have been shown to synthesize Epo when exposed to low O_2 tensions.
This hepatic Epo is both bioactive and immunoreactive (22, 23, 46).

DISCUSSION

Blood-borne Epo originates mainly from cells in the cortex of the kidney. The
primary parameter controlling the production of Epo is the O_2 content of the

arterial blood, which depends on both the O_2 carrying capacity and the O_2 tension. There is some evidence to assume that the kidney is better able than other organs to sense the O_2 content of the blood. The O_2 supply of the kidneys remains relatively constant over a wide range of changes in cardiac output and arterial blood pressure because of the autoregulation of the renal blood flow. In addition, a moderate decrease in renal blood flow elicits a proportional reduction in renal O_2 consumption. In fact, the autoregulation of the renal blood flow seems to be favorable to O_2 sensing because the lowering of the O_2 content of the arterial blood is not compensated for by an increase in the flow rate (36, 53).

Erslev et al. (7) have raised the interesting question as to why the production of Epo is not stimulated in severe erythrocytosis with hematocrit values as high as 0.8, in association with increased blood viscosity and impaired blood flow. The authors have explained this phenomenon by the fact that O_2 consumption decreases with lowered blood flow in the kidney. According to Erslev et al. (7), the unique relationshp between renal O_2 consumption and blood flow prevents the development of a vicious cycle, with erythrocytosis causing further erythrocytosis. Along these lines, however, one may ask why extrarenal sites do not respond with enhanced production of Epo in erythrocytosis.

Several pieces of evidence indicate that a renal O_2 sensor is involved in the control of the production of Epo. The level of Epo in the blood increases to some extent when the O_2 supply of the kidney is reduced by constricting the renal arteries. Isolated kidneys release Epo during hypoxemic perfusion. As noted, there is some evidence that suggests that prostanoids play an essential role in the mechanisms by which hypoxia initiates the synthesis of Epo in the kidney.

It still remains to be elucidated whether the production of Epo in the kidney is exclusively under the control of a renal O_2 sensing system. In contrast to a lowered whole body O_2 supply, the reduction of renal blood flow in rats resulted only in a moderate increase in the plasma level of the hormone, even when the O_2 tension of renal venous blood was extremely low. Another incompletely understood finding is the lack of stimulation of the production of Epo during "anemic" perfusion of isolated rat kidneys. Note that Reissmann and Nomura (55) made very similar observations in earlier studies with isolated rabbit kidneys. On the other hand, the production of Epo increases in isolated perfused rat kidneys when the O_2 tension of the perfusion medium is reduced. Thus, both the results of our in vivo studies in which renal blood flow was reduced and the studies in isolated perfused kidneys suggest that the relevant O_2 sensing cells must be related to the arterial, rather than the venous side of the capillary network of the kidney cortex.

Hence, the possibility should be reconsidered that the renal synthesis of Epo is partially under the control of extrarenal O_2 sensitive mechanisms involving nervous or humoral factors. Halvorsen (26) earlier assigned an important role to the hypothalamus in erythropoiesis. The plasma level of Epo is much lower in hypophysectomized than in sham-operated control animals during hypoxic stress (27, 54). Furthermore, the peripheral autonomic nervous system plays a modulating role in the production of Epo (11).

ACKNOWLEDGMENTS

This work was partially supported by grant DFG Je 95/6 from the Deutsche Forschungsge-meinschaft. The excellent secretarial assistance of Gisela Thaler is gratefully acknowledged.

REFERENCES

1. BERU, N., J. McDONALD, C. LACOMBE, AND E. GOLDWASSER. Expression of the erythropoietin gene. *Mol. Cell. Biol. 6*:2571–2575, 1986.
2. BONDURANT, M. C., AND M. J. KOURY. Anemia induces accumulation of erythropoietin mRNA in the kidney and liver. *Mol. Cell. Biol. 6*:2731–2733, 1986.
3. BOURGOIGNIE, J. J., N. I. GALLAGHER, H. M. PERRY, L. KURZ, M. A. WARNECKE, AND R. M. DONATI. Renin and erythropoietin in normotensive and in hypertensive patients. *J. Lab. Clin. Med. 71*:523–536, 1968.
4. CARO, J., J. HICKEY, AND A. J. ERSLEV. Erythropoietin production by an established kidney proximal tubule cell line (LLCPK₁). *Exp. Hematol. 12*:357, 1984.
5. COOPER, G. W., AND M. R. NOCENTI. Unilateral renal ischemia and erythropoietin. *Proc. Soc. Exp. Biol. Med. 108*:546–549, 1961.
6. ERSLEV, A. J. In vitro production of erythropoietin by kidneys perfused with a serum-free solution. *Blood 44*:77–85, 1974.
7. ERSLEV, A. J., J. CARO, AND A. BESARAB. Why the kidney? *Nephron 41*:213–216, 1985.
8. ERSLEV, A. J., J. CARO, E. KANSU, AND R. SILVER. Renal and extrarenal erythropoietin production in anaemic rats. *Br. J. Haematol. 45*:65–72, 1980.
9. ERSLEV, A. J., R. W. SOLIT, R. C. CAMISHION, S. AMSEL, J. ILDA, AND W. F. BALLINGER. II. Erythropoietin in vitro. III. Perfusion of a lung-kidney preparation. *Am. J. Physiol. 208*:1153–1170, 1965.
10. ESCHBACH, J. W., J. C. EGRIE, M. R. DOWNING, J. K. BROWNE, AND J. W. ADAMSON. Correction of the anemia of end-stage renal disease with recombinant human erythropoietin. *N. Engl. J. Med. 316*:73–78, 1987.
11. FINK, G. D., AND J. W. FISHER. Role of the sympathetic nervous system in the control of erythropoietin production. In: *Kidney Hormones, vol. II. Erythropoietin,* ed. J. W. Fisher. New York: Academic Press, 1977, pp. 387–413.
12. FISHER, J. W. Control of erythropoietin production. *Proc. Soc. Exp. Biol. Med. 173*:289–305, 1983.
13. FISHER, J. W., AND B. J. BIRDWELL. The production of an erythropoietic factor by the in situ perfused kidney. *Acta Haematol. 26*:224–232, 1961.
14. FISHER, J. W., D. B. KNIGHT, AND C. COUCH. Influence of several diuretic drugs on erythropoietin formation. *J. Pharmacol. Exp. Ther. 141*:113–121, 1963.
15. FISHER, J. W., AND J. W. LANGSTON. The influence of hypoxemia and cobalt on erythropoietin production in the isolated perfused dog kidney. *Blood 29*:114–125, 1967.
16. FISHER, J. W., AND J. W. LANGSTON. Effects of testosterone, cobalt and hypoxia on erythropoietin production in the isolated perfused dog kidney. *Ann. N.Y. Acad. Sci. 149*:75–87, 1968.
17. FISHER, J. W., AND A. I. SAMUELS. Relationship between renal blood flow and erythropoietin production in dogs. *Proc. Soc. Exp. Biol. Med. 125*:482–485, 1967.
18. FISHER, J. W., R. SCHOFIELD, AND D. D. PORTEOUS. Effects of renal hypoxia on erythropoietin production. *Br. J. Haematol. 11*:382–388, 1965.
19. FOLEY, J. W., D. M. GROSS, P. K. NELSON, AND J. W. FISHER. The effects of arachidonic acid on erythropoietin production in exhypoxic polycythemic mice and the isolated perfused canine kidney. *J. Pharmacol. Exp. Ther. 207*:402–409, 1978.
20. FRIED, W. Erythropoietin and the kidney. *Nephron 15*:327–349, 1975.
21. FRIED, W., J. BARONE-VARELAS, AND M. BERMAN. Detection of high erythropoietin titers in renal extracts of hypoxic rats. *J. Lab. Clin. Med. 97*:82–86, 1981.
22. GOLDBERG, M. A., S. P. DUNNING, AND H. F. BUNN. Regulation of the erythropoietin gene: evidence that the oxygen sensor is a heme protein. *Science 242*:1412–1415, 1988.
23. GOLDBERG, M. A., G. A. GLASS, J. M. CUNNINGHAM, AND H. F. BUNN. The regulated expression of erythropoietin by two human hepatoma cell lines. *Proc. Natl. Acad. Sci. (USA) 84*:7972–7976, 1987.
24. GROSS, D. M., V. M. MUJOVIC, W. JUBIZ, AND J. W. FISHER. Enhanced erythropoietin and prostaglandin E production in the dog following renal artery constriction. *Proc. Soc. Exp. Biol. Med. 151*:498–501, 1976.
25. GRÜTZMACHER, P., AND W. SCHOEPPE. Renal artery stenosis and renal polyglobulia. In:

Erythropoietin, ed. W. Jelkmann and A. J. Gross. Heidelberg, Berlin, New York: Springer-Verlag, 1989 (in press).

26. HALVORSEN, S. The central nervous system in regulation of erythropoiesis. *Acta Haematol. 35*:65–79, 1966.

27. HALVORSEN, S., B. L. ROH, AND J. W. FISHER. Erythropoietin production in nephrectomized and hypophysectomized animals. *Am. J. Physiol. 215*:349–352, 1968.

28. HUDGSON, P., J. M. S. PEARCE, AND W. K. YEATES. Renal artery stenosis with hypertension and high haematocrit. *Br. Med. J. 1*:18–21, 1967.

29. JACOBSON, L. O., E. GOLDWASSESR, W. FRIED, AND L. PLZAK. Role of the kidney in erythropoiesis. *Nature 179*:633–634, 1957.

30. JEKLMANN, W. Temporal pattern of erythropoietin titers in kidney tissue during hypoxic hypoxia. *Pflügers Arch. 393*:88–91, 1982.

31. JELKMANN, W. Renal erythropoietin: properties and production. *Rev. Physiol. Biochem. Pharmacol. 104*:139–215, 1986.

32. JELKMANN, W., AND C. BAUER. Demonstration of high levels of erythropoietin in rat kidneys following hypoxic hypoxia. *Pflügers Arch. 392*:34–39, 1981.

33. JEKLMANN, W., J. BROOKINS, AND J. W. FISHER. Indomethacin blockade of albuterol-induced erythropoietin production in isolated perfused dog kidneys. *Proc. Soc. Exp. Biol. Med. 162*:65–70, 1979.

34. JELKMANN, W., A. KURTZ, AND C. BAUER. In vitro production of erythropoietin. In: *Kidney Hormones,* ed. J. W. Fisher. London, New York, San Francisco: Academic Press, 1986, pp. 559–583.

35. JELKMANN, W., N. MARIENHOFF, S. GIESSELMANN, AND L. BUSCH. Lowered plasma erythropoietin in hypoxic rats with kidney tubule lesions. *Blut 57*:317–321, 1988.

36. KIIL, F. Blood flow and oxygen utilization by the kidney. In: *Kidney Hormones,* ed. J. W. Fisher. London, New York: Academic Press, 1971, pp. 1–30.

37. KOURY, S. T., M. C. BONDURANT, AND M. J. KOURY. Localization of erythropoietin synthesizing cells in murine kidneys by in situ hybridization. *Blood 71*:524–527, 1988.

38. KURATOWSKA, Z., B. LEWARTOWSKI, AND E. MICHALAK. Studies on the production of erythropoietin by isolated perfused organs. *Blood 18*:527–534, 1961.

39. KURTZ, A., W. JELKMANN, F. SINOWATZ, AND C. BAUER. Renal mesangial cell cultures as a model for study of erythropoietin production. *Proc. Natl. Acad. Sci. (USA) 80*:4008–4011, 1983.

40. LACOMBE, C., J. L. DA SILVA, P. BRUNEVAL, J. G. FOURNIER, F. WENDLING, N. CASADEVALL, J. P. CAMILLERI, J. BARIETY, B. VARET, AND P. TAMBOURIN. Peritubular cells are the site of erythropoietin synthesis in the murine hypoxic kidney. *J. Clin. Invest. 81*:620–623, 1988.

41. LOZZIO, B. B., T. P. McDONALD, AND R. D. LANGE. Erythropoietin formation in rats bearing congenital hydronephrosis. *Isr. J. Med. Sci. 7*:1001–1006, 1971.

42. MALGOR, L. A., AND J. W. FISHER. Effects of testosterone on erythropoietin production in isolated perfused kidneys. *Am. J. Physiol. 218*:1732–1736, 1970.

43. McDONALD, T. P., D. H. MARTIN, M. L. SIMMONS, AND R. D. LANGE. Preliminary results of erythropoietin production by bovine kidney cells in culture. *Life Sci. 8*:949–954, 1969.

44. MUJOVIC, V. M., AND J. W. FISHER. The effects of indomethacin on erythropoietin production in dogs following renal artery constriction. I. The possible role of prostaglandins in the generation of erythropoietin by the kidney. *J. Pharmacol. Exp. Ther. 191*:575–580, 1974.

45. NAETS, J. P. Erythropoiesis in nephrectomized dogs. *Nature 181*:1134–1135, 1958.

46. NIELSEN, O. J., S. J. SCHUSTER, R. KAUFMAN, A. J. ERSLEV, AND J. CARO. Regulation of erythropoietin production in a human hepatoblastoma cell line. *Blood 70*:1904–1909, 1987.

47. OGLE, J. W., R. D. LANGE, AND C. D. R. DUNN. Erythropoiesis-stimulating factor production by rabbit kidney cultures from "programmed" rabbits. *Blood 52*:233–239, 1978.

48. OZAWA, S. Erythropoietin from the kidney cells cultured in vitro. *Keio J. Med. 16*:193–203, 1967.

49. PAGEL, H., W. JELKMANN, AND C. WEISS. A comparison of the effects of renal artery constriction and anemia on the production of erythropoietin. *Pflügers Arch. 413*:62–66, 1988.

50. PAGEL, H., W. JELKMANN, AND C. WEISS. O_2-supply to the kidneys and the production of erythropoietin. *Respir. Physiol. 77*:111–118, 1989.

51. PAUL, P., S. A. ROTHMANN, AND R. C. MEAGHER. Modulation of erythropoietin production by adenosine. *J. Lab. Clin. Med. 112*:168–173, 1988.

52. PAVLOVIC-KENTERA, V., D. P. HALL, C. BRAGASSA, AND R. D. LANGE. Unilateral renal hypoxia and production of erythropoietin. *J. Lab. Clin. Med. 65*:577–588, 1965.

53. PENINGTON, D. G. Erythropoietin in tissues. Features of the renal erythropoietin-producing system. In: *Hormones and the Kidney,* ed. P. Williams. New York: Academic Press, 1963, pp. 201–219.

54. PESCHLE, C., I. A. RAPPAPORT, M. C. MAGLI, G. MARONE, F. LETTIERI, C. CILLO, AND A. S. GORDON. Role of the hypophysis in erythropoietin production during hypoxia. *Blood* 51:1117–1124, 1978.

55. REISSMANN, K. R., AND T. NOMURA. Erythropoietin formation in isolated kidneys and liver. In: *Erythropoiesis,* ed. L. O. Jacobson, and M. Doyle. New York: Grune & Stratton, 1962, pp. 71–77.

56. REISSMANN, K. R., T. NOMURA, R. W. GUNN, AND F. BROSIUS. Erythropoietic response to anemia or erythropoietin injection in uremic rats with or without functioning renal tissue. *Blood* 16:1411–1423, 1960.

57. SCHMID, R., AND A. S. GILBERTSEN. Fundamental observations on the production of compensatory polycythemia in a case of patent ductus arteriosus with reversed blood flow. *Blood* 10:247–251, 1955.

58. SCHUREK, H. J., AND J. M. ALT. Effect of albumin on the function of perfused rat kidney. *Am. J. Physiol.* 240:F569–F576, 1981.

59. SCHUSTER, S. J., J. H. WILSON, A. J. ERSLEV, AND J. CARO. Physiologic regulation and tissue localization of renal erythropoietin messenger RNA. *Blood* 70:316–318, 1987.

60. STOHLMAN, F., C. E. RATH, AND J. C. ROSE. Evidence for a humoral regulation of erythropoiesis. *Blood* 9:721–733, 1954.

61. TAKAKU, F., K. HIRASHIMA, AND K. NAKAO. Studies on the mechanism of erythropoietin production. I. Effect of unilateral construction of the renal artery. *J. Lab. Clin. Med.* 59:815–820, 1962.

62. TARAZI, R. C., E. D. FROHLICH, H. P. DUSTAN, R. W. GIFFORD, AND I. H. PAGE. Hypertension and high hematocrit. *Am. J. Cardiol.* 18:855–858, 1966.

63. WINEARLS, C. G., D. O. OLIVER, M. J. PIPPARD, C. REID, M. R. DOWNING, AND P. M. COTES. Effect of human erythropoietin derived from recombinant DNA on the anaemia of patients maintained by chronic hemodialysis. *Lancet ii*:1175–1178, 1986.

64. ZANGHERI, E. O., H. CAMPANA, F. PONCE, J. C. SILVA, F. O. FERNANDEZ, AND J. R. E. SUAREZ. Production of erythropoietin by anoxic perfusion of the isolated kidney of a dog. *Nature* 199:572–573, 1963.

5

Hypoxia and Erythropoietin Production

JAMES W. FISHER, M. UENO, J. NAKASHIMA,
AND BARBARA BECKMAN

Hypoxia is known to be the fundamental stimulus for the control of erythropoietin production (13, 14, 20, 31). Several external messenger substances are released during hypoxia, which activate adenylate cyclase, and increase the generation of the second messenger cyclic AMP, which is involved in the regulation of erythropoietin (Ep) production (14, 20). Some of the factors that are known to be released during hypoxia and seem to be involved in the regulation of Ep production are adenosine (37), oxygen-derived metabolites (38), eicosanoids (26), and beta$_2$-adrenergic agonists (12). These external messenger substances can act alone or in concert to trigger receptors that activate stimulatory G proteins in the membrane of a renal Ep-producing cell, and increase adenylate cyclase and cyclic AMP. Cyclic AMP causes the dissociation of the regulatory subunit from the catalytic head of protein kinase A. Important phosphoproteins are generated by kinase A in the kidney, which may lead to increased biosynthesis of Ep at the level of transcription of messenger RNA or the translation of Ep in the renal cell. In addition, phosphoproteins could be involved with the actual release process for Ep in the cell. Atrial natriuretic factor (ANF) is known to be released during hypoxia (2, 3) and to increase Ep secretion in renal carcinoma cells in culture through an ANF receptor mechanism coupled to guanylate cyclase (39). The purpose of this presentation is to review the regulatory factors that may be involved in hypoxic stimulation of kidney production of Ep.

METHODS

Exhypoxic Polycythemic Mouse Assay

CD-1 strain female mice (Charles River Breeding Laboratories, Wilmington, MA) were exposed in a hypobaric chamber at 0.42 atm for 22 hours per day for 14 days according to a modification of the method of Cotes and Bangham (8). The mice were allowed free access to food and water. At time 0 and each consecutive day of exposure to hypoxia, five mice were selected at random in an initial group and were weighed, anesthetized with ether, and exsanguinated by cardiac puncture. Blood was removed for the determination of microhematocrit and serum Ep concentration. Blood samples for the Ep assay were allowed to clot for approximately 1 hour and after centrifugation, the serum was removed and stored at $-70°C$ until assayed for Ep using our sensitive radioimmunoassay (RIA) (22, 32). The remaining mice were kept at normal atmospheric pressure. Hematocrit and serum levels of Ep were determined in five mice on each posthypoxic day up to the 10th day. The total duration of this study was 24 days. Chromium-51 red cell mass was determined at days 0, 7, 14 during exposure to hypoxia and on the 10th posthypoxic day.

Radioimmunoassay for Erythropoietin

Highly purified human recombinant Ep ($>160,000$U/mg) produced by a baby hamster kidney transfected cell according to the method of Powell et al. (30) was labeled with ^{125}I by the chloramine T method, which we have previously described (22, 32). Purified human recombinant Ep was also used as the immunogen and Ep antisera was raised in mixed breed rabbits. This antiserum was used in a dilution of 1 : 128,000. The separation of bound from free-labeled antigen was carried out using a second antibody (goat antirabbit gamma globulin). Mouse Ep produced by murine erythroleukemia cells (Hyclone Labs., 4 U/mg) was used for the preparation of the Ep standard curve for the RIA.

The Renal Carcinoma Cell Culture System

Renal carcinoma (RC) cells obtained from a lung metastasis in a patient with erythrocytosis were serially transplanted into BALB/c athymic nude mice. The RC cells were prepared in a monolayer cell culture maintained in Eagle's MEM supplemented with 10% fetal bovine serum (FBS), 0.1 mM nonessential amino acids, 1 mM sodium pyruvate, 100 U/ml penicillin G, and 100 μg/ml streptomycin in a humidifed atmosphere of 5% CO_2 and 95% air at 37°C and passaged every 3 weeks. After at least five passages of the subculture, the cells were harvested by trypsinization and dispersed into 4.5 cm^2 multiwells at a concentration of 2×10^5 cells/ml culture medium. The Ep activity was determined by RIA as described previously (22, 32). The spent culture medium was frozen at $-80°C$ until used in the Ep assay. Figure 5.1 shows the correlation between the growth of the RC cells and the Ep levels in the culture medium. The cells reached confluent density in 6 days and saturation density in 18 days after seeding. The culture medium with 10% FBS contained undetectable levels of Ep. Renal carcinoma cells in early confluency, which was from the sixth to the ninth day after seeding, when Ep activity should be less than 50 mU/ml/24 hour (Fig. 5.1), were used in the present studies. The details of our monolayer cell culture system have been described previously (16). The cells appeared to be epitheliallike when examined under a phase contrast microscope, and electron microscopically the cells retained ultrastructural characteristics similar to the original tumor cells showing tight junctions, cell surface microvilli, a cytoplasm with diffusely scattered glycogen particles, sparse lipid droplets, and an infolding nucleus showing the presence of heterochromatin.

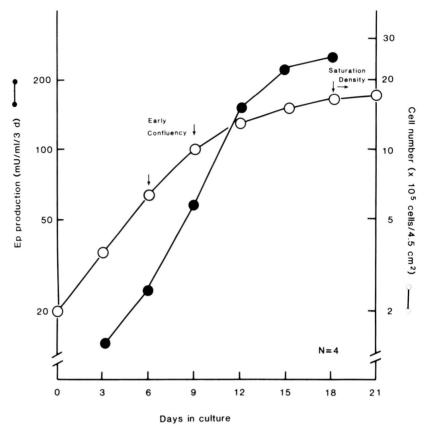

FIGURE 5.1. Correlation between the growth of renal carcinoma (RC) cells (○—○) and erythropoietin (Ep) (●—●) levels in 3 days spent culture media, determined by a sensitive radioimmunoassay (RIA). The cells grew exponentially with an approximate population doubling time of 3.5 to 4.0 days. The RC cells reach confluency in 6 days after seeding (2.0 × 10⁵ cells/4.5 cm²-well) and saturation density after 18 days. The RC cells were studied during the first 3 days when they were in a confluent phase, which is termed *early confluency*.

RESULTS

As noted in Fig. 5.2, serum Ep concentrations in control mice (day 0) were 2.35 ± 0.33 mU/ml. Exposure of mice to hypoxia in a hypobaric chamber for 22 hours on the first day resulted in a significant ($P<0.05$) increase in serum Ep titers to a mean value of 122.9 ± 63.5 mU/ml. The highest serum Ep level was reached after 3 days of hypoxia (394.4 ± 132.6 mU/ml) and then gradually declined to a concentration of 36.5 ± 11.4 mU/ml after 14 days of hypoxia (Fig. 5.2). Serum Ep levels during the 10 posthypoxic days were below detectable levels in our RIA. The reason for the large variations in serum Ep levels during exposure to hypoxia in each group is not known, but may be related to variations in age, weight, and biologic variation in response to hypoxia.

The mean hematocrit value for the control untreated normoxic mice was 40 ± 0.84%. Exposure of mice to hypoxia in the hypobaric chamber produced a significant increase in hematocrit values after 4 days of exposure ($P<0.05$)

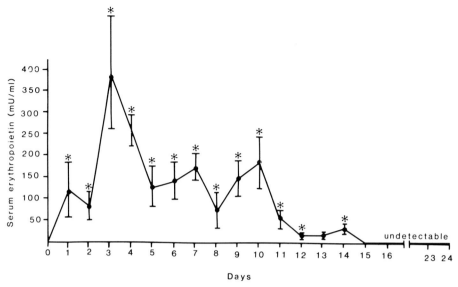

FIGURE 5.2. Serum erythropoietin concentrations in mice exposed to hypoxia (0.42 atm, 22 hours/day) for 14 days and during the 10-day posthypoxic period. *Significantly different from the 0 day control value (P<0.05). Line over each point is ± SEM. *n* = 5.

(Fig. 5.3). A further gradual increase in the hematocrit was seen after each consecutive day of exposure to hypoxia, and reached 72.2 ± 1.53% after 14 days. When the mice were returned to ambient pressure, there was a gradual decline in hematocrit, although the mean hematocrit value for each day of the posthypoxic period up to the 10th day out of the hypobaric chamber (60.2 ± 1.98%) was significantly (P<0.15) higher than baseline values.

The eicosanoids (26) and the beta$_2$-adrenergic agonists (3) probably play some role in severe pathophysiologic hypoxic stimulation. We have only been

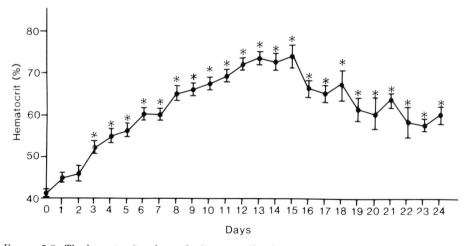

FIGURE 5.3. The hematocrit values of mice exposed to hypoxia (0.42 atm, 22 hours/day) for 14 days followed by 10 posthypoxic days at ambient pressure. *Significantly different from day 0 control (P<0.05). Line over each point is ± SEM. *n* = 5.

able, however, to partially block the effects of hypoxia on Ep production with cyclooxygenase inhibitors (26), such as meclofenamate or indomethacin, or beta$_2$-adrenergic blockers, such as propranolol (β_1, β_2) or butoxamine (β_2) (3); therefore, we have searched for other messenger substances that could be released during hypoxia to regulate kidney production of Ep. In considering other agents that could be involved, adenosine and oxygen-derived metabolites (H_2O_2, superoxide and the hydroxyl radical), probably are produced by an ischemic or posthypoxic reoxygenation type of stimulus (15, 24) for Ep production (38).

Adenosine is known to be increased in the kidney during ischemic hypoxia (25). It has recently been demonstrated that adenosine (ADE) modulates renin secretion in rat kidney slices (7), and the effects of ADE seem to be associated with the activation of specific A_1 and A_2 receptors. The most potent selective A_1 receptor agonist in suppressing adenylate cyclase leading to a decrease in cyclic AMP is probably N^6-cyclohexyladenosine (CHA) (9). In contrast, $5'$-N-ethyl-carboxamideadenosine (NECA), a selective A_2 receptor agonist, stimulates adenylate cyclase. We have previously reported that cyclic AMP may be important in the regulation of Ep production both in polycythemic mice (33) and in an Ep-producing renal carcinoma cell line (18). In addition, albuterol, a selective beta$_2$-adrenergic agonist, is known to activate adenylate cyclase and to stimulate Ep production in rabbits (11).

Hypoxia increases the degradation of ATP due to limited oxygen availability, resulting in the formation of ADE and other nucleosides (23). The production of nucleosides has been reported to be markedly enhanced during renal ischemia and histochemical studies revealed that ADE is localized in renal proximal tubules (36). Thus, there is a possibility that the erythropoietic effects of hypoxia may result from the effects of ADE on endogenous cyclic AMP levels. Heretofore, however, there have been no reports concerned with ADE and Ep production. In the present studies, the role of ADE on Ep production in polycythemic mice in response to hypoxia was investigated using selective and specific ADE receptor agonists that have a slower rate of metabolism than ADE and are not taken up by the cell.

Percent ^{59}Fe incorporation in red cells in exhypoxic polycythemic mice treated with ADE in concentrations of 400 and 1600 nmol/kg and exposed to 4 hours of hypoxia were significantly ($P<0.05$) increased to 12.26 $\pm$ 1.28 and 13.38 $\pm$ 1.53, respectively, and significantly ($P<0.05$) higher than vehicle controls (7.18 $\pm$ 0.67) (Fig. 5.4). On the other hand, when the dose of ADE was increased to 6400 nmol/kg, the radioiron incorporation was not significantly elevated above the hypoxic controls. NECA, the A_2 agonist, also produced a significant ($P<0.05$) increase in radioiron incorporation in a dose-dependent manner in a dose range of 25 to 100 nmol/kg. NECA, however, caused a much smaller increase in radioiron at 200 nmol/kg than with the 100 nmol/kg dose. NECA produced a significantly greater increase in radioiron incorporation than ADE. NECA appeared to be toxic when administered in concentrations higher than 400 nmol/kg. On the other hand, CHA did not produce a significant change in radioiron incorporation even when mice were treated with doses of CHA up to 1600 nmol/kg. The possibility that the test substances may affect the response to Ep or may protect Ep from degradation cannot be excluded.

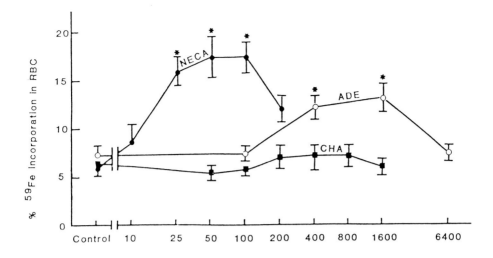

DOSE (nmol/kg/day, i.v.)

FIGURE 5.4. Effects of ADE (○) [100 to 6400 nmol/kg/day, i.v.], CHA (□) [50 to 1600 nmol/kg/day, i.v.], NECA (●) [10 to 200 nmol/kg/day, i.v.] on radioiron incorporation in red cells in response to 4 hours to hypoxia on the sixth posthypoxic day. The control value is the radioiron incorporation for untreated mice exposed to reduced atmospheric pressure (0.42 atm) for 4 hours on posthypoxic day 6. Each value represents the mean ± SEM of 11 to 34 mice. *Indicates significantly different from control (P<0.05). Values in parentheses represent the hematocrits of mice in each group. The mean hematocrit for the control nonhypoxic mice was 60.5 ± 0.9 (n = 35). The mean hematocrit values for all of the treatment groups ranged between 61.3 and 64.1 and were not significantly different.

Theophylline has been postulated to be a specific antagonist of ADE receptors and is known to antagonize ADE receptor activation in concentrations that do not inhibit phosphodiesterase (27). As seen in Table 5.1, theophylline in a concentration of 80 mg/kg produced a significant (P<0.05) increase in radioiron incorporation from a control level of 5.04 ± 0.68% with hypoxia alone to 8.68 ± 1.37% with hypoxia plus theophylline. In spite of this enhancement of

TABLE 5.1. Effects of ADE and NECA on Radioiron Incorporation in Response to Erythropoietin

Drugs[a]	Ep (Units)[b]		
	0	0.2	0.8
Saline	0.54 ± 0.06 (9)	5.48 ± 0.73 (9)	25.07 ± 1.46 (9)
ADE, 1600 nmol/kg	1.18 ± 0.61 (9)	7.18 ± 1.24 (10)	23.14 ± 1.13 (9)
NECA, 100 nmol/kg	2.33 ± 0.56 (8)[c]	9.55 ± 1.48 (9)[c]	24.14 ± 1.83 (8)

[a]Drugs were administered i.v. on posthypoxic days 3, 4, 5, and 6.
[b]Ep was administered subcutaneously on posthypoxic days 6 and 7.
[c]Significantly different from control (saline) group (P<0.05).
Each percent ^{59}Fe incorporation value represents the mean ± SEM.
Numbers in parentheses indicate number of samples. ADE, adenosine hemisulfate; NECA, 5'-N-ethyl-carboxamideadenosine.

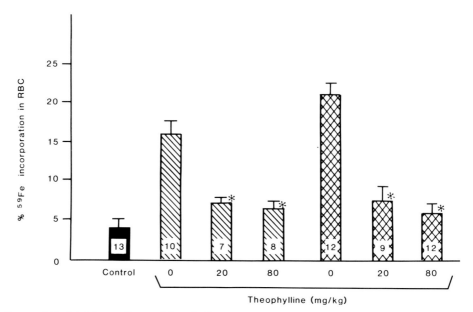

FIGURE 5.5. Inhibitory effects of theophylline (20 and 80 mg/kg/day, i.p.) on the enhancement of radioiron incorporation in red cells induced by ADE (▨ : 1600 nmol/kg/day, i.v.) and NECA (▩ : 100 nmol/kg/day, i.v.) in combination with 4 hours of hypoxia. Each value represents the mean ± SEM of 7 to 13 mice. The number of mice is at the bottom of each bar. Mean percent ^{59}Fe incorporation in red cells when standard erythropoietin (Ep) was administered at 200 mU/mouse and 800 mU/mouse in these experiments was 5.48 ± 0.73 and 25.07 ± 1.46, respectively. The asterisk (*) over each bar indicates that this group is significantly different from ADE or NECA alone (P<0.05). The mean hematocrit values ranged between 60.6 and 63.7% and the hematocrit values were not significantly different in any of the groups.

radioiron incorporation by theophylline (20 and 80 mg/kg) alone, a significant inhibition was seen in the enhancement induced by ADE (1600 nmol/kg) and NECA (100 nmol/kg) (Fig. 5.5). In addition, the ADE enhancement of radioiron was not attenuated by dipyridamole (25 and 100 mg/kg, i.p.), which is known to be an inhibitor of nucleoside uptake by cells in culture and in vivo in mice (26). Throughout the present studies, there was no significant difference in the mean hematocrit values of any of the groups studied as indicated in Figs. 5.4 and 5.5 and Table 5.1.

To study the role of oxygen-derived metabolites on Ep production after the renal carcinoma cells reached confluency, they were incubated with 10^{-5}M xanthine and increasing concentrations of xanthine oxidase (8×10^{-7} to 5×10^{-4} U/ml) for 24 hours at 37°C. This xanthine–xanthine oxidase system was previously shown to generate O_2, H_2O_2, and hydroxyl radicals (15, 24). As seen in Fig. 5.6, the xanthine–xanthine oxidase ($\leq 4 \times 10^{-6}$ U/ml) system produced a dose-related increase (twofold) in Ep production by the RC cells, whereas xanthine alone had no effect on Ep production. Catalase, a scavenger of H_2O_2, significantly (P<0.05) inhibited the enhancement of Ep production induced by xanthine–xanthine oxidase (5×10^{-4} U/ml) in concentrations of ≥ 50 µg/ml (Fig. 5.7), but had no effect on the basal levels of Ep in the culture medium in

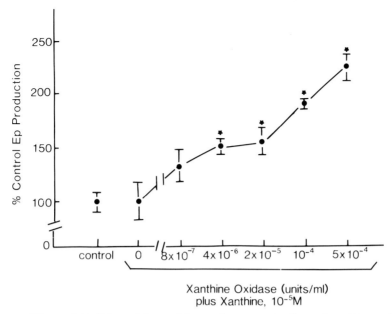

FIGURE 5.6. Effects of 10^{-5}M xanthine and increasing concentrations of xanthine oxidase on erythropoietin (Ep) production by renal carcinoma (RC) cells in culture. RC cells were incubated for 24 hours in culture media in *early confluency*. After incubation, the viable cells were counted and the culture media assayed for Ep (RIA). The values are expressed as the percentage of the basal level of Ep that equals 100% and represents the mean $\pm$ SEM of 6 different samples. *P<0.05.

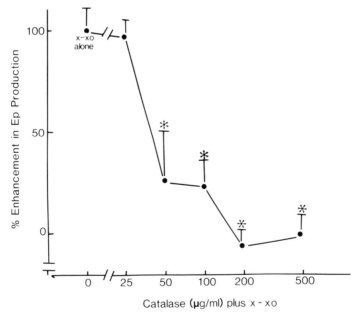

FIGURE 5.7. Inhibitory effects of catalase on the increased erythropoietin (Ep) production induced by 10^{-5}M xanthine plus 5×10^{-4} U/ml xanthine oxidase. The renal carcinoma (RC) cells were incubated with several concentrations of catalase (specific activity 17,000 U/mg) plus xanthine–xanthine oxidase (x–xo) for 24 hours in *early confluency*. Values are expressed as percentage of the enhancement level of Ep production induced by x–xo and represent the mean $\pm$ SEM of 6 to 12 different samples. 0% represents the basal level of Ep production.

concentrations of 200 µg/ml. In contrast, superoxide dismutase (SOD) (2 to 50 µg/ml) produced a significant increase in Ep production up to 142.3 ± 11.4% and 152.9 ± 14.6% at 10 µg/ml and 50 µg/ml, respectively.

Glucose oxidase is known to produce H_2O_2 directly, without affecting O_2 production. The concentration of glucose, a substrate for glucose oxidase, in our culture medium was 1000 mg/L. Figure 5.8 indicates that glucose oxidase significantly increased Ep production in concentrations of 0.032 mU/ml up to 4 mU/ml. As noted in Fig. 5.9, treatment of our cells with H_2O_2 itself produced a significant dose-dependent ($4 \times 10^{-6}M$ to $10^{-4}M$) (approximately fourfold over control levels) increase in Ep production, with a maximum enhancement at a concentration of $2 \times 10^{-5}M$. Hydrogen peroxide, however, has been reported to be cytotoxic and could produce some nonspecific effect on the cultured cells, causing leakage of cytoplasmic hormones. Therefore, a 24-hour ^{51}Cr release assay was carried out to assess the possibility that the reactive oxygen metabolites may have caused cellular damage. Glucose oxidase and H_2O_2 were shown to be cytotoxic to RC cells in concentrations of ≥ 40 mU/ml and $\geq 2 \times 10^{-3}M$, respectively. On the other hand, xanthine–xanthine oxidase was not cytotoxic to our cells at a concentration up to 5×10^{-2} U/ml. Viable cells, excluding trypan blue, were counted in each experiment after 24 hours of incubation and no cytotoxic effect was seen on the number and growth of the RC cells by any of the chemical agents in the concentrations used in these studies.

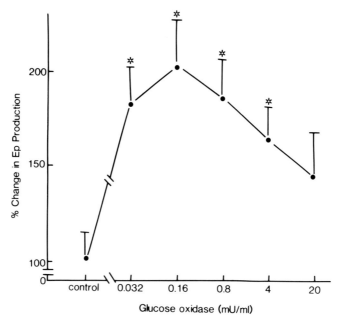

FIGURE 5.8. Effects of glucose oxidase on erythropoietin (Ep) production in renal carcinoma (RC) cell cultures. RC cells in *early confluency* were incubated for 24 hours. The values are expressed as the percentage of the basal level of Ep that equals 100% and represent the mean ± SEM of 6 different samples. *P<0.05.

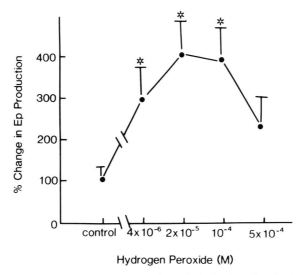

FIGURE 5.9. Effects of hydrogen peroxide on erythropoietin (Ep) production by renal carcinoma (RC) cells. RC cells in *early confluency* were incubated for 24 hours in culture medium. The values are expressed as percentage of basal levels of Ep that equals to 100% and represents the mean ± SEM of 6 different samples. *$P<0.05$.

DISCUSSION

In our present study, we have determined several parameters of erythropoiesis in mice in response to daily exposure to hypoxia over a 14-day period and for 10 posthypoxic days (34). Serum Ep levels were significantly increased over the first 22 hours of hypoxia and peak levels were seen after 3 days of hypoxia. Increased Ep production results in enhanced red blood cell formation in bone marrow, which caused an elevation in red blood cell mass and hematocrit. The early rise in red blood cell production is probably due to the effects of Ep on the later erythroid progenitor cells. The increase in red blood cell mass exerts a feedback inhibition on Ep production, which could explain the decline in serum Ep concentrations observed after 4 days of exposure to hypoxia. Continued exposure of mice to hypoxia results in a further increase in red blood cell mass and hematocrit and a further decline in Ep production up to the 14th day. The increase in red blood cell mass, despite the decrease in Ep concentrations, is probably related to the wave of erythropoiesis that has already developed in the bone marrow due to Ep as well as other factors that affect early erythroid progenitor cells. Discontinuation of hypoxia resulted in a marked decline of Ep production. Beginning 1 day after removal of mice from the hypobaric chamber, and up to the 10th posthypoxic day, serum Ep levels in the mice were nondetectable by RIA. This marked inhibition in Ep production is probably due to the removal of the hypoxic stimulus and to the feedback inhibitory mechanisms exerted by the increased red blood cell mass. Prolonged exposure of the mice to hypoxia resulted in loss of body weight up to the ninth day, then a slight return toward normal body weight was seen during the last few days of the hypoxic period. The loss in body weight is probably caused by reduced food intake due to the stress of hypoxia. The decrease in body weight is not likely to be responsible for the decline in Ep production during hypoxia. The highest serum Ep levels were seen on the third day of exposure to hypoxia when the body weight of the mice was significantly lower than that of the control mice, and there was no significant correlation between Ep levels and body weight (34).

In the present studies, ADE itself and selective ADE agonists were shown to affect radioiron incorporation in polycythemic mice in response to hypoxia. There was no significant change in hematocrits of mice in any of the experiments, suggesting that the enhancement of radioiron incorporation induced by ADE or selective agonists was not associated with a change in hematocrit. Most mice that were treated with CHA at a dosage of 3200 nmol/kg/day or with NECA at a dosage of 400 nmol/kg/day for 4 consecutive days died. On the other hand, no observable toxic effects were seen in mice treated with high doses (6400 nmol/kg/day) of ADE. Therefore, dosages of ADE and ADE agonists were selected that were relatively nontoxic. NECA, an A_2 agonist, increased radioiron incorporation at 25 to 100 nmol/kg/day, suggesting that enhancement of cyclic AMP through A_2 receptor activation may be responsible for the increase in Ep production. A similar increase in radioiron incorporation was observed when ADE was administered under the same conditions in a higher dose range. ADE was less effective than NECA in increasing radioiron incorporation, which may be due to the inactivation of ADE in vivo by ADE deaminase.

In the present studies, xanthine–xanthine oxidase increased Ep production in a dose-dependent manner, possibly through the generation of reactive oxygen metabolites. This enhancement of Ep production was completely blocked by catalase, a scavenger of H_2O_2. Superoxide dismutase (SOD), a scavenger of O_2^- did not produce a significant inhibition of the increased Ep production induced by xanthine–xanthine oxidase; on the other hand, SOD produced a more marked increase in Ep production than xanthine–xanthine oxidase alone indicating that H_2O_2 may be associated with Ep biosynthesis. Neoplastic cells have been reported to possess less superoxide dismutase activity than normal cells (10, 29). Although the SOD activity in our cultured cells was not monitored, it is possible that these RC cells have a lower amount of SOD. Significant amounts of H_2O_2, however, are still generated from O_2^- by a nonenzymatic mechanism. On the other hand, it is still possible that O_2^- reacted with some cellular component and that SOD by inhibiting the reaction using superoxide could have stimulated H_2O_2 production. Therefore, the addition of exogenous SOD plus xanthine–xanthine oxidase in our RC cells should result in a greater increase in the formation of H_2O_2 than xanthine–xanthine oxidase alone, thus producing a further increase in Ep production.

More directly, glucose oxidase is well known to generate H_2O_2 without producing O_2^- as an intermediate (28). These results provide further evidence for a key role of H_2O_2 in Ep production. Both H_2O_2 and O_2^-, however, have been reported to produce cytotoxicity (40) and could damage the cultured cells resulting in an increase in membrane permeability to large molecules. Therefore, a ^{51}Cr release assay (1, 40) was carried out to determine whether the agents generating reactive oxygen metabolites enhance ^{51}Cr released from our cells. The results of our studies failed to reveal any significant cytotoxicity in the doses used in our experiments on Ep secretion in RC cells; therefore, we con-

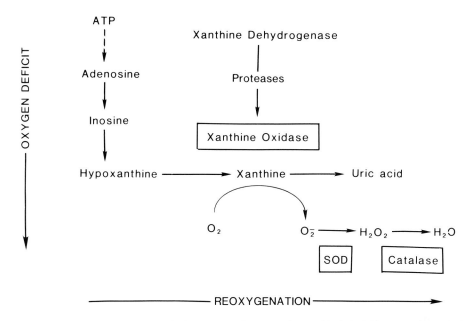

FIGURE 5.10. Model for the role of adenosine and oxygen-free radicals in kidney erythropoietin production during hypoxia and reperfusion. Modified from Grisham, M.B. et al. In: *Superoxide and Superoxide Dismutase in Chemistry, Biol. and Med.* New York: Elsevier Sc. Pub., 1988, pp. 571–575.

clude that the enhancement of Ep production induced by H_2O_2 is not caused by nonspecific leakage of Ep from our RC cells in culture. Hydrogen peroxide has also been demonstrated to mimic the action of insulin on rat fat cells without damaging these cells (21).

Although in the present studies we did not investigate the mechanism by which H_2O_2 increased Ep production, Shah (35) reported that increased prostaglandin production, especially PGE_2, might be induced by H_2O_2 in isolated glomeruli. We also reported that sodium meclofenamate, a cyclooxygenase inhibitor, inhibited Ep production by the RC cells in culture (17). Moreover, other investigators have reported that H_2O_2 triggers the secretion of eicosanoids in vitro (5, 6, 19); therefore, H_2O_2 could increase Ep production either by increased synthesis of eicosanoids or by other external messengers to increase adenylate cyclase activity. In addition, H_2O_2 could activate adenylate cyclase directly to increase cyclic AMP levels. Further studies are necessary to elucidate the mechanism of Ep enhancement of H_2O_2 and to determine whether the magnitude of the effects seen in vitro are sufficient to increase renal Ep production after hypoxia and reoxygenation.

It is of interest to note that McCord (24) demonstrated that reactive oxygen metabolites accumulate after reperfusion and reoxygenation of hypoxic tissues. It is also worth noting that Barger and Herd (40) showed that during stress, there is a regional redistribution of blood flow in the kidney. It is quite possible that there is a reduction in renal blood flow at various cortical sites in the kidney followed by reperfusion (a waxing and waning of flow) that could provide the oxygen-derived metabolites for Ep production after an hypoxic stimulus. We have found in our experience that intermittent hypoxia is more effective in stimulating Ep production than continuous hypoxia. In addition, the xanthine–xanthine oxidase system has been reported to produce an increase in the cyclic AMP content of rat kidney cells (35).

Figure 5.10 shows our proposed model for the role of adenosine and oxygen free radicals in Ep production and hypoxia-induced Ep production, which is a modification of the model of Grisham et al. (15) for the hypoxic heart model. An oxygen deficit leads to the breakdown of ATP and eventually an increase in adenosine, resulting in higher levels of hypoxanthine and xanthine in the kidney. We propose that there is an early increase in adenosine levels in the kidney after exposure to an hypoxic stimulus that is important in triggering selective adenosine A_1 and A_2 receptors in the kidney to regulate Ep production very early. Hypoxanthine and xanthine are acted upon by xanthine oxidase, which is produced by an action of proteases during hypoxia. It is well known that hypoxia increases cytosolic levels of calcium in the cell; this increase of calcium activates proteases during hypoxia and generates xanthine oxidase. During reoxygenation the xanthine oxidase generated acts on xanthine to produce oxygen-derived metabolites. It is well known that blood flow in the cortex of the kidney during stress, such as hypoxia, waxes and wanes. This could explain the effect of hypoxia on adenosine and the reoxygenation that only occurs with types of hypoxic stimuli, like ischemic hypoxia, as well as the production of O_2-derived metabolites.

ACKNOWLEDGMENTS

This study was supported by U.S.P.H.S. grant DK 13211.

REFERENCES

1. AGER, A., AND J. L. GORDON. Differential effects of hydrogen peroxide on indices of endo-thelial cell function. *J. Exp. Med. 159*:592–603, 1984.
2. BAERTSCHI, A. J., J. M. ADAMS, AND M. P. SULLIVAN. Acute hypoxemia stimulates atrial natriuretic factor secretion in vivo. *Am. J. Physiol. 255*:H295–H300, 1988.
3. BAERTSCHI, A. J., C. HAUSMANINGER, R. S. WALSH, R. M. MENTZER JR., D. A. WYATT, AND R. A. PENCE. Hypoxia-induced release of atrial natriuretic factor (ANF) from the isolated rat and rabbit heart. *Biochem. Biophs. Res. Comm. 140*:427–433, 1986.
4. BARGER, A. C., AND J. A. HERD. The renal circulation. *N. Engl. J. Med. 284*:482–490, 1971.
5. BAUD, L., J. HAGEGE, J. E. SPAER, J. RONDEAU, R. PEREZ, AND J. ARDAILLOU. Reactive oxygen production by cultured rat glomerular mesangial cells during phagocytosis is associ-ated with stimulation of lipoxygenase activity. *J. Exp. Med. 158*:1836–1852, 1983.
6. BAUD, L., M. P. NIVEZ, D. CHANSEL, AND R. ARDAILLOU. Stimulation by oxygen radicals of prostaglandin production by rat renal glomeruli. *Kidney Int. 20*:332–339, 1981.
7. CHURCHILL, P. C., AND J. CHURCHILL. A_1 and A_2 adenosine receptor activation inhibits and stimulates renin secretion of rat renal cortical slices. *J. Phar. Exper. Ther. 232*(3):589–594, 1985.
8. COTES, M., AND D. R. BANGHAM. Bioassay of erythropoietin in mice made polycythemic by exposure to air at a reduced pressure. *Nature 191*:1065–1067, 1961.
9. DALY, J. W. Adenosine receptors: characterization with radioactive ligands. In: *Physiology and Pharmacology of Adenosine Derivates*, eds. J. W. Daly, Y. Kuroda, J. W. Phillis, H. Shimizu, and M. Ui. New York: Raven Press, 1983, pp. 59–70.
10. DIONISI, O., T. GALEOTTI, T. TERRANOVA, AND A. AZZI. Superoxide radicals and hydrogen

peroxide formation in mitochondria from normal and neoplastic tissues. *Biochem. Biophys. Acta 403*:292–300, 1975.

11. FINK, G. D., AND J. W. FISHER. Stimulation of erythropoiesis by beta adrenergic agonists. II. Mechanism of action. *J. Pharmacol. Exp. Ther. 202*:199–208, 1977.

12. FINK, G. D., L. G. PAULO, AND J. W. FISHER. Effects of beta-adrenergic blocking agents on erythropoietin production in rabbits exposed to hypoxia. *J. Pharmacol. Exp. Ther. 193*:176–181, 1975.

13. FISHER, J. W. Control of erythropoietin production. *Proc. Soc. Exp. Biol. Med. 173*:289–305, 1983.

14. FISHER, J. W. Pharmacologic modulation of erythropoietin production. *Ann. Rev. Pharmacol. Toxicol. 28*:101–122, 1988.

15. GRISHAM, M. B., AND J. M. McCORD. *Superoxide and Superoxide Dismutase in Chemistry, Biol. and Med.* Amsterdam, New York: Elsevier, 1988, pp. 571–575.

16. HAGIWARA, M., I. CHEN, R. McGONIGLE, B. S. BECKMAN, F. H. KASTEN, AND J. W. FISHER. Erythropoietin production in a primary culture of human renal carcinoma cells maintained in nude mice. *Blood 63*:828–835, 1984.

17. HAGIWARA, M., D. B. McNAMARA, I. CHEN, AND J. W. FISHER. Role of endogenous prostaglandin E in erythropoietin production and dome formation by human renal carcinoma cells in culture. *J. Clin. Invest. 74*:1251–1261, 1984.

18. HAGIWARA, M., S. M. PINCUS, I. -L. CHEN, B. S. BECKMAN, AND J. W. FISHER. Effects of dibutyryl adenosine 3', 5'-cyclic monophosphate on erythropoietin production in human renal carcinoma cell cultures. *Blood 66*(3):714–717, 1985.

19. HARLAN, J. M., AND K. S. CALLAHAN. Role of hydrogen peroxide in the neutrophil-mediated release of prostacyclin from cultured endothelial cell. *J. Clin. Invest. 74*:442–448, 1984.

20. JELKMANN, W. Renal erythropoietin: properties and production. *Rev. Physiol. Biochem. Pharmacol. 104*:139–215, 1986.

21. LIPKIN, E. W., D. C. TELLER, AND C. DE HAEN. Dynamic aspects of insulin action: synchronization of oscillatory glycolysis in isolated perfused rat fat cells by insulin and hydrogen peroxide. *Biochem 22*:792, 1983.

22. MASON-GARCIA, M., B. S. BECKMAN, J. W. BROOKINS, J. S. POWELL, W. LANHAM, S. BLAISDELL L. KEAY, S.C. LI, AND J. W. FISHER, Development of a New Radioimmunoassay for Erythropoietin Using Recombinant Erythropoietin. *Kid. Int.* (in press), 1990.

23. McCORD, J. M. Mechanisms of disease. *N. Engl. J. Med. 312*:159–163, 1985.

24. McCORD, J. M. Oxygen-derived free radicals in postischemic tissue injury. *N. Engl. J. Med. 312*:159–163, 1985.

25. MILLER, W. L., R. A. THOMAS, R. M. BERNE, AND R. RUBIO. Adenosine production in the ischemic kidney. *Circ. Res. 43*:390–397, 1978.

26. NELSON, P. K., J. BROOKINS, AND J. W. FISHER. Erythropoietic effects of prostacyclin (PGI_2) and its metabolite 6-keto-prostaglandin E ($6KPGE_1$). *J. Pharmacol. Exp. Ther. 226*:493–499, 1983.

27. NELSON, J. A., AND S. DRAKE. Potentiation of methotrexate toxicity by dipyridamole. *Cancer Res. 44*:2493–2496, 1984.

28. NILSSON, R., F. M. PICK, AND R. C. BRAY. EPR studies on reduction of oxygen to superoxide by some biochemical oxidase. *Biochim. Biophys. Acta 192*:145–148, 1969.

29. OBERLY, L. W., AND G. R. BUETTNER. Role of superoxide dismutase in cancer: a review. *Cancer Res. 39*:1141–1149, 1979.

30. POWELL, J. W., K. L. BERKNER, R. V. LEBO, AND J. W. ADAMSON. Human erythropoietin gene: high level expression in stably transfected mammalian cells and chromosome localization. *Proc. Natl. Scad. Sci. 83*:6465–6469, 1986.

31. REISSMAN, K. R. Studies on the mechanism of erythropoietic stimulation of parabiotic rats during hypoxia. *Blood 5*:372–380, 1950.

32. REGE, A. B., J. BROOKINS, AND J. W. FISHER. Radioimmunossay for erythropoietin. Serum levels in human subjects and patients with hemopoietic disorders. *J. Lab. Clin. Med. 100*:829–843, 1982.

33. RODGERS, G. M., J. W. FISHER, AND W. J. GEORGE. The role of renal adenosine 3', 5'-monophosphate in the control of erythropoietin production. *Am. J. Med. 58*:31–38, 1975.

34. SEFERYNSKA, I., J. BROOKINS, J. C. RICE, AND J. W. FISHER. Erythropoietin production in the exhypoxic polycythemic mouse assay system. *Am. J. Physiol. 256*:C925–C929, 1989.

35. SHAH, S. V. Effect of enzymatically generated reactive oxygen metabolites on the cyclic nucleotide content in isolated rat glomeruli. *J. Clin. Invest. 74*:393–401, 1984.

36. SPIELMAN, W. S. Antagonistic effect of theophylline on the adenosine-induced decrease in renin release. *Am. J. Physiol. 247*:F246–F251, 1984.

37. UENO, M., J. BROOKINS, B. S. BECKMAN, AND J. W. FISHER. A_1 and A_2 adenosine receptor regulation of erythropoietin production. *Life Sci. 43*:229–237, 1988.

38. UENO, M., J. BROOKINS, B. S. BECKMAN, AND J. W. FISHER. Effects of reactive oxygen metabolites on erythropoietin production in renal carcinoma cells. *Biochem. Biophy. Res. Comm.* *154*(2):773–780, 1988.
39. UENO, M., I. RONDON, B. S. BECKMAN, J. BROOKINS, J. NAKASHIMA, E. F. COLE, AND J. W. FISHER. Increased secretion of erythropoietin in response to atrial natriuretic factor (ANF) in renal carcinoma cell cultures. *Am. J. Physiol.* (in press), 1990.
40. WEISS, S. J., J. YOUNG, A. F. LOBUGLIO, A. SLIVKA, AND N. F. NIMEH. Role of hydrogen peroxide in neutrophil-mediated destruction of cultured endothelial cells. *J. Clin. Invest.* *68*:714–721, 1981.

6

Regulating Mechanisms Involved in the Expression of the Erythropoietin Gene

JAIME CARO, STEPHEN SCHUSTER, BASSAM FRAIJ,
AND SYLVIA RAMIREZ

Under physiologic conditions, the circulating red blood cell mass is maintained at a size optimal for oxygen transport by appropriate adjustments in the rate of red blood cell production. Early clues to how adjustments in erythropoiesis are made were provided by observations in high altitude dwellers (6). The work of Jourdanet (15) and Viault (24) in the nineteenth century and, among many, Hurtado et al. (11) in this century, led to the conclusion that a low arterial oxygen tension stimulated erythropoiesis. Erythropoiesis, however, is also stimulated by anemia despite normal arterial oxygen tension. These apparent contradictory observations are reconciled by the hypothesis that it is the tissue oxygen tension, as determined by the supply and demand of oxygen, that regulates red blood cell production, rather than arterial oxygen pressure per se (9). The link between tissue oxygen tension and erythropoiesis is provided by the polypeptide growth factor erythropoietin. This hormone is primarily produced in the kidney and acts as the mediator in the feedback circuit that regulates red blood cell production (Fig. 6.1). This basic feedback system operates under physiological conditions to maintain the red blood cell mass at an optimal size and also provides the mechanisms to respond to anemia or hypoxia.

Although defined experimentally by Erslev in 1953 (5), erythropoietin was not purified until 1977 by Miyake et al. (19). The recent cloning of the human erythropoietin gene (13) has now revealed its complete molecular structure. Comparison of the deduced amino acid sequence from a human complementary DNA with the N-terminal sequence of human urinary erythropoietin suggests that the complementary DNA encodes a hydrophobic 27-amino acid leader sequence followed by an 166-amino acid mature protein. The deduced molecular weight of the protein backbone is 18,398 daltons. It has three N-linked and one O-linked glycosylation sites, which brings the total molecular weight to about 34,000 daltons. The function of this high carbohydrate content is not known, although it is suspected to contribute to the stability and solubility of the molecule.

To date, no significant amino acid sequence homology has been found between erythropoietin and other growth factors. There appears to be only one gene for erythropoietin in the human genome and its locus appears to be located on chromosome 7 (20). The erythropoietin messenger RNA is encoded by five exons. Comparative analysis between the human, mouse, and monkey

63

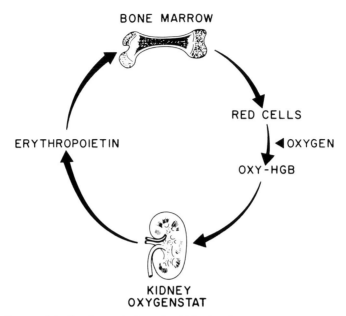

FIGURE 6.1. Proposed feedback regulation of red blood cell production that maintains the red blood cell mass at an optimal size for oxygen transport.

genes has revealed more than 80% homology in the protein sequences between the three species. There is also a high degree of homology at the putative 5′ and 3′ regulatory sequences suggesting that the control mechanism of gene expression is also highly conserved between species (18, 23).

Erythropoietin acts in the bone marrow on stem cells already committed to erythroid development. Studies using in vitro clonal culture systems have defined two classes of progenitor cells able to form distinct colonies in semi-solid media, the more immature and highly proliferative BFU-E and the more mature CFU-E (12). Erythropoietin acts as a mitogenic growth factor, stimulating proliferation of both BFU-E and CFU-E and also probably as a differentiation factor to the terminal erythroblast compartment (Fig. 6.2).

In 1957, Jacobson and co-workers (14) established the kidney as the major source of erythropoietin in the adult mammal. Extrarenal sources of erythropoietin also exist in adults, but they probably account for no more than 10 to 15% of the total erythropoietin production (7). Anephric individuals maintained by chronic hemodialysis have very low levels of erythropoietin despite their severe degree of anemia (3). Indeed, the anemia of chronic renal failure is in large part the result of insufficient erythropoietin production as indicated by the successful correction of the anemia with the use of exogenous recombinant erythropoietin (8, 25). That the kidney is, in fact, the site of erythropoietin synthesis and not merely involved in the activation of a prohormone was recently confirmed by the finding of specific erythropoietin messenger RNA in kidneys from hypoxic-stimulated animals (1, 2, 21). The precise cells in the kidneys responsible for erythropoietin production still remain a matter of controversy. Experiments using in situ hybridization techniques, however, point to cortical interstitial cells as the more likely candidates (16, 17 and Chapter

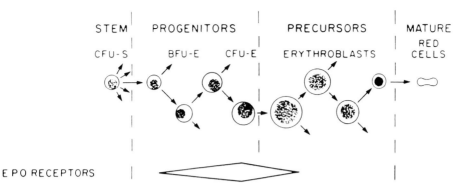

STEM | PROGENITORS | PRECURSORS | MATURE
RED
CFU-S | BFU-E | CFU-E | ERYTHROBLASTS | CELLS

E PO RECEPTORS

FIGURE 6.2. Proposed action of erythropoietin (Epo) on erythroid progenitor cells. Erythropoietin acts by surface receptors as a growth factor for BFU-E and CFU-E and as a differentiating
factor for CFU-E and erythroblasts.

7). The kidneys are also involved in the mechanism of oxygen sensing, which
controls erythropoietin production, as more erythropoietin is produced by isolated kidneys perfused in hypoxic as compared with normoxic conditions (4).
It is unknown, however, whether the same cell that senses hypoxia is the one
that produces erythropoietin.

Exposure to acute hypoxia promotes a rapid synthesis of erythropoietin
that is detectable in the kidneys at approximately 1 hour after induction of the
hypoxic stimuli (Fig. 6.3). Plasma levels lag slightly behind kidney levels and
significant increases in erythropoietin levels are detected at about 2 hours af-

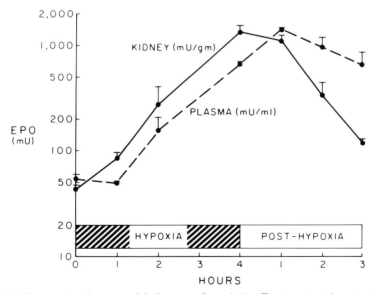

FIGURE 6.3. Changes in plasma and kidney erythropoietin (Epo) content in rats at various
times after onset of hypoxia and during the posthypoxic period. Epo levels in plasma and kidney homogenates were measured by a sensitive radioimmunoassay. Results are expressed as
the mean ± SE of two or three independent measurements.

EPO mRNA KINETICS

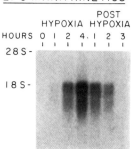

FIGURE 6.4. Northern blot analysis of RNA from rat kidneys obtained at various times after the onset of hypoxia and during the posthypoxic period. PolyA⁺ RNAs were prepared for each time point and hybridized with a complementary strand RNA probe for erythropoietin (Epo) mRNA.

ter stimulation. After discontinuation of the hypoxic stimulus, there is a rapid decline in kidney and plasma erythropoietin. Simultaneous measurement of specific erythropoietin messenger RNA using Northern blot hybridization shows that erythropoietin messenger RNA starts to accumulate at about 1 hour after initiation of the hypoxic stimulus and disappears very rapidly after cessation of stimulation (Fig. 6.4). Thus, it appears that renal erythropoietin synthesis is regulated by the level of its specific messenger RNA, and these levels are highly sensitive to variation in tissue oxygenation (21). The mechanism that regulates the accumulation of erythropoietin messenger RNA in response to hypoxia has been studied by measuring the rate of transcription of the erythropoietin gene in isolated nuclei from kidneys of animals stimulated with hypoxia (22). As shown in Fig. 6.5, transcription rates from nuclear "run-on" assays show a marked increase in transcription of the erythropoietin gene in hypoxic nuclei compared with normal controls. Transcription was completely abolished in the presence of low concentrations of alpha amanitin, a specific inhibitor of polymerase II. It has also been found, although not shown here, that this stimulation of transcription is almost completely suppressed by

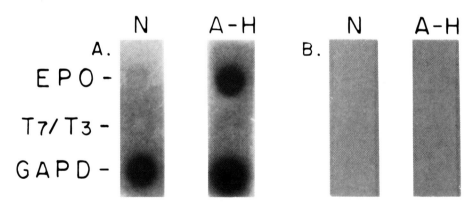

FIGURE 6.5. Effect of hypoxia on transcription of the erythropoietin gene in isolated rat kidney nuclei. Nuclei prepared from kidneys of normal (N) and hypoxia (A-H) rats were allowed to incorporate α-³²P UTP without (A) or with (B) α-amanitin. The ³²P-labeled transcripts were hybridized with filter-bound immobilized plasmids containing a mouse erythropoietin genomic fragment (Epo), the mouse glyceraldehyde-3-phosphate dehydrogenase cDNA (GAPD), or the cloning vector T7/T3 α-19. The filters were washed, digested with RNase A, and exposed to x-ray film for 72 hours.

the addition of cycloheximide, an inhibitor of protein synthesis, suggesting that new protein synthesis is necessary for hypoxia-induced transcription stimulation of the erythropoietin gene.

The mechanisms by which hypoxia is sensed and the mechanisms that mediate this hypoxic stimulation of transcription of the erythropoietin gene are still unknown. Recent work by Goldberg and co-workers (10), however, suggests the possible role of a heme protein in hypoxic sensing and transduction.

REFERENCES

1. BERU, N., J. McDONALD, C. LACOMBE, AND E. GOLDWASSER. Expression of the erythropoietin gene. *Mol. Cell. Biol.* 6:2571, 1986.
2. BONDURANT, M., AND M. KOURY. Anemia induces accumulation of erythropoietin mRNA in the kidneys and liver. *Mol. Cell. Biol.* 6:2731, 1986.
3. CARO, J., S. BROWN, O. MILLER, T. MURRAY, AND A. J. ERSLEV. Erythropoietin levels in uremic nephric and anephric patients. *J. Lab. Clin. Med.* 93:449, 1979.
4. CARO, J., AND A. J. ERSLEV. Erythropoietin assays and their use in the study of anemias. In: *Treatment of Renal Anemia with Recombinant Human Erythropoietin,* eds. K. M. Koch, K. K. Kuhn, B. Nonnast-Daniel, and F. Scigalla. Basel: Karger, 1988, pp. 54–62.
5. ERSLEV, A. J. Humoral regulation of red cell production. *Blood* 8:349, 1953.
6. ERSLEV, A. J. Blood and mountains. In: *Blood, Pure and Eloquent,* ed. M. M. Wintrobe. New York: McGraw-Hill, 1980, pp. 257–280.
7. ERSLEV, A. J., J. CARO, E. KANSU, AND R. SILVER. Renal and extrarenal erythropoietin production in anemic rats. *Br. J. Haematol.* 45:65, 1980.
8. ESCHBACH, J. W., J. C. EGRIE, M. R. DOWNING, J. K. BROWN, AND J. W. ADAMSON. Correction of the anemia of end-stage renal disease with recombinant human erythropoietin: results of a phase I and II clinical trial. *N. Engl. J. Med.* 316:73, 1987.
9. FRIED, W., L. PLZAK, L. O. JACOBSON, AND E. GOLDWASSER. Studies on erythropoiesis. III. Factors controlling erythropoietin production. *Proc. Soc. Exp. Biol. Med.* 94:237, 1957.
10. GOLDBERG, M., S. P. DUNNING, AND F. BUNN. Regulation of erythropoietin gene: evidence the oxygen sensor is a heme protein. *Science* 242:1412, 1988.
11. HURTADO, A., C. MERINO, AND E. DELGADO. Influence of anoxemia on the hemopoietic activity. *Arch. Intern. Med.* 75:284, 1945.
12. ISCOVE, N. N., AND F. SIEBER. Erythroid progenitors in mouse bone marrow detected by macroscopic colony formation in culture. *Exp. Hematol.* 3:32, 1975.
13. JACOBS, K., C. SHOEMAKER, R. RUDERSDORF, S. D. NEILL, R. J. KAUFMAN, A. MUFSON, J. SEEHRA, S. S. JONES, R. HEWICK, E. F. FRITSCH, M. KAWAKITA, T. SHIMIZU, AND T. MIYAKE. Isolation and characterization of tenomic and cDNA clones of human erythropoietin. *Nature* 313:806, 1985.
14. JACOBSON, L. O., E. GOLDWASSER, W. FRIED, AND L. PLZAK. Role of the kidney in erythropoiesis. *Nature* 179:633, 1957.
15. JOURDANET, D. *De l'anemie des altitudes et de l'anemie en geneal dans ses rapports avec la pression de l'atmosphere.* Paris: Bailliere, 1863.
16. KOURY, S. T., M. C. BONDURANT, AND M. J. KOURY. Localization of erythropoietin synthesizing cells in murine kidneys by in situ hybridization. *Blood* 71:524, 1988.
17. LACOMBE, C., J.-L. DaSILVA, P. BRUNEVAL, J. G. FOURNIER, F. WENDLING, N. CASADEVALL, J.-P. CAMILLERI, J. BARIETY, B. VARET, AND P. TAMBOURIN. Peritubular cells are the site of erythropoietin synthesis in the murine hypoxic kidney. *J. Clin. Invest.* 81:620, 1988.
18. McDONALD, J. D., F. K. LIN, AND E. GOLDWASSER. Cloning, sequencing and evolutionary analysis of the mouse erythropoietin gene. *Mol. Cell. Biol.* 6:842, 1986.
19. MIYAKE, T., C. K. H. KUNG, AND E. GOLDWASSER. Purification of human erythropoietin. *J. Biol. Chem.* 252:5558, 1977.
20. POWELL, J. S., K. L. BERKNER, R. V. LEBO, AND J. W. ADAMSON. Human erythropoietin gene: high level expression in stably transfected mammalian cells and chromosome localization. *Proc. Natl. Acad. Sci. (USA)* 83:6465, 1986.
21. SCHUSTER, S. J., J. H. WILSON, A. J. ERSLEV, AND J. CARO. Physiologic regulation and tissue localization of renal erythropoietin messenger RNA. *Blood* 70:316, 1987.
22. SCHUSTER, S. J., E. V. BADIAVAS, P. COSTA-GIOMI, R. WEINMANN, A. J. ERSLEV, AND J. CARO. Stimulation of erythropoietin gene transcription during hypoxia and cobalt exposure. *Blood* 73:13, 1989.

23. SHOEMAKER, C. B., AND L. D. MITSOCK. Murine erythropoietin gene: cloning, expression, and human gene homology. *Mol. Cell. Biol. 6*:849, 1986.
24. VIAULT, P. Sur l'augmentation considerable du nombre de globules rangés dans le sang chez les habitants des hautes plateaux de l'Amerique du sud. *CR Acad. Sci. (Paris) 119*:917, 1890.
25. WINEARLS, C. G., D. O. OLIVER, M. J. PIPPARD, C. REID, M. R. DOWNING, AND P. M. COTES. Effect of human erythropietin derived from recombinant DNA on the anaemia of patients maintained by chronic haemodialysis. *Lancet ii*:1175, 1986.

7

Expression of the Erythropoietin Gene in the Kidney and the Liver of the Anemic Mouse

C. LACOMBE, J. L. DA SILVA, P. BRUNEVAL, C. CHESNE,
A. GUILLOUZO, J. P. CAMILLERI, J. BARIETY,
B. VARET, AND P. TAMBOURIN

Erythropoeitin (Ep) is the glycoprotein hormone that controls red blood cell production in mammals. Erythropoietin synthesis is regulated by feedback mechanisms involving tissue oxygen tension. Since the work of Jacobson et al. (12), the kidney was known to be the major site of Ep production (see Ref. 13). Within the kidney, the identity of the cells responsible for Ep production has remained controversial. Immunofluorescence data (8), and glomerular (3, 4) and mesangial (15) culture studies supported a glomerular origin for the renal Ep-producing cells. On the contrary, a nonglomerular origin, that is, tubular or interstitial, was suggested for the Ep-producing cells based on studies of renal tissue fractions (19). Using in situ hybridization techniques, we recently demonstrated that the renal Ep-producing cells were peritubular cells in the murine hypoxic kidney cortex (16).

To a much lesser extent anemia or cobalt injection induced accumulation of Ep messenger RNA (mRNA) also in the liver (1, 2). Accordingly, using in situ hybridization in the liver, we could not detect any significant Ep mRNA signal above the background. Therefore, we performed cellular fractionation of anemic mouse liver cells, and showed that nonparenchymal cells were probably producing Ep.

METHODS

Induction of Erythropoietin Production in Mice

To increase the amount of Ep mRNA synthesis, ICFW mice were made profoundly anemic by 6-gray irradiation followed 24 hours later by an intraperitoneal injection of phenylhydrazine (60 mg/kg body wt). Nine days later (hematocrit < 10%), mice were bled for serum Ep titration and different organs were removed. One kidney of each mouse was frozen in liquid nitrogen for subsequent in situ hybridization, and the second one was processed for poly(A)$^+$ RNA isolation. The Ep level in the plasma of these anemic mice was shown to be between 6 and 10 IU/ml by an in vitro bioassay using murine CFU-

E-derived colonies in plasma clot and by an in vivo bioassay using ^{59}Fe-incorporation in polycythemic mice (normal values, 20 to 30 mU/ml).

Cellular Separation of Liver Cells

At day 9 after phenylhydrazine injection, 10 anemic mice were anesthetized. The livers were perfused in situ by portal vein catheterism with HEPES-buffered saline (flow rate 4 ml/min) for 10 minutes, then with HEPES-buffered saline containing 0.07% collagenase (flow rate, 2 ml/min) for 15 minutes at 37°C. The livers were then excised, and the cells dispersed in L15 Leibovitz medium. The cell suspension was then centrifuged through a 30% metrizamide cushion at 1400 g for 15 minutes. The pellet contained the parenchymal cells, whereas the band at the top of the tube contained the nonparenchymal cells (21).

Probes

A genomic Ep probe was used (18). This probe was a 243 bp PstI-XhoII restriction fragment encompassing the second exon of the mouse Ep gene that was inserted at the PstI and BamHI sites of a pUC18 vector. A 265-bp Ep-insert/pUC18 PstI-EcoRI purified fragment was derived from this construct.

To better characterize the liver cellular fractions, a rat albumin probe, a v-fms probe (6), and a mouse CSF-1 probe (17) were also used. The rat glyceraldehyde-3-phosphate-deshydrogenase probe was used to quantify RNA samples.

Northern Blot Analysis

Ribonucleic acids were extracted from crushed organs of hypoxic mice, from healthy mouse kidneys, and from the liver cellular fractions using the guanidium–cesium chloride technique (5).

Total RNAs from the different organs were purified by oligo (dT) affinity chromatography to obtain poly(A)$^+$ RNA-enriched preparations. Five micrograms of poly(A)$^+$ RNAs were used for electrophoresis of each sample, except for the liver cellular fractions, where 20 µg of total RNA per sample were electrophoresed.

After glyoxal denaturation and transfer to Gene Screen membranes, the RNAs were hybridized with ^{32}P-labeled probes (specific activity, 3 to 4 $\times$ 10^8 cpm/µg DNA). The filters were washed at 60°C for 0.5 hours in 2 $\times$ standard saline citrate (SSC)–1% sodium dodecylsulfate (SDS), then at 60°C for 0.5 hours in 0.5 $\times$ SSC–0.5% SDS followed by two washes in 0.1 $\times$ SSC for 0.5 hours at room temperature. The filters were exposed at -70°C with an intensifying screen.

In situ Hybridization

Five-micron thick sections of frozen kidneys from six anemic and two control mice were prepared. They were fixed in 4% formaldehyde in 0.1 M phosphate buffer saline pH 7.4 for 20 minutes and dehydrated in alcohols. The procedure for in situ hybridization has been previously described (16). The tissue sections were immersed in HCl 0.2N for 10 minutes. They were then incubated in 15 μg/ml proteinase K (protease XI, Sigma) in 20 mM Tris-HCl, pH 7.4, and 2 mM calcium chloride at 37°C for 15 minutes. Tissue sections were then hybridized under a sealed coverslip for 24 hours at 37°C in 15 μl of a solution containing 50% deionized formamide, 10 mM Tris-HCl, pH 7.4, 1 mM EDTA, 600 mM NaCl, 0.02% Ficoll, 0.02% polyvinylpyrrolidone, 0.02% bovine serum albumine, 10% dextran sulfate, 2 mg/ml yeast *t*-RNA (Sigma), 400 μg/ml salmon sperm DNA (Sigma), 400 μg/ml herring sperm DNA (Sigma), 10 mM dithiothreitol, and 0.2 μg/ml of the radiolabeled probe previously denatured at 100°C for 2 min. The probes were labeled by the random primer elongation method (7), with a commercially available kit (Amersham International, U.K.). Using [35]S dCTP (400 Ci/mmol), the specific activity of the probes was 2.10^8 cpm/μg of DNA.

The slides were then washed at room temperature with gentle agitation successively in 50% formamidein-4 × SSC for 1 hour, followed by two washes in 2 × SSC for 0.5 hours, and finally in 2 × SSC overnight. Sections were then dehydrated in alcohols and covered with Kodak NTB2 emulsion for autoradiography. After 10 to 12 days of exposure, the slides were developed in Kodak D19, fixed with Kodak A44, and stained with hematoxylin and eosin.

Three control procedures were performed to assess the specificity of the in situ hydridization labeling: (1) treatment of tissue sections with 50 μg/ml ribonuclease A (type III, Sigma) in 2 × SSC for 30 minutes at 37°C, then rinsed for 30 minutes in 2 × SSC, and followed by hybridization with the Ep probe; (2) hybridization with a ^{35}S-labeled pUC18 vector without the Ep probe; and (3) hybridization of nonanemic tissue kidney sections with the specific Ep probe.

Immunohistochemistry
Frozen kidney sections of a normal and an anemic mouse were fixed in cold acetone. Rabbit polyclonal antihuman Willebrand factor antibody (DAKO-PATTS, Copenhagen, Denmark) was used at a dilution of 1/100 in 0.1M phosphate buffer saline at pH 7.4. Indirect immunofluorescence was performed using a goat fluorescent antirabbit antibody (Institut Pasteur Production, Paris, France) at a dilution of 1/50. The monoclonal anti-F4/80 antibody, which recognizes a membrane antigen specific for murine monocyte–macrophage (11) was kindly provided by G. Milon (Institut Pasteur, Paris, France) and was used at a dilution of 1/32. Another antimouse monocyte–macrophage monoclonal antibody, M1/70 (10) was commercially available (Serotec, Realef., Paris, France), and used at a dilution of 1/20. These two monoclonal antibodies were revealed using a peroxidase-conjugated antirat immunoglobulin antibody at a dilution of 1/200 (Biosys, Compiègne, France). For positive controls, F4/80 and M1/70 antibodies were, respectively, tested in mouse liver and mouse spleen sections.

Electron Microscopy
Small blocks of tissue from anemic and normal mouse kidneys were fixed by immersion in 2.5% glutaraldehyde phosphate-buffered saline buffer 0.1M (pH 7.4). After postfixation in 2% osmium tetroxide, the tissue samples were routinely processed for electron microscopy.

RESULTS

Expression of the Erythropoietin Gene in Organs of Hypoxic Mice

Northern blots containing similar amounts of poly(A)$^+$ RNAs from hypoxic mice and hybridized with the Ep probe revealed a strong 1.8-kb Ep signal in the kidneys, and a lower signal in the liver after 72 hours of exposure. Other organs, including brain, testes, and salivary glands, were all negative even after a longer exposure of the film (15 days). In healthy mouse kidney, basal Ep expression was detected as a very faint signal (Fig. 7.1).

In situ Hybridization of Anemic Mouse Kidney Sections

Renal specimen of all the mice showed normal structure without any interstitial inflammatory infiltrates, as assessed by light microscopy in hematoxylin and eosin stained frozen sections.

Using in situ hybridization of anemic mouse kidney sections, we detected an intense signal in many cells of the renal cortex and the outer medulla. The positive cells were clearly located outside of the glomeruli and outside of the tubules, which remained both entirely negative (Fig. 7.2). The labeled cells were found in a peritubular location, some of them lining capillary vascular lumens. The nuclei of these cells were prominent between the tubules. Arteries and veins were negative. No signal was detected in the inner medulla. Similar results were obtained in all hypoxic kidneys. In control procedures, positive cells could be detected neither in ribonuclease-treated sections, nor in sections hybridized with the pUC18 plasmid. In kidney sections of healthy mice, no signal was detected after in situ hybridization with the Ep probe.

Immunohistochemical studies exhibited similar results in kidneys from both anemic and healthy mice. When using an antihuman Willebrand factor antibody, a strong labeling was observed in endothelial cells lining peritubular capillaries and larger vessels in the renal cortex and the medulla (Fig. 7.3).

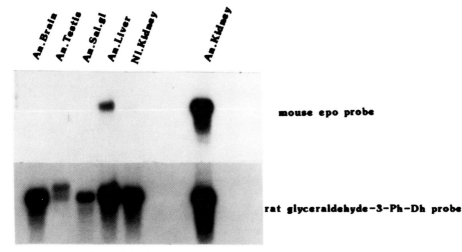

FIGURE 7.1. Northern blot of poly (A)$^+$ RNAs extracted from different organs of hypoxic mice and from normal mouse kidney. Poly (A)$^+$ RNA (5 μg) were electrophoresed and probed with (1) mouse Ep probe and (2) rat glyceraldehyde-3-phosphate-deshydrogenase probe.

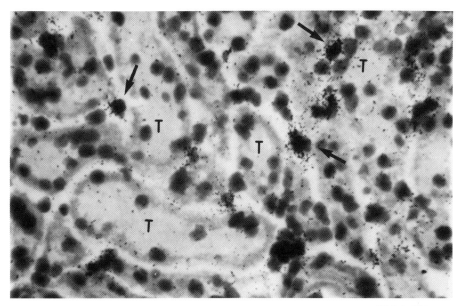

FIGURE 7.2. In situ hybridization of a hypoxic mouse kidney section using a ^{35}S-labeled mouse Ep probe. Positive cells are in a peritubular location (*arrows*) and the tubular cells (T) are negative (X800).

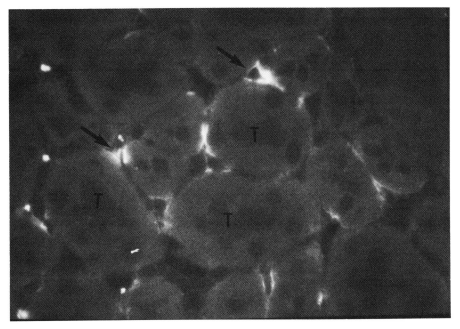

FIGURE 7.3. Indirect immunofluorescence with antihuman Willebrand factor antibody in anemic mouse kidney sections showing the labeled areas of the peritubular capillary endothelial cells (X800).

Antimouse monocyte–macrophage antibodies F4/80 and M1/70 showed no labeling in most of the kidney sections or scanty labeled cells in rare sections, whereas both monoclonal antibodies strongly labeled Kupffer cells and mononuclear cells in the mouse liver and in the mouse red pulp spleen, respectively.

Ultrastructural study of the anemic mouse kidneys showed that most of the peritubular cells in the renal cortex and the outer medulla were capillary endothelial cells. No inflammatory interstitial cells were observed. When compared with the healthy mouse kidney, the peritubular capillary endothelial cells of the anemic mouse kidneys exhibited prominent rough and smooth reticulum, Golgi apparatus, and free polyribosomes.

Erythropoietin Expression in the Anemic Mouse Liver

To characterize the efficiency of the liver cellular fractionation and the nature of the different fractions, the same Northern blot was sequentially hybridized with the Ep probe, the albumin probe, the v-fms probe, the CSF-1 probe, and with the housekeeping gene glyceraldehyde-3-phosphate-deshydrogenase (GAPDH) probe (Figs. 7.4 A and B). The band densities from the films were measured with a densitometer, and curves were corrected for unequal amounts of RNA loaded using the results from the GAPDH probe (Fig. 7.5). The albumin probe did not detect any signal in the nonparenchymal cellular fraction, indicating that nonparenchymal cells were free of parenchymal cells after separation on the metrizamide cushion. The nonparenchymal cells were enriched for macrophages, fibroblasts, and endothelial cells, based on the very strong signals observed on this cellular fraction when v-fms and CSF-1 probes were used to hybridize the same Northern blot.

On the other hand, parenchymal cells were still contaminated by one or several types of nonparenchymal cells and especially by CSF-1-producing cells. Using the Ep probe, an Ep mRNA expression was observed in all fractions, particularly in the nonparenchymal cellular fraction.

DISCUSSION

As previously shown by others (1, 2), we also found that an Ep mRNA accumulation occurred in the kidney and liver of adult rodents placed under hypoxic conditions.

We described that the renal cells producing Ep under hypoxic conditions were peritubular cells of the cortex and the outer medulla (16). Neither the glomeruli nor the tubules were involved in Ep mRNA synthesis. The nature of these peritubular cells producing Ep mRNA were more precisely determined by immunohistochemical techniques. Because bone marrow macrophages have been described to produce Ep in culture, we used two antimacrophage antibodies to evaluate the number of macrophages in these sections. We found very few macrophages in contrast with the high number of Ep-producing cells. On the other hand, when using an endothelial marker, labeled cells were found in the same peritubular location as the Ep-producing cells. To further demon-

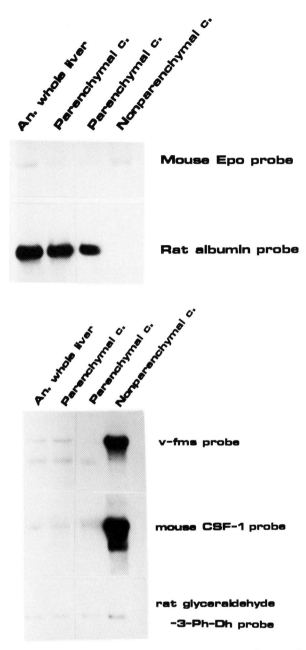

FIGURE 7.4. Northern blot of total RNAs extracted from the whole hypoxic liver and from the different cellular fractions. This blot was probed sequentially with the mouse Ep probe and the rat albumin probe (**A**), and then with the v-fms, mouse CSF-1, and rat GAPDH probes (**B**).

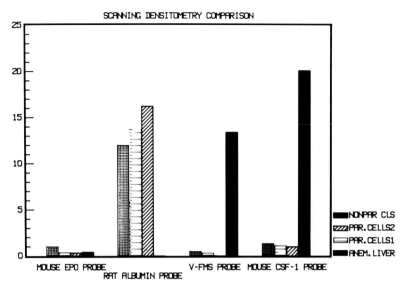

FIGURE 7.5. Scanning densitometry comparison deduced from the results of Figures 7.4A and B. Calculated areas were corrected for unequal amounts of RNA loaded according to the results obtained with the GAPDH probe.

strate that peritubular cells, which produced Ep, were endothelial cells, double labeling with the Ep probe and an anti-Willebrand factor antibody should be performed.

The cells producing Ep in the adult hypoxic liver are still not identified. Our experiments using liver cellular fractionation demonstrated that nonparenchymal cells synthesize Ep. Erythropoietin expression was also detected in the parenchymal cellular fraction, which may be due either to contaminating nonparenchymal cells or to Ep production by the hepatocytes themselves.

Finally, there was no correlation between the levels of CSF-1 receptor expression in nonparenchymal cells, as detected with the v-fms probe and Ep expression in the same tissues. Our data suggest that liver cells belonging to the mononuclear phagocytic lineage and expressing fms (20) are probably not responsible for the detectable Ep signal observed in the nonparenchymal fraction.

Other methods of liver cells fractionation should allow a better identification of the cells involved in Ep production.

In summary, in the mouse hypoxic kidney, we (16) and another group (14) demonstrated that peritubular capillary cells produce Ep. Because in situ hybridization is not a very sensitive technique, basal Ep production by the tubular cells themselves cannot be ruled out. Similarly, in the hypoxic liver, which accounts for about 15% of the Ep production, nonhepatocytic cells seem to be responsible for Ep synthesis, although the production of some Ep mRNA by parenchymal cells cannot be formally excluded. Further studies aimed at defining a specific receptor involved in the oxygen-sensing mechanism (9) and borne by these peritubular and nonparenchymal cells are indicated.

ACKNOWLEDGMENTS

We thank E. Goldwasser for providing the murine Ep gene probe, P. Bucau-Varlet for excellent technical assistance, C. Fournet for expert typing, and M. Sitbon for critical reading of the manuscript.

REFERENCES

1. BERU, N., J. MCDONALD, C. LACOMBE, AND E. GOLDWASSER. Expression of the erythropoietin gene. *Mol. Cell. Biol.* 6:2571–2575, 1986.
2. BONDURANT, M. C., AND J. M. KOURY. Anemia induces accumulation of erythropoietin mRNA in the kidney and the liver. *Mol. Cell. Biol.* 6:2731–2733, 1986.
3. BURLINGTON, H., E. P. CRONKITE, U. REINIKE, AND E. D. ZANJANI. Erythropoietin production in cultures of goat renal glomeruli. *Proc. Natl. Acad. Sci. (USA)* 69:3547–3550, 1972.
4. BUSUTTIL, R. W., B. L. ROH, AND J. W. FISHER. Localization of erythropoietin in the glomerulus of the hypoxic dog kidney using a fluorescent antibody technique. *Acta Haematol.* 47:238, 1972.
5. CHIRGWIN, J. M., R. J. PRZYBYLA, R. J. MCDONALD, AND W. J. RUTTER. Isolation of biologically active ribonucleic acid from sources enriched in ribonuclease. *Biochem.* 18:5294–5299, 1979.
6. DONNER, L., L. A. FEDELE, C. F. GARON, S. J. ANDERSON, AND C. J. SHERR. McDonough feline sarcoma virus: characterization of the molecularly cloned provirus and its feline oncogene (v-fms). *J. Virol.* 41:489–500, 1982.
7. FEINBERG, A. P., AND B. VOLGELSTEIN. A technique for radiolabelling DNA restriction endonuclease fragments to high specific activity. *Ann. Biochem.* 132:6–13, 1983.
8. FISCHER, J. W., G. TAYLOR, AND D. D. PORTEOUS. Localization of erythropoietin in glomeruli of sheep kidney by fluorescent antibody technique. *Nature* 205:611–612, 1965.
9. GOLDBERG, M. A., S. P. DUNNING, AND H. F. BUNN. Regulation of the erythropoietin gene: evidence that the oxygen sensor is a heme protein. *Science* 242:1412–1414, 1988.
10. HO, M. K., AND T. A. SPRINGER. Macl antigen: quantitative expression in macrophage populations and tissues, and immunofluorescent localization in spleen. *J. Immunol.* 128:2281–2286, 1982.
11. HUME, D. A., AND S. GORDON. Mononuclear phagocyte system of the mouse defined by immunohistochemical localization of antigen F4/80. *J. Exp. Med.* 157:1704–1709, 1983.
12. JACOBSON, L. O., E. GOLDWASSER, W. FRIED, AND L. PIZAK. Role of the kidney in erythropoiesis. *Nature* 179:633–634, 1957.
13. JELKMANN, W. Renal erythropoietin: properties and production. *Rev. Physiol. Biochem. Pharmacol.* 104:140–215, 1986.
14. KOURY, S. T., M. C. BONDURANT, AND M. J. KOURY. Localization of erythropoietin synthesizing cells in murine kidneys by *in situ* hybridization. *Blood* 71:524–527, 1988.
15. KURTZ, A., W. JELKMANN, F. SINOWATZ, AND C. BAUER. Renal mesangial cell cultures as a model for study of erythropoietin production. *Proc. Natl. Acad. Sci. (USA)* 80:4008–4011, 1983.
16. LACOMBE, C., J. L. DA SILVA, P. BRUNEVAL, J. G. FOURNIER, F. WENDLING, N. CASADEVALL, J. P. CAMILLERI, J. BARIETY, B. VARET, AND P. TAMBOURIN. Peritubular capillary cells are the site of erythropoietin synthesis in the murine hypoxic kidney. *J. Clin. Invest.* 81:620–623, 1988.
17. LARDNER, M. B., G. A. MARTIN, J. A. NOBLE, V. P. WITTMAN, M. K. WARREN, M. MCGROGAN, AND E. R. STANLEY. cDNA cloning and expression of murine macrophage colony-stimulating factor from L929 cells. *Proc. Natl. Acad. Sci. (USA)* 85:6706–6710, 1988.
18. MCDONALD, J. D., F. K. LIN, AND E. GOLDWASSER. Cloning sequencing, and evolutionary analysis of the mouse erythropoietin gene. *Mol. Cell. Biol.* 6:842–848, 1986.
19. SCHUSTER, S. J., J. H. WILSON, A. J. ERSLEV, AND J. CARO. Physiologic regulation and tissue localization of renal erythropoietin messenger RNA. *Blood* 70:316–318, 1987.
20. SHERR, C. J., C. W. RETTENMIER, R. SACCA, M. F. ROUSSEL, A. T. LOOK, AND E. R. STANLEY. The c-fms proto-oncogene product is related to the receptor for the mononuclear phagocyte growth factor, CSF-1. *Cell* 41:665–676, 1985.
21. STEFFAN, A. M., J. L. GENDRAULT, R. S. MCCUSKEY, P. A. MCCUSKEY, AND A. KIRN. Phagocytosis, an unrecognized property of murine endothelial liver cells. *Hepatology* 6:830–836, 1986.

III

CELL BIOLOGY AND FUNCTIONS OF PERIPHERAL CHEMORECEPTORS

8

Oxygen Sensing by Arterial Chemoreceptors

ASHIMA ANAND AND A. S. PAINTAL

The physiology of arterial chemoreceptors, as well as other aspects relating to them, has been presented relatively recently in an authoritative review by Eyzaguirre et al. (11). This chapter reveals that from the very beginning, arterial chemoreceptors have been believed to detect the chemical composition of the blood, specifically the partial pressure of oxygen in the blood and also possibly the partial pressure of carbon dioxide. The oxygen content of the blood was ruled out as an important factor because Comroe and Schmidt (8) found that these chemoreceptors were apparently not stimulated when the oxygen content of the blood was reduced. From this finding, it followed that the dissolved oxygen in the plasma was enough for their metabolic needs (8). A few years later, Landgren and Neil (26) showed that the carotid chemoreceptors were also markedly stimulated after hemorrhage. Neil (32) advanced the view that stagnation led to the accumulation of some excitatory substance (metabolites) that constituted the excitatory substance of the chemoreceptors. The local concentration of the metabolite that constituted the stimulus for the chemoreceptors determined the degree of stimulation of these chemoreceptors. This concentration depended on the level of oxygen tension in the blood and the rate at which it was removed from the blood circulating through the sinusoids (32). Then came the classic paper by Daly et al. (9) showing that the oxygen consumption by the carotid body was not small, as assumed, but very large—even greater than that of the cerebral cortex—and that the blood flow through the carotid body was also large. This was consistent with its large rate of oxygen consumption. These two new findings should have resulted in the revision of the metabolite hypothesis; but, possibly, this was not done because just 2 years earlier Duke et al. (10) had shown that the chemoreceptors were not stimulated by reducing the oxygen content to as low as 25% of normal by administering carbon monoxide (CO), an observation that they felt was consistent with the earlier views of Comroe and Schmidt (8).

By this time a tradition had developed among physiologists that the carotid body constituted the ideal preparation for studying the physiology of chemoreceptors. Sophistication in this field of research was carried one step further when Eyzaguirre and Lewin (14) developed the superfused carotid body preparation and the metabolite hypothesis of Neil (32) was strengthened further by the well-known "in-series carotid body preparation" leading to the view that acetylcholine (Ach) was the metabolite, also referred to as the transmitter (13).

At about the same time, at the Wates Symposium held in 1966 (48), it was revealed from experiments done on aortic chemoreceptors (35) that the stimulation of the chemoreceptors could not be dependent on a metabolite that was washed away by the blood flow, as aortic chemoreceptors showed clear evidence of adaptation after circulatory standstill. This adaptation could not happen if the metabolite was the stimulus as it would accumulate with time. Even more convincing was the fact that there was no increase in discharge when circulatory standstill was produced while ventilating the cat with nitrogen; that is, at a time when the local Po_2 in the vicinity of the chemoreceptors must have fallen to 0 mm Hg. These observations, thus, showed that the actual stimulus must be the fall in local Po_2 in the aortic body. The observations were also consistent with the fact that the oxygen consumption of the chemoreceptor complex was high (16). (Indeed the high rate of oxygen consumption is well illustrated by the fact that a fall in blood pressure by about 40 mm Hg causes an increase in discharge that occurs within about 4 seconds (5).) Simultaneously it was shown that aortic chemoreceptors were stimulated clearly by ventilating the cat with CO such that the oxygen content fell to 4 vol % (34). This was confirmed by Mills and Edwards (30). These observations including the ones showing that the carotid and aortic chemoreceptors were stimulated by reduction in blood pressure (2, 26, 27, 34) led to the conclusion that the stimulation of the chemoreceptors was determined by the local tissue Po_2 (sensed by the local Po_2 oxygen sensor) and that the tissue Po_2 itself depended on the oxygen available as determined by the oxygen content of the blood and blood flow through the chemoreceptor tissue (34).

The question that was raised at the Wates Symposium (48) was: Why did the carotid chemoreceptors not respond in the same way?; that is, why were they not stimulated by reducing the oxygen content of the blood (see Ref. 23). At that time (35) it was suggested by experiments on the carotid chemoreceptors that the preparation of the nerve for recording impulses involved exposure of the carotid body to air and, therefore, oxygen from the air could flow to the chemoreceptors particularly to the ones located near the surface of the carotid body. That the gases in the external environment could effectively influence the activity of carotid chemoreceptors was well demonstrated in the superfused carotid body preparation (11, 13, 14). Cooling the surface of the carotid body could also reduce the effect of CO, as reducing body temperature abolishes the excitatory effect of CO on aortic chemoreceptors (42).

It is interesting to note that although it was clearly demonstrated that the external environment could effectively influence the activity of chemoreceptors, this was ignored by several groups of investigators. Indeed for more than 20 years many groups of investigators have carried out experiments on carotid chemoreceptors with the carotid bodies exposed to varying degrees (depending on the "cleanliness" of the preparation). Certainly work on the carotid body has led to wide differences in observations such as the effect of hypotension or hemorrhage.

EFFECT OF HYPOTENSION

Initially Landgren and Neil (26) showed that withdrawing blood (20 ml) caused a marked increase in the activity of chemoreceptors. In fact, as shown consistently by them, the degree of activity was equivalent to ventilating a cat with 4.5% oxygen in nitrogen. It is noteworthy that although the blood pressure was low in most of the experiments, the activity was still considerable even when the blood pressure was about 70 mm Hg. These observations, however, were not confirmed subsequently by Biscoe et al. (6), who unlike Landgren and Neil (26) used few fiber preparations or single fiber preparations instead of recording from the entire carotid nerve. Recording from whole nerve would not require a long length of nerve. Because Biscoe et al. (6) needed a longer length of nerve, it is possible that they needed to dissect closer to the carotid body to get the required length and thus removed more of the tissue around the carotid body. If this was the case, then they exposed the carotid body to more air than was done in the case of the preparation used by Landgren and Neil (26). Alternatively, it is possible that the few fibers that Biscoe et al. (6) sampled were from chemoreceptors that were near the surface of the carotid body and that oxygen flowed to them from outside when they reduced the blood pressure in their cats. Could the same thing have taken place in the experiments of Mitchell and McCloskey (31) and Lahiri et al. (25) who reported markedly lower effect of hypotension on carotid chemoreceptors than on aortic chemoreceptors when both were recorded simultaneously. If this is not so, then the conclusion that follows is that the metabolic usage of oxygen by the glomus tissue of the carotid body is less than that of the aortic bodies, which is highly unlikely. It needs to be mentioned here that because it is conclusively established from superfusion experiments that oxygen must flow into the carotid body from outside, one is forced to the conclusion that even the high rate of oxygen consumption calculated by Daly et al. (9) must have been an underestimate as the oxygen coming from the fluid around the carotid body (although not superfused) would not have been taken into account in the arterovenous difference measurements by them (9). This must also apply to the measurement done by others, such as Purves (46).

CHEMOEXCITATORY FACTORS IN HYPOTENSION

The excitatory effect of hypotension (due to hemorrhage or partial obstruction of venous return) on chemoreceptor activity depends not only on the degree of fall in perfusion pressure leading to a reduction of oxygen availability (Fig. 8.1), but also on the degree of reflex glomeral vasoconstriction produced by the sympathetic outflow to them. It must be remembered, however, that the primary cause of the fall in tissue Po_2 (which is the actual stimulus) is the activity of the metabolic cells (Fig. 8.1) in the absence of which there would be no fall in tissue Po_2 and, hence, no excitation of chemoreceptors would be produced by hemorrhagic hypotension.

Some quantitative information is now available about the effect of hypotension on aortic chemoreceptor activity. For instance, lowering the blood pres-

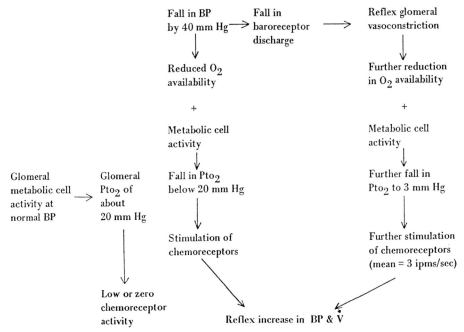

FIGURE 8.1. Role of glomeral metabolic cell activity in stimulation of chemoreceptors during hypotension (P_tO_2 = local tissue Po_2).

sure by about 37 mm Hg caused aortic chemoreceptor activity to increase to 3.2 impulses/sec (see Fig. 2A in Ref. 5), that is, to about 33% of a maximum activity of 9 impulses/sec, which appears during circulatory arrest when the tissue Po_2 would be 0 mm Hg (see Ref. 37). As will be shown by the predicted curve in Fig. 8.3A, this level of activity (33%) would be expected to occur at a tissue Po_2 of 3 mm Hg, which would also occur when the arterial Po_2 is reduced to about 35 mm Hg.

CONTRIBUTION OF SYMPATHETIC OUTFLOW

During hypotension the sympathetic outflow may increase or decrease depending on how the hypotension is produced. This has been clearly demonstrated in recent experiments showing that when the hypotension is produced by impeding blood flow into the heart (equivalent to hemorrhage), the increase in activity occurs quickly and can be considerable, presumably also because of the constriction of the glomeral vessels owing to sympathetic activity that is known to occur during hemorrhage. Indeed this was seriously considered by Landgren and Neil (26) in their observations on carotid chemoreceptors. On the other hand, if the reduction in blood pressure is caused by reducing the sympathetic outflow (e.g., by injecting a barbiturate or veratridine), then instead of an increase of activity, there is an initial reduction in chemoreceptor activity (Fig. 8.2). The opposite is obtained when the blood pressure rises after occlusion of the common carotid arteries due to increased sympathetic outflow, then there is a stimulation of the aortic chemoreceptors (Table 8.1). On the

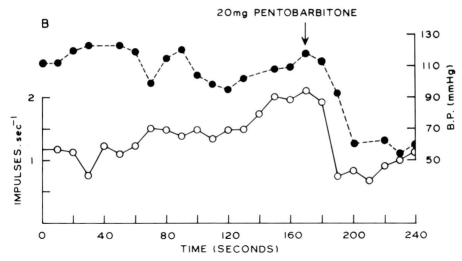

FIGURE 8.2. Effect of injecting 20 mg of sodium pentabarbitone at arrow on the average activity of four aortic chemoreceptors whose activity increased after ventilating the cat with 6.7% CO_2 gas mixture. Note that the activity ($-\bigcirc-\bigcirc-$) fell instead of increasing after the blood pressure ($-\bullet-\bullet-$) fell by 50 mm Hg (5).

other hand, if the aortic blood pressure is made to rise passively by occlusion of the thoracic aorta, then there is relative reduction of chemoreceptor activity (3, 27), not only due to increased perfusion pressure, but also due to the reflex reduction of sympathetic outflow owing to stimulation of carotid and aortic baroreceptors leading to the reduction of chemoreceptor activity. The opposite will happen when the aortic blood pressure falls after releasing the occlusion of the descending aorta. Here aortic chemoreceptor activity would increase not only because of the reduction of the perfusion pressure but also because of sympathetically mediated glomeral vasoconstriction due to the precipitous de-

TABLE 8.1. Effect of Different Maneuvers Causing a Rise (↑) or Fall (↓) in Aortic Blood Pressure on Aortic Chemoreceptor Activity

		Effect On	
Maneuver	Aortic Blood Pressure	Sympathetic Outflow to Glomeral Vessels	Aortic Chemoreceptor Activity
Hemorrhage Obstructions of venous return }	↓	↑	↑

Injection of barbiturate
  during hypoxia or
  hypercapnia
	↓	↓	↑
			delayed

Occlusion of common carotid arteries	↑	↑	↑
Occlusion of descending aorta	↑	↓	↓
Release of occlusion on common carotid arteries	↓	↓	↑ delayed (predicted)

crease in baroreceptor stimulation. All these effects of rise and fall in blood pressure are summarized in Table 8.1 and referring to this table would be useful in interpeting the observations of Lee et al. (27), as in their experiments the carotid nerves were intact and the variations in the baroreceptor and carotid chemoreceptor activity due to raising or lowering the blood presure altered the sympathetic outflow to the aortic glomeral vessels.

It is worthwhile recalling the hypothesis of Lee et al. (27) that "the sympathetic innervation must be of physiological importance at least in tending to maintain a constant sensitivity of the receptors in the face of an increased blood pressure." This hypothesis could account for the effect of raising the blood pressure on the aortic chemoreceptor activity (by occlusion of the common carotid arteries) no doubt by increasing sympathetic activity. It should be noted, however, that occlusion of the common carotid arteries actually mimicks a hemorrhage, which, as already been shown (27), leads to an increase in sympathetic activity. In the case of hypotension, the hypothesis of Lee et al. (27) cannot apply because the hypotension is accompanied by an increase in sympathetic activity, that is, the sympathetic activity is now not keeping the chemoreceptor discharge constant but is tending to increase the activity by positive feedback. Presumably this positive feedback would accelerate the reflex rise in blood pressure and this could be an important function of the sympathetic outflow to the aortic and carotid bodies.

OTHER EFFECTS OF THE SYMPATHETIC OUTFLOW

Although the role of the sympathetic outflow has been inferred in the case of the increased activity of aortic chemoreceptors during hypotension, it should be remembered that the direct excitatory effect of stimulating sympathetic preganglionic fibers has been unequivocally demonstrated by Mills (29), as also in the case of the carotid chemoreceptors (see Ref. 11). The excitatory effects of noradrenaline have also been demonstrated (11). It has also been shown that it is through the sympathetic outflow that activity of aortic chemoreceptors is increased on stimulating intestinal receptors by squeezing or pressing the small intestines of the cat (3). Increased sympathetic outflow is also involved in enhancing the activity of aortic chemoreceptors during hypoxia. In some experiments this factor (i.e., sympathetic activity) seems to have been the major factor in increasing the activity of certain chemoreceptors during acute hypoxia, apparently by reducing oxygen availability through glomeral vasoconstriction (5). Finally, involvement of the sympathetic outflow is also seen during hypercapnia, as described later (Fig. 8.2).

EFFECT OF HYPERCAPNIA

It is possible that most physiologists still assume that CO_2 is the second natural stimulus for chemoreceptors. It is for this reason that attempts are made to look for oscillations in the chemoreceptor discharge of carotid chemoreceptors (see Ref. 11). It is assumed that the oscillations are due to the cyclical respiratory variations in the Pa_{CO_2}, whereas variations in the Pa_{O_2} are not causal. The excitatory effect of CO_2 has been suspected or assumed for more than 30 years and evidence for this has been presented from time to time (see Ref. 48). It is against this background that one has to consider why little attention was paid to the observations of Paintal and Riley (45) showing that CO_2 had no demonstrable excitatory effect on aortic chemoreceptors. In fact, even after the results had been confirmed by Sampson and Hainsworth (47) and supported to some extent by the observations of Fitzgerald and Dehghani (18), no particular note was taken of the lack of clear stimulation of aortic chemoreceptors by CO_2. The paper by Lahiri et al. (24) had an important influence on the thinking of the investigators in this field (see Ref. 11). Notice was taken of the conclusion that although the excitatory effect of hypercapnia on carotid chemoreceptors was clear, there was also some excitatory effect on aortic chemoreceptors (24). This led to the conclusion that aortic chemoreceptors did not differ from carotid chemoreceptors. From this a theory about the excitation of arterial chemoreceptors based on both low Pa_{O_2} and high Pa_{CO_2} being the natural excitatory stimuli was advanced by Lahiri and his co-workers (11). More recently, however, it has been demonstrated that even the small excitatory effect of CO_2 on aortic chemoreceptors observed by Lahiri et al. (24) is not attributable to CO_2 itself but to the increased sympathetic outflow that occurs on administering hypercapnic mixtures to the cat (5). Indeed, as shown in Fig. 8.2, the excitatory effect of CO_2 can be abolished by reducing the sympathetic outflow by injecting a dose of sodium pentobarbital. It has been pointed out that the differing excitatory effects of CO_2 observed by different investigators could be partly attributed to differing levels of sympathetic activity obtained in the experiments (5).

At present, therefore, it is helpful to conclude that CO_2 does not have a direct excitatory effect on aortic chemoreceptors. It definitely does have a dynamic excitatory effect on carotid chemoreceptors, however, and possibly some static effect. It is important to explain this difference between the two groups of receptors. One possibility is that the regenerative region [where drugs produce their excitatory effects (33)] of carotid chemoreceptors is more sensitive to CO_2 than the regenerative region of aortic chemoreceptors. Such a plausible assumption has the merit of allowing one to assume further that there is only one natural stimulus sensed by the chemoreceptor complex, that is, the level of the local tissue P_{O_2}. This would be sensed by the oxygen sensor and the information then transduced into nerve impulses.

THE OXYGEN SENSOR AND OXYGEN SENSING

At present it is generally assumed that the type I cell is probably the one responsible for the high rate of usage of oxygen, that is, it is the metabolic cell. Thus, the local tissue P_{O_2} is determined by two factors: (1) the oxygen available through the blood (oxygen content plus blood flow) and (2) the metabolic rate of the type I cell (34, 37, 39). Most investigators, however, believe that the same cell (type I cell) is also the one that senses the level of the local P_{O_2} (see Ref. 11). If that is true, then the question that arises is: Can a cell be both a sensor of a stimulus as well as a generator of a stimulus? One could draw a parallel with the muscle spindle wherein the level of stretch (the sensory stimulus) is partly determined by the state of contraction of the intrafusal fibers (28). This is only true, however, if the central connections with the spinal cord are intact, not if the muscle nerve is severed. And it is the severed nerve condition that one is concerned with when one considers the mechanisms of sensing at the sensory receptor complex. Thus, there is no example of a receptor system wherein the sensing mechanism also determines (along with other determinants) the level of the stimulus that is being sensed. It was, therefore, proposed that there must be another cell that serves as the oxygen sensor, and it was suggested that the type II cell was probably the oxygen sensor (34).

One important question that has not been satisfactorily answered so far is: What is the level of local Po_2 for any given level of oxygen availability? In an attempt to answer this question the local tissue Po_2 was measured with oxygen microelectrodes mainly by two groups of investigators (1, 49, 50). Both groups, however, reported markedly differing values for the local Po_2 at different depths of the carotid body. In any case all the values obtained relating to the carotid body must have been influenced by the oxygen in the air. Whalen and Nair (49, 50) have also provided observations showing the fall in the local tissue Po_2 after stopping blood flow. One would expect this from the rate of increase of chemoreceptor activity. Indeed, one could have used the amount of chemoreceptor activity as a guide to the arterial Po_2 had the metabolic rate of the carotid body been zero or very low. Actually one could have done the same thing as in the case of pulmonary stretch receptors, that is, estimate the volume of the lungs from measurements of the frequency of discharge once the volume–frequency of discharge curve had been plotted (see Fig. 6 in Ref. 2). In spite of the high metabolic usage of oxygen, it should still be possible to estimate the value of the local tissue Po_2 from the level of chemoreceptor activity. Indeed, this has been attempted by assuming that (1) the only stimulus for the chemoreceptors was the local tissue Po_2, (2) that maximal stimulation would occur at zero tissue Po_2, and (3) that if the metabolism of the aortic body could be reduced to zero, then the arterial Po_2 would correspond to the local tissue Po_2 in the glomus (43).

To get an actual plot of the stimulus–response relationship it was assumed that the stimulus–response relation when expressed as a percentage of maximum activity essentially remains the same when the temperature is lowered, as occurs in other sensory receptors such as the muscle spindle, carotid baroreceptors, and pulmonary stretch receptors (Fig. 8.3C and D). The difference between the responses at 36.5 and 26.5°C in Fig. 8.3A and at 38.0 and 27.3°C in Fig. 8.3B can be justifiably attributed to the effect of the high rate of metabolism that causes the local tissue Po_2 (which is the stimulus) to be lowered to a much lower level than the arterial Po_2 at normal body temperature. From these results it was concluded that at threshold activity of aortic chemoreceptors, the local tissue Po_2 would be about 15 to 20 mm Hg and that when the activity was about 10% of maximum the local tissue Po_2 would be about 5 to 9 mm Hg, and that when the arterial Po_2 was about 20 mm Hg at normal body temperature, the tissue Po_2 in the aortic body would be in the range of 1 to 2 mm Hg. Figure 8.3C shows the interesting observation that at 27.3°C the ac-

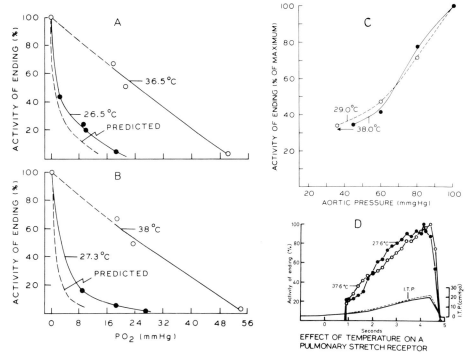

FIGURE 8.3. Stimulus–response relationship of two chemoreceptors (**A** and **B**) at normal temperatures and at about 27°C. The abscissa for these two sets of curves in A and B represents
the measured Po_2 of the arterial blood. The ordinate represents the activity of the ending as a
percentage of maximum activity. The *interrupted line* represents the predicted relation between the activity of the chemoreceptor (ordinate) and the near actual stimulus to it, i.e., the
local tissue Po_2; the abscissa, therefore, represents the tissue Po_2 for the predicted curves. The
derivation of these curves is described in Ref. 43. The stimulus–response relation of a rabbit
aortic baroreceptor (**C**) and a pulmonary stretch receptor of a cat (**D**) at normal and reduced
temperatures. Note the stimulus–response (expressed as percentage of maximum activity on
the ordinate) relationship remains the same on lowering the temperature. **C** was obtained from
Ref. 43 and **D** from Ref. 37.

tivity at an arterial Po_2 of about 4 mm Hg (ventilating with 2% O_2) was about
45% of maximal at 0 mm Hg (i.e., maximum activity after circulatory arrest).

It is likely that the predicted curves shown in Fig. 8.3A and B are actually
obtained in the aortic body, because in the brain cortex Cater et al. (7) recorded
a Po_2 of 2.5 mm Hg when the arterial Po_2 was about 20 mm Hg.

MECHANISMS OF IMPULSE GENERATION AT CHEMORECEPTORS

When considering the mechanisms of impulse generation, sensory physiologists assume without saying so, either that all sensory receptors must have
the same basic mechanisms for generating impulses or the alternative, that is,
they assume that sensory receptors may differ basically in the events involved
in impulse generation at sensory receptors. Some receptors may involve the
participation of a chemical transmitter and others may not (40). The latter

assumption implies that in the same mammalian system sensory neurons may specialize differently. For example, in the case of chemoreceptors, the vast majority of investigators, although accepting that no chemical transmitters are involved at the muscle spindle, the Ruffini endings, and the pacinian corpuscle, assume that in the case of chemoreceptors a chemical transmitter is involved. They tacitly assume that in the petrosal ganglion of the IX nerve the biopolar ganglion cells must be of two types, one type belonging to baroreceptors in which the nerve fiber terminal is specialized to produce a generator potential through mechanical deformation of the terminal (Fig. 8.4), and a second type of bipolar cell belonging to chemoreceptors whose terminals are specialized for being acted upon by chemical substances released from the type I cells. The petrosal ganglion is the equivalent of the dorsal root ganglion system, which is not designed to convey sensory information from areas, such as the skin, the muscles, and the joints, through the action of chemical substances on its nerve terminals, supposedly liberated by the sensory meter that is made of nonneural elements. Figure 8.4 shows schematically how the numerous mechanoreceptor systems in the skin, muscles, joints, and viscera work. All known sensory receptors function basically according to this scheme; there are some specific variations in the organization of the sensory meter (Fig. 8.4), which is the actual sensor and converts the external stimulus into a suitable mechanical event that deforms the generator region (3 in Fig. 8.4) to produce a generator current that results in producing a propagated impulse when the generator current attains suprathreshold levels (20, 21). In the case of the hair cells of the auditory sensory receptor system, which are the most sensitive mechanoreceptors, it has been proposed, entirely on the basis of electron microscopic evidence of synapselike structures, that the information from the sensory meter (i.e., the hair cell) is not transmitted mechanically to the auditory nerve terminals, but through a chemical transmitter, which, so far, has not been found (38). The same scheme is presumed to operate at chemoreceptors—again based on ultrastructural evidence of the existence of synapselike contacts between the type I cells and the sensory nerve terminals, and the presence of granules in the type I cells that look as if they contain transmitter material. It is pertinent to recall that the slowly adapting type I cutaneous receptor of the Merkel cell contains dense-cored granules (presumably transmitter). It has been shown (4) that this receptor continues to generate high frequency discharge after largely depleting the dense-cored granules (killing the cat by ventilating it with nitrogen and ensuring no entry of oxygen to the receptor from the environment). Thus, transmission of information through a chemical transmitter now seems very unlikely. This does not imply, however, that the many chemical substances shown to exist in or outside the Merkel cell or type I cell (see Ref. 11) are without function. These could, among other functions, be concerned in the modulation of generator and regenerative processes, just as certain modulators are known to function at central synapses.

One should remember that synaptic transmission stops within a few minutes if the animal is killed by hypoxia (ventilating with nitrogen). In the absence of oxygen, transmitters are not produced by nerve terminals that are specialized to do so. On the other hand, in the case of aortic chemoreceptors, the generation of impulses at submaximal frequency of about 2 to 5 impulses

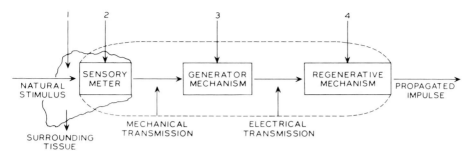

FIGURE 8.4. Mechanisms involved in the generation of impulses at sensory receptors. Note the theory of chemical transmission at chemoreceptors requires that a chemical transmitter between 2 and 3 activates the generator mechanism, whereas there is usually mechanical transmission at all the known mechanoreceptors. The present authors hypothesize that in the case of the chemoreceptors also there is mechanical transmission involved (34,39,44).

can continue for more than 30 minutes. This is the typical behavior of all sensory receptors that have been designed to operate under several restrictions of life-support systems. The gastric stretch receptors that have nonmedullated fibers and, hence, the finest sensory nerve terminals, continue to discharge impulses during gastric distention up to 30 minutes after the cat has been killed by nitrogen ventilation, thereby ensuring that the local oxygen tension is 0 mm Hg (41). In the case of the chemoreceptors, it follows that the oxygen sensor cannot be dependent on the presence of oxygen to function as a local Po_2 meter.

THE SEARCH FOR A TRANSMITTER

Although the existence of a metabolite that was responsible for stimulating chemoreceptors but was washed away by the bloodstream had been rendered unlikely by the observations on the effects of circulatory arrest (34), the possibility that chemoreceptors were stimulated by a chemical transmitter in the way that chemical transmitters generate impulses at neurons (by producing an excitatory postsynaptic potential) was considered. Eyzaguirre and his coworkers (13) were the first to propose from their superfusion experiments, involving the Loewi-type preparation, that Ach was the transmitter. This conclusion was shown to be untenable as it was impossible for the upstream carotid body to produce the required amounts of Ach in the "in-series" preparation (36). There are many other reasons, however, why Ach cannot be the transmitter, even if it is accepted that a transmitter exists (see Ref. 11). One of the important reasons is that Ach is known to produce its excitatory effects at sensory receptors by acting on their regenerative region (33), and it follows that it should do the same in the case of chemoreceptors. Because it had been postulated that it was the transmitter at chemoreceptors, however, it was to be expected that Ach would, in this special case, produce its excitatory effect by acting not on the regenerative region but on the generator region. Thus, as the endings of medullated fibers and of nonmedullated fibers responded equally to hypoxic stimuli (34, 45), it followed that Ach should act *equally* on the generator regions of chemoreceptors with both medullated and nonmedullated fibers and, therefore, Ach should, for a given dose, produce activity of equal intensity in chemoreceptors of both types of fibers. This was not found to be the case, however, for it was shown unequivocally that Ach had much greater excitatory effects on the endings with nonmedullated fibers; in fact some chemoreceptors with medullated fibers were not stimulated at all by Ach (34). Thus, Ach appeared to act in the same way as it acted on other sensory receptors, that is, at the regenerative region and not on the generator region (34).

In view of the importance of this conclusion, Fidone and Sato (17) repeated the experiments on carotid chemoreceptors using a nonconventional method of measuring the conduction velocities of medullated fibers, and they came to almost the opposite conclusion. The validity of their technique for measuring the conduction velocities of medullated fibers in the carotid sinus nerve was tested on vagal nerve fibers. In a preliminary report (38), it was pointed out that their method of measuring conduction velocities yielded absurdly high conduction velocity values. Unfortunately no attention was paid to this observation (38) and, therefore, the earlier observations on the differential effects of Ach (34) were ignored. Because of this and because Ach became a less favored transmitter candidate in the subsequent years, a number of other substances were proposed as possible transmitters and research in this area increased greatly (see Ref. 11). Recently (44), however, it was established beyond doubt that the observations of Fidone and Sato (17) on the conduction velocities of chemoreceptors with medullated fibers could not be correct. Furthermore, the observations of Kirkwood et al. (22) and of Gallego and Belmonte (19) suggest that the conduction velocities of the medullated fibers of chemoreceptors in the carotid nerve were similar to those in the aortic nerve and nowhere as large as the values obtained by Fidone and Sato (17). Moreover, it was shown clearly (44) that it was not possible to justify the number of medullated fibers found electrophysiologically by Fidone and Sato (17) with the histological data of Eyzaguirre and Uchizono (15). Thus, the conclusion that followed was that most of the A fibers of Fidone and Sato (17) were in fact nonmedullated fibers. Therefore, the earlier conclusion that the endings of nonmedullated fibers are far more sensitive to Ach than the endings of medullated fibers is valid and, therefore, Ach could not be a transmitter (34). It was finally concluded that any candidate transmitter can be seriously entertained as a transmitter at chemoreceptors only if it excites equally the endings of both medullated and nonmedullated fibers (44). The aortic chemoreceptors are best suited for such studies. In addition to the search for a candidate transmitter, it would be helpful to also design experiments to test the other hypothesis, that is, the mechanical hypothesis of transduction at chemoreceptors (34, 37, 39, 44).

CONCLUSION

The responses of aortic and carotid chemoreceptors at different temperatures, blood pressures, and blood oxygen content have shown that the local tissue P_{O_2} must be the *actual* natural stimulus for the chemoreceptors. The gross natural stimulus is oxygen availability, which is determined by the blood oxygen content and the blood flow. The local P_{O_2} is determined by the metabolic cell depending on the level of oxygen availability. Accordingly, hypotension constitutes a major mechanism of stimulation of chemoreceptors. In fact, a fall in blood pressure by 40 mm Hg leads to about 33% of maximum activity. As predicted from arterial P_{O_2} response curves at normal and reduced body temperatures, this level of activity should result from a local tissue P_{O_2} of about 3 mm Hg. It is important to realize that the chemoreceptors do not sense the level of arterial P_{O_2} as is generally assumed.

REFERENCES

1. ACKER, H., D. W. LUBBERS, AND M. J. PURVES. Local oxygen tension field in the glomus caroticum of the cat and its change at changing arterial P_{O_2}. *Pflugers Arch. ges Physiol* 329:136–155, 1971.
2. ADRIAN, E. D. Afferent impulses in the vagus and their effect on respiration. *J. Physiol. (London)* 79:332–358, 1933.
3. ANAND, A. Reflex stimulation of aortic chemoreceptors and the role of vascular receptors. *Respir. Physiol.* 38:59–69, 1979.
4. ANAND, A., A. IGGO, AND A. S. PAINTAL. Lability of granular vesicles in Merkel cells of the type I slowly adapting cutaneous receptors. *J. Physiol. (London)* 296:19P, 1979.
5. ANAND, A., AND A. S. PAINTAL. The influence of the sympathetic outflow on aortic chemoreceptors of the cat during hypoxia and hypercapnia. *J. Physiol. (London)* 395:215–231, 1988.
6. BISCOE, T. J., G. W. BRADLEY, AND M. J. PURVES. The relation between carotid body chemoreceptor discharge, carotid sinus pressure and carotid body venous flow. *J. Physiol. (London)* 208:99–120, 1970.
7. CATER, D. B., D. W. HILL, P. J. LINDOP, J. F. NUNN, AND I. A. SILVER. Oxygen washout studies in the anesthetized dog. *J. Appl. Physiol.* 18:888–894, 1963.
8. COMROE, J. H. JR., AND C. F. SCHMIDT. The part played by reflexes from the carotid body in the chemical regulation of respiration in the dog. *Am. J. Physiol.* 121:75–97, 1938.
9. DALY, M. DE BURGH, C. J. LAMBERTSEN, AND A. SCHWEITZER. Observations on the volume of blood flow and oxygen utilization of the carotid body in the cat. *J. Physiol. (London)* 125:67–89, 1954.
10. DUKE, H. N., J. H. GREEN, AND E. NEIL. Carotid chemoreceptor impulse activity during inhalation of carbon monoxide mixtures. *J. Physiol. (London)* 118:520–527, 1952.
11. EYZAGUIRRE, C., R. S. FITZGERALD, S. LAHIRI, AND P. ZAPATA. Arterial chemoreceptors. In: *Handbook of Physiology. The Cardiovascular System III. Peripheral Circulation and Organ Blood Flow*, Part 2., ed. J. T. Shepherd and F. M. Abboud. Baltimore: Williams & Wilkins, 1983, pp. 557–621.
12. EYZAGUIRRE, C., AND A. GALLEGO. An examination of de Castro's original slides. In: *The Peripheral Arterial Chemoreceptors*, ed. M. J. Purves. London: Cambridge Univ. Press, 1975, pp. 1–23.
13. EYZAGUIRRE, C., H. KOYANO, AND J. R. TAYLOR. Presence of acetylcholine and transmitter release from carotid body chemoreceptors. *J. Physiol. (London)* 78:463–476, 1965.
14. EYZAGUIRRE, C., AND J. LEWIN. Effect of different oxygen tensions on the carotid body *in vitro*. *J. Physiol. (London)* 159:238–250, 1961.
15. EYZAGUIRRE, C., AND K. UCHIZONO. Observations on the fibre content of nerves reaching the carotid body of the cat. *J. Physiol. (London)* 159:268–281, 1961.
16. FAY, F. S. Oxygen consumption of the carotid body. *Am. J. Physiol.* 218:518–523, 1970.
17. FIDONE, S. J., AND A. SATO. A study of chemoreceptor and baroreceptor A and C-fibers in the cat carotid nerve. *J. Physiol. (London)* 205:527–548, 1969.
18. FITZGERALD, R. S., AND G. A. DEHGHANI. Neural responses of the cat carotid and aortic bodies to hypercapnia and hypoxia. *J. Appl. Physiol.* 52:596–601, 1982.
19. GALLEGO, R., AND C. BELMONTE. Chemoreceptor and baroreceptor neurones in the petrosal ganglion. In: *The Peripheral Arterial Chemoreceptors*, ed. D. J. Pallot. London: Croom Helm, 1984, pp. 1–7.
20. GRAY, J. A. B. Mechanical into electrical energy in certain mechanoreceptors. *Prog. Biophys. Biophys. Chem.* 9:285–324, 1959.
21. KATZ, B. Depolarization of sensory terminals and the initiation of impulses in the muscle spindle. *J. Physiol. (London)* 111:261–282, 1950.
22. KIRKWOOD, P. A., N. NISIMARU, AND T. A. SEARS. Carotid sinus nerve afferent discharges in the anesthetized cat. *J. Physiol. (London)* 360:44P, 1985.

23. LAHIRI, S. Role of arterial O_2 flow in peripheral chemoreceptor excitation. *Federation Proc. 39*:2648–2652, 1980.

24. LAHIRI, S., E. MULLIGAN, T. NISHINO, AND A. MOKASHI. Aortic body chemoreceptor responses to changes in PCO_2 and PO_2 in cat. *J. Appl. Physiol. 47*:858–866, 1979.

25. LAHIRI, S., T. NISHINO, A. MOKASHI, AND E. MULLIGAN. Relative responses of aortic body and carotid body chemoreceptors to hypotension. *J. Appl. Physiol. 48*:781–788, 1980.

26. LANDGREN, S., AND E. NEIL. Chemoreceptor impulse activity following hemorrhage. *Acta Physiol. Scand. 23*:158–167, 1951.

27. LEE, K. D., R. A. MAYOU, AND R. W. TORRANCE. The effect of blood pressure upon chemoreceptor discharge to hypoxia, and the modification of this effect by the sympathetic-adrenal system. *Quart. J. Exper. Physiol. 49*:171–183, 1964.

28. MATHEWS, P. B. C. *Mammalian Muscle Receptors and Their Central Actions.* London: Edward Arnold, 1972.

29. MILLS, E. Activity of aortic chemoreceptors during electrical stimulation of the stellate ganglion in the cat. *J. Physiol. (London) 199*:103–114, 1968.

30. MILLS, E., AND M. W. EDWARDS. Stimulation of aortic and carotid chemoreceptors during carbon monoxide inhalation. *J. Appl. Physiol. 25*:494–502, 1968.

31. MITCHELL, J. H., AND D. I. McCLOSKEY. Chemoreceptor responses to sympathetic stimulation and changes in blood pressure. *Respir. Physiol. 20*:297–302, 1974.

32. NEIL, E. Chemoreceptor areas and chemoreceptor circulatory reflexes. *Acta Physiol. Scand. 22*:54–65, 1951.

33. PAINTAL, A. S. Effects of drugs on vertebrate mechanoreceptors. *Pharmacol. Rev. 16*:361–380, 1964.

34. PAINTAL, A. S. Mechanism of stimulation of aortic chemoreceptors by natural stimuli and chemical substances. *J. Physiol. (London) 189*:63–84, 1967.

35. PAINTAL, A. S. Some considerations relating to studies on chemoreceptor responses. In: *Arterial Chemoreceptors,* ed. R. W. Torrance. Oxford: Blackwell, 1968, pp. 253–260.

36. PAINTAL, A. S. Further evidence that acetylcholine is not a transmitter at chemoreceptors. *J. Physiol. (London) 204*:94–95, 1969.

37. PAINTAL, A. S. The responses of chemoreceptors at reduced temperatures. *J. Physiol. (London) 217*:1–18, 1971.

38. PAINTAL, A. S. Action of drugs on sensory nerve endings. *Rev. Pharmacol. 11*:231–240, 1971.

39. PAINTAL, A. S. Vagal sensory receptors and their reflex effects. *Physiol Rev. 53*:159–227, 1973.

40. PAINTAL, A. S. Natural and paranatural stimulation of sensory receptors. In: *Sensory Functions of the Skin,* ed. Y. Zotterman. Oxford: Pergamon Press, 1976, pp. 3–12.

41. PAINTAL, A. S. Mechanical transmission of sensory information at chemoreceptors. In: *Morphology and Mechanisms of Chemoreceptors,* ed. A. S. Paintal. Delhi: V. P. Chest Inst., 1976, pp. 121–129.

42. PAINTAL, A. S. The effect of reduction of temperature on the responses of aortic chemoreceptors during administration of carbon monoxide. In: *Morphology and Mechanisms of Chemoreceptors,* ed. A. S. Paintal. Delhi: V. P. Chest Inst., 1976, pp. 335–339.

43. PAINTAL, A. S. A functional estimate of the local PO_2 at aortic chemoreceptors. In: *Chemoreception in the Carotid Body,* ed. H. Acker, S. Fidone, D. Pallot, C. Eyzaguirre, D. W. Lubbers, and R. W. Torrance. Berlin: Springer-Verlag, 1977, pp. 250–255.

44. PAINTAL, A. S. The responses of chemoreceptors with medullated and non-medullated fibres to chemical substances and the mechanical hypothesis. *Prog. Brain Res. 74*:161–168, 1988.

45. PAINTAL, A. S., AND R. L. RILEY. Responses of aortic chemoreceptors. *J. Appl. Physiol. 21*:543–548, 1966.

46. PURVES, M. J. The effect of hypoxia, hypercapnia and hypotension upon carotid body blood flow and oxygen consumption in the cat. *J. Physiol. (London) 209*:395–416, 1970.

47. SAMPSON, S. R., AND R. HAINSWORTH. Responses of aortic body chemoreceptors of the cat to physiological stimuli. *Am. J. Physiol. 222*:953–958, 1972.

48. TORRANCE, R. W. *Arterial Chemoreceptors.* Oxford: Blackwell Scientific Publ., 1968.

49. WHALEN, W. J., AND P. NAIR. Some factors affecting tissue PO_2 in the carotid body. *J. Appl. Physiol. 39*:562–566, 1975.

50. WHALEN, W. J., AND P. NAIR. Factors affecting the tissue PO_2 in the carotid body. In: *Morphology and Mechanisms of Chemoreceptors,* ed. A. S. Paintal. Delhi: V. P. Chest Inst., 1976, pp. 91–100.

9

Oxygen Biology of Peripheral Chemoreceptors

SUKHAMAY LAHIRI

The focus of this chapter is on "adaptive" response of aortic and carotid body chemoreceptors to chronic hyperoxia, which generates an overwhelming excess of oxygen-related free radicals (13). Prolonged normobaric hyperoxia would allow the organism to develop responses and adaptation that may not be expressed during acute hyperbaric hyperoxia. This chapter deals with two aspects of chemoreceptive functions. First, the hypothesis that aortic chemoreceptor responses to chronic hyperoxia would be different from those of carotid chemoreceptors because of a possible difference in oxygen flow to the two chemoreceptor organs (18). If proven, the results would further add to the evidence that aortic body chemoreceptors monitor combined state of systemic circulatory and respiratory oxygen flow and carotid body chemoreceptors monitor respiratory oxygen flow (18, 22). Accordingly, the two chemoreflexes from the two chemoreceptor organs are designed to perform two separate but complementary functions related to oxygen transport to tissues. The second aspect concerns the mechanism of adaptive response of peripheral chemoreceptors to chronic hyperoxia.

The rationale for the experimental study was that hyperoxia induced by breathing 100% oxygen at sea level would generate more oxygen-related free radicals in the tissues with higher blood flow and O_2 metabolism, and those tissues in consequence might express an appropriate adaptive response that is necessarily time dependent. In the case of oxygen sensing tissues, the chemical mechanism by which oxygen is sensed would react with the oxygen species and show changes in structure and function. The adaptive response might involve oxygen metabolism or membrane transport function, or both, in the peripheral chemoreceptors.

Previously we reported that an appropriate administration of metabolic inhibitors to the carotid body attenuated its chemosensory response to hypoxia (27, 29). The results appeared to support the hypothesis that oxygen metabolism is the basis of oxygen chemoreception in the carotid body. Chronic hyperoxia is known to affect pulmonary cellular and mitochondrial structures (10, 13). A similar effect on carotid body cells might alter oxygen chemosensing involving neurotransmitter release according to the metabolic hypothesis. Besides, an absence of oxygen stimulus might eliminate the related trophic effect and desensitize the receptors. There are reasons to believe that trophic func-

95

tion may play an important role in carotid body structure and function (see Ref. 8 for review).

EXPERIMENTAL DESIGN AND METHODS

Cats were exposed to 100% O_2 for 17 to 67 hours. They were anesthetized with sodium pentobarbital (30 to 40 mg/kg initially) and carotid chemoreceptor and aortic chemoreceptor afferents were prepared according to the methods described previously (21). The cats either breathed spontaneously or were paralyzed and artificially ventilated. In either case, hypoxic and hypercapnic tests were performed by altering the inspired gases and maintaining the end-tidal Po_2 and Pco_2 at predetermined levels for 3 to 5 minutes for steady-state effects.

The chemoreceptor afferents were further tested against pharmacological agents, such as cyanide, nicotine, and dopamine (intravenous dose), to further distinguish between the responses that are dependent on and independent of oxygen chemosensing, consistent with the metabolic hypothesis (17, 26, 27). Cyanide, as a metabolic inhibitor of oxidative phosphorylation, is expected to show transient synergistic effect with hypoxia but would block the response to hypoxia in a steady-state application.

Carotid bodies were also fixed by perfusion with glutaraldehyde fixative, and ultrastructures were studied with transmission electron microscopy (25).

A similar experimental protocol was applied to the control cats for structure and function studies of the carotid and aortic bodies.

RESULTS

Chemosensory Response to Hypoxia

Responses to hypoxia of the carotid and aortic body chemoreceptors from the same cat that was exposed to 100% O_2 for 65 hours are shown in Fig. 9.1. Carotid chemosensory discharge did not change with hypoxia (Fig. 9.1A), whereas aortic chemoreceptors were stimulated (Fig. 9.1B).

The results from six cats are summarized in Fig. 9.2, showing that the carotid chemoreceptor responses were significantly lower than those of aortic chemoreceptors. Normally, carotid chemoreceptor responses to hypoxia are more vigorous than those of aortic chemoreceptors.

Chemosensory Responses to Hypercapnia

Responses of carotid chemoreceptors to hypercapnia were augmented although those to hypoxia were blunted (Fig. 9.3). Aortic chemoreceptor responses remained normal. It is known that normal aortic chemoreceptor responses to CO_2

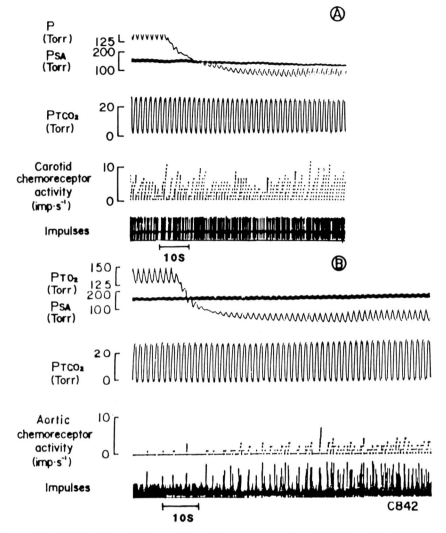

FIGURE 9.1. Effect of chronic hyperoxia on the responses of carotid (**A**) and aortic (**B**) body chemoreceptor responses to the onset of hypoxia. Carotid chemoreceptors were not stimulated, whereas aortic chemoreceptors clearly responded. Tracings from top are tracheal Po_2 (PTo_2), systemic arterial blood pressure (P_{SA}), tracheal Pco_2 ($PTco_2$); chemoreceptor activity (impulses per second and impulses).

are relatively weak (see Refs. 7, 8 for review) but the reasons for the difference are not established.

Effects of Pharmacologic Agents

Carotid chemoreceptor responses to cyanide were severely attenuated in the chronically hyperoxic cats, whereas those to nicotine (excitatory) and to dopamine (inhibitory) were normal (20). Aortic chemoreceptor responses to all three agents were normal (unpublished observations).

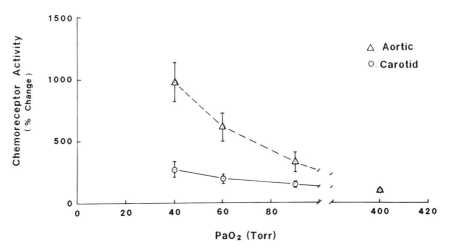

FIGURE 9.2. Attenuated response of carotid chemoreceptors to steady-state hypoxia relative to that of aortic chemoreceptors in chronically hyperoxic cats. The chemoreceptor activities are expressed as percent of their respective control during hyperoxia. (Mean ± SEM; $n = 6$.)

Carotid Body Structure

Ultrastructures of carotid bodies from chronically hyperoxic (62 hours) and control cats are shown in Fig. 9.4. The visible changes are in the mitochondrial structures, mostly in the glomus cells, although some similar changes were seen in the nerve endings in synaptic apposition with the glomus cells. Sustentacular cells (type II) did not show these changes.

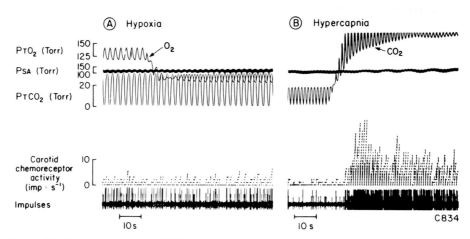

FIGURE 9.3. Comparison of carotid chemoreceptor responses to hypoxia (A) and to hypercapnia (B) in a cat that was exposed to chronic hyperoxia. The responses to hypercapnia were vigorous, whereas those to hypoxia were absent. Tracings from top are the same as in Fig. 9.1.

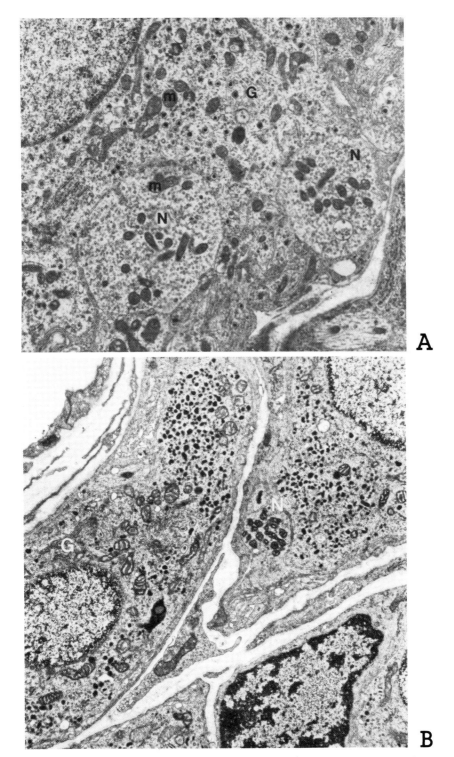

FIGURE 9.4. Morphological characteristics of carotid body cells and nerve endings in the control cat (**A**) and in the chronically hyperoxia cat (**B**). Note that there are subtle changes in the mitochondrial (m) morphology in glomus cells (G) and nerve (N) endings in the carotid body from the cat that was exposed to inspired Po_2 of 700 mm Hg for 62 hours.

DISCUSSION

The relevant effects of chronic normobaric hyperoxia (NH) in the cat are summarized in Table 9.1. The scores represent relative responses to those of the controls with the respective chemoreceptors.

The results (Table 9.1) show that aortic chemosensory responses were not affected by NH, whereas carotid chemosensory responses were attenuated only to hypoxia and cyanide. A further subtle effect of NH was that the carotid chemosensory response to hypercapnia was augmented even in the absence of arterial hypoxemia.

Let us first focus on the differential responses between aortic and carotid body chemoreceptors. There is already a consensus that aortic chemoreceptors vigorously respond to any maneuver that decreases arterial O_2 flow even at the normal arterial Po_2 (see Ref. 18). Moderate carboxyhemoglobinemia, anemia, and hypotension stimulate aortic chemoreceptors but not carotid chemoreceptors. The present results add to the differential responses in that chronic hyperoxia affected carotid chemoreceptors but not aortic chemoreceptors. These characteristics are summarized in Table 9.2.

The stimulatory effects of anemia, carboxyhemoglobinemia, and hypotension are explained partly by the reasoning that aortic body oxygen flow is limiting because of its circulatory architecture—normally supplied by a relatively long and slender secondary blood vessel (15, 28). Physiological evidence is derived from the fact that the latency of response of aortic chemoreceptors to a blood-borne agent is long relative to those of carotid chemoreceptors, although the blood vessels to the aortic bodies are located nearer to the heart (28).

The fact that aortic chemosensory responses to any of the agents, particularly to hypoxia, were not altered by chronic hyperoxia strongly indicated that the factor that attenuated carotid chemoreceptor response to hypoxia was not present in the aortic body. Our interpretation is that the concentration of oxygen-related free radicals were relatively low in the aortic body tissue. This is presumably due to its low blood flow, preventing a great rise in its tissue Po_2 and hence concentration of O_2 free radicals during hyperoxia.

Some 35 years ago carotid body tissue blood flow was first measured and reported to be very high (3), a finding that was later disputed (4). More recently we measured cat carotid body blood flow by the microsphere technique and found that it was indeed very high, about 1500 ml/min per 100 g (1). Accord-

TABLE 9.1. Effects of Normobaric Hyperoxia on Chemoreceptor Responses

Agents with Known Chemosensory Effects	Chemosensory Responses After NH	
	Carotid	Aortic
Hypoxia (excitatory)	−	+
Hypercapnia (excitatory)	+ +	+
Cyanide (excitatory)	−	+
Nicotine (excitatory)	+	+
Dopamine (inhibitory)	+	+

TABLE 9.2. Chemoreceptor Response to Stimuli

| Experimental Maneuver | Chemosensory Responses | |
	Carotid	Aortic
Anemia	−	+
Carboxyhemoglobinemia	−	+
Hypotension	−	+
Chronic hyperoxia	+	−

ingly we believe that the effect of chronic hyperoxia on the carotid body was dependent on this high tissue blood and oxygen flow. By the same reasoning, we conclude that aortic body did not show the effect because of its relatively low blood flow. This conclusion is consistent with the preponderant responses of aortic chemoreceptors to anemia, carboxyhemoglobinemia, and hypotension.

Oxygen-derived free radicals are known to affect many cellular processes, particularly membranes of cells and subcellular particles (10, 13). There are reports that mitochondrial structures of pulmonary cells are significantly affected by hyperoxia (10, 13) and by the metabolic state (14). Our ultrastructural studies of the carotid body also showed some subtle changes, particularly of the glomus cell mitochondria. This change may or may not be causally linked with the attenuated chemosensory function. There is a striking resemblance, however, between the effects of chronic hyperoxia and of mitochondrial metabolic inhibitor, such as antimycin A and oligomycin, on carotid chemosensory responses to hypoxia and hypercapnia. It is well known that acute administration of mitochondrial metabolic inhibitors briefly stimulate carotid and aortic body chemoreceptor afferents (see Ref. 7 for review). Further administration of the inhibitors attenuated the chemosensory responses to hypoxia, up to a point, without blocking those to hypercapnia, nicotine, and dopamine (27, 29). This information, expressed in terms of their responses relative to the control, is outlined in Table 9.3.

Thus, it appears that oligomycin, which blocks ATP synthesis, also blocks the response to arterial hypoxia and to further administration of the metabolic inhibitors. Because similar results were obtained with antimycin A (inhibitor of electron transport chain and retards reduction of O_2) and carbonylcyanide-p-trifluoromethoxyphenylhydrazone (uncoupler that augments O_2 reduction and does not block energy utilization for certain function, such as mitochon-

TABLE 9.3. Effect of Oligomycin on Chemoreceptor Responses

| Potential Stimulus | Chemosensory Responses | After Oligomycin |
	Carotid Body	Aortic Body
Hypoxia	−	±
Hypercapnia	+ +	+ +
Cyanide	−	±
Nicotine	+	+
Dopamine	+	+

drial Ca^{2+} transport, but prevents energy capture in the form of ATP), we concluded that it was ultimately the phosphorylation potential that is linked with the hypoxic response of the peripheral chemoreceptors (27). Hypoxia that normally influences oxygen metabolism (30) is unable to exert the same influence during the metabolic blockade, and hence shows a lack of chemosensory response. The general scenario of the hypoxic effect is that a decrease in the phosphorylation potential or a related function could change influx of Ca^{2+}, which in turn leads to appropriate neurotransmitter release. The neurotransmitters then act on the respective membrane receptors, activating ionic channels, and depolarizing and generating propagated action potentials. How cellular Ca^{2+} signals O_2 chemoreception is not clear, however, because voltage-sensitive calcium-channel blockers actually stimulate chemosensory discharge (5). A reduction of external Ca^{2+} initially stimulated carotid chemosensory discharge (see Ref. 7), whereas hypoxic response has been reported to be dependent on normal concentration of Ca^{2+} in the external medium (see Ref. 7 for review). Also, hypoxia has been reported to decrease K^+ conductance without affecting Ca^{2+} conductance of isolated glomus cells of the carotid body (24). Thus, the literature on the questions of Ca^{2+} in O_2 chemoreception is rather uncertain.

The mechanism of hypercapnic excitation of chemoreceptors is obviously different from that of hypoxic stimulation (25), although arterial hypoxia normally augments the response of single chemoreceptor afferents to hypercapnia and decreases the threshold of CO_2 stimulus in a cooperative fashion (see Ref. 8 for review). Although the hypoxic stimulation of carotid chemoreceptors was nearly eliminated by chronic hyperoxia and by oligomycin (20, 27, 29), the augmentation of hypercapnic stimulation is reminiscent of the cooperative hypoxic effect. Thus, the common effect of chronic hyperoxia and oligomycin is to create a stable cellular hypoxialike effect that augments the effect of hypercapnia. The site and mechanism of these effects are unknown, but the phenomenon clearly indicates that the responses to the two stimuli are interactive at the cellular level.

Hypotheses

The effects of chronic hyperoxia on carotid chemoreceptors seem to be explained by the mitochondrial metabolic effects. Crucial tests involving metabolic and metabolite measurements, however, have yet to be accomplished. Measurement of ATP level alone of the entire carotid body without paying attention to the cellular redox state may yield misleading results.

The results so far have not ruled out the chromophore hypothesis of chemoreception that states that a membrane protein, ion channel, or otherwise, reversibly binds with O_2 in the physiological Po_2 range that initiates chemoreception. It is possible that this protein is chemically altered by oxygen-related free radicals during sustained chronic hyperoxia and that the chromophore loses its normal properties and hence oxygen sensing.

Recent studies have shown that glomus cells are excitable (6, 24), and that hypoxia decreases outward K^+ current during glomus cell excitation. It has been proposed that oxygen directly binds with K^+-channel protein, implementing oxygen chemoreception (24). The details of the model have not been spelled out and tested.

Another well-known oxygen-sensing system involves erythropoietin release and production in the kidney and the liver (2, 12, also see Chapters 4 through 7). The cellular site of erythropoietin synthesis and its mechanism of release currently provide an exciting guide to the questions of cellular oxygen sensing and response. Because inhibition of oxidative phosphorylation does not stimulate erythropoietin production (see Refs. 2, 12), it has been suggested that the effect of hypoxia may not be mediated by oxidative metabolism. Blocking of oxidative phosphorylation, however, also blocks oxygen chemosensing in the carotid body (17, 26, 27, 29); therefore, blockade of oxygen chemosensing by cyanide need not stimulate erythropoietin production except for a brief initial transient period. Thus, evidence against oxidative phosphorylation playing a role in erythropoietin production may not be conclusive. Not withstanding the objection, the proposal that a hemoprotein that reversibly binds with oxygen controls erythropoietin production is attractive (12).

Di Giulio et al. (5) recently found that cobalt and nickel in low concentrations (micromoles) delivered into the carotid arterial blood (less than 1 millimolar) promptly and reversibly stimulated carotid chemosensory discharge, without diminishing the hypoxic effect. Chronic cobalt administration increased carotid body growth along with increased erythropoiesis (unpublished observations), mimicking the effect of hypoxia. Thus, the effect of cobalt fits into a general model of hypoxic effects on a chromophore protein that may initiate oxygen sensing. Originally, the chromophore hypothesis of oxygen chemoreception in the peripheral chemoreceptors was proposed by Lloyd et al. (23). Subsequently we pointed out similarities between O_2–CO_2 stimulus interaction in the carotid chemosensory discharge and the equilibrium curve of a chromophore protein with the Bohr effect in favor of the hypothesis (see Ref. 19). Lloyd et al. (23) hypothesized that CO if administered during hypoxia would bind with the chromophore protein and turn off the chemosensory discharge and respiratory chemoreflex, as CO binds with hemoprotein. They tested the hypothesis in human respiratory control and obtained supportive evidence. We also found a transient decrease in the peripheral chemoreceptor activity during CO administration (unpublished observations). The response, however, could be linked to a concomitant rise in arterial Po_2 due to O_2 displacement by CO in the blood (9). It seems that the crucial experiment testing the chromophore hypothesis with CO has not been performed and reported. The experiment needs a hemoglobin-free perfused carotid body preparation or isolated carotid body cells, perhaps glomus cell, showing that at an appropriate level, CO diminishes hypoxic effects. It is known, however, that at a very high Pco carotid chemosensory discharge shows photolabile excitation (16). This effect of CO is attributed to its reversible reaction with cytochrome oxidase.

Carbon monoxide (Pco, 70 mm Hg) has also been reported to decrease the effect of hypoxia (Po_2, 7 mm Hg) on erythropoietin production by cultured hepatic cell line (12). The observation has been used to support the chromophore hypothesis of oxygen sensing in erythropoietin production.

Carbon monoxide has also been used to test oxygen sensing by smooth muscle cells of the aorta (11). It is possible that CO binds with the heme of membrane-bound guanylate cyclase, initiating a cascade of molecular events and relaxation of the smooth muscle. A similar reaction may occur in the peripheral chemoreceptor due to hypoxia.

The metabolic inhibitors, such as oligomycin and antimycin A, avidly bind with protein. The observations made with these so-called mitochondrial inhibitors on whole carotid body need not be entirely due to their effects on energy metabolism. They could still interrupt the chromophore function by binding with the protein. They certainly show more than one effect on chemosensory discharge. For example, oligomycin in small graduated doses initially stimulates, then reversibly attenuates the oxygen effect, and finally stops the chemosensory discharge.

Thus, it is reasonable to state that the mechanisms by which chronic hyperoxia modifies carotid chemosensory responses are not known, but that natural oxygen in excess mimics the effects of unnatural inhibitors of oxidative phosphorylation. The hypothesis that the common effects are actually mediated by mechanisms other than metabolic events is testable both at the levels of the integrated whole carotid body and in single cells. Cellular studies should also include capillary endothelial cells of carotid body because they appear to be specialized (11) and show growth response during chronic hypoxia (see Ref. 7) and chronic cobalt treatment (unpublished observations).

SIGNIFICANCE

This chapter amply demonstrated that oxygen chemoreception mechanism is labile, and exposure to a greater than normal oxygen pressure could attenuate the carotid chemosensory chemoreflex responses to hypoxia. Aortic chemoreceptors, however, may continue to respond to hypoxia normally and elicit normal chemoreflex responses. This differential response of chemoreceptors at the two-organ levels yet illustrates the importance of the integrative physiological functions, although the molecular mechanisms of oxygen chemoreception may be the same in the cells of the two organs.

Whether chronic hyperoxia affects erythropoietin production and release is not known. It is unlikely to do so on the ground that the P_{O_2} in these tissues is not high because they respond to anemia and carboxyhemoglobinemia. The effect on carotid body oxygen sensing, however, appears to be specific, and provides a model for further studies in understanding the molecular mechanism of cellular oxygen sensing.

ACKNOWLEDGMENT

This chapter is based on the experimental studies in which many of my colleagues, including Dr. Eileen Mulligan, Dr. Machiko Shirahata, Dr. Takashi Nishino, and Anil Mokashi participated. The studies were supported in part by grants from the National Institute of Health (HL-19737, HL-07027, and NS-21068).

REFERENCES

1. BARNETT, S., E. MULLIGAN, L. C. WAGERLE, AND S. LAHIRI. Measurement of carotid body blood flow in cats by use of radioactive microspheres. *J. Appl. Physiol.* 65:2484–2489, 1988.

2. BAUER, C., AND A. KURTZ. Oxygen sensing in the kidney and its relation to erythropoietin production. *Ann. Rev. Physiol. 51*:845–856, 1989.

3. DALY, M. DEB., C. J. LAMBERSTSEN, AND A. SCHWEITZER. Observations on the volume of blood flow and oxygen utilization of the carotid body in the cat. *J. Physiol. (London) 125*:67–89, 1954.

4. DEGNER, F., AND H. ACKER. Mathematical analysis of tissue Po_2 distribution in the cat carotid body. *Pfluegers Arch. 407*:305–311, 1986.

5. DI GIULIO, C., W-X. HUANG, S. LAHIRI, A. MOKASHI, AND D. G. BUERK. Cobalt stimulates carotid body chemoreceptors. *J. Appl. Physiol. 68*:1844–1849, 1990.

6. DUCHEN, M. R., K. W. T. CADDEY, G. C. KIRBY, D. L. PATTERSON, J. PONTE, AND T. J. BISCOE. Biophysical studies of the cellular elements of the rabbit carotid body. *Neuroscience 26*:291–311, 1988.

7. EYZAGUIRRE, C., R. S. FITZGERALD, S. LAHIRI, AND P. ZAPATA. Arterial chemoreceptor. In: *Handbook of Physiology—Peripheral Circulation and Organ Blood Flow,* ed. J. T. Shepherd, and F. M. Abboud. Bethesda, MD: Am. Physiol. Soc., 1983, sect. 2, vol. III, pt. 2, chapt. 16, pp. 557–621.

8. FITZGERALD, R. S., AND S. LAHIRI. Reflex responses to chemoreceptor stimulation. In: *Handbook of Physiology—The Respiratory System,* ed. N. S. Cherniack and J. G. Widdicombe. Bethesda, MD: Am. Physiol. Soc., 1986, sect. 3, vol. II, pt. 1, chapt. 10, pp. 313–362.

9. FOLGERING, H., AND P. C. G. NYE. A breath of carbon monoxide raises arterial Po_2. *J. Physiol. (London) 319*:89P, 1980.

10. FREEMAN, B. A., AND J. D. CRAPO. Hyperoxia increases oxygen radical production in rat lungs and lung mitochondria. *J. Biol. Chem. 256*:10986–10992, 1981.

11. FURCHGOT, R. F., AND D. JOTHIANANDAN. Endothelium-independent relaxation of rabbit aorta by carbon monoxide. *FASEB. J. 3*:A1177, 1989.

12. GOLDBERG, M. A., S. P. DUNNING, AND H. F. BUNN. Regulation of the erythropoietin gene: evidence that oxygen sensor is a heme protein. *Science 242*:1412–1415, 1988.

13. GRISHAM, M. B., AND D. N. GRANGER. Metabolic sources of reactive oxygen metabolites during oxidant stress and ischemia with reperfusion. *Clin. Chest Med. 10*:71–81, 1989.

14. HACKENBROCK, C. R. Ultrastructural bases for metabolically linked mechanical activity in mitochondria. *J. Cell Biol. 30*:269–296, 1966.

15. HOWE, A. The vasculature of the aortic bodies in the cat. *J. Physiol. (London) 134*:311–318, 1956.

16. JOELS, N., AND E. NEIL. The action of high tensions of carbon monoxide on the carotid chemoreceptors. *Arch. Int. Pharmocodyn. Ther. 139*:528–534, 1962.

17. KRYLOV, S. S., AND S. V. ANICHKOV. The effect of metabolic inhibitors on carotid chemoreceptor. In: *Arterial Chemoreceptors,* ed. R.W. Torrance. Oxford: Blackwell, 1968, pp. 103–109.

18. LAHIRI, S. Role of arterial O_2 flow in peripheral chemoreceptor excitation. *Federation Proc. 39*:2648–2652, 1980.

19. LAHIRI, S. Chemical modification of carotid body chemoreception by sulfhydryls. *Science 212*:1065–1066, 1981.

20. LAHIRI, S., E. MULLIGAN, S. ANDRONIKOU, M. SHIRAHATA, AND A. MOKASHI. Carotid body chemosensory function in prolonged normobaric hyperoxia in the cat. *J. Appl. Physiol. 62*:1924–1931, 1987.

21. LAHIRI, S., E. MULLIGAN, T. NISHINO, AND A. MOKASHI. Aortic body chemoreceptor responses to changes in Pco_2 and Po_2 in the cat. *J. Appl. Physiol. 47*:858–866, 1979.

22. LAHIRI, S., T. NISHINO, E. MULLIGAN, AND A. MOKASHI. Relative latency of responses of chemoreceptor afferents from aortic and carotid bodies. *J. Appl. Physiol. 48*:262–269, 1980.

23. LLOYD, B. B., D. J. C. CUNNINGHAM, AND R. C. GOODE. Depression of hypoxic hyperventilation in man by sudden inspiration of carbon monoxide. In: *Arterial Chemoreceptors,* ed. R. W. Torrance. Oxford: Blackwell, 1988, pp. 145–147.

24. LÓPEZ-BARNEO, J., J. R. LÓPEZ-LÓPEZ, J. UREÑA, AND C. GONZÁLEZ. Chemotransduction in the carotid body: K^+ current modulated by Po_2 in type I chemoreceptor cells. *Science 241*:580–582, 1988.

25. MCDONALD, D. M. Peripheral chemoreceptors: structure–function relationship of the carotid body. In: *Regulation of Breathing,* ed. T. F. Hornbein. New York: Marcel Dekker, 1981, vol. 17, pt. II, chapt. 12, pp. 773–843.

26. MULLIGAN, E., AND S. LAHIRI. Dependence of carotid chemoreceptor stimulation by metabolic inhibitors on Pao_2 and $Paco_2$. *J. Appl. Physiol. 50*:884–891, 1981.

27. MULLIGAN, E., S. LAHIRI, AND B. STOREY. Carotid body O_2 chemoreception and mitochondrial oxidative phosphorylation. *J. Appl. Physiol. 51*:438–446, 1981.

28. NONIDEZ, J. F. Observations on the blood supply and the innervation of the aortic paragan-
glion of the cat. *J. Anat. (London)* 70:215–224, 1936.
29. SHIRAHATA, M., S. ANDRONIKOU, AND S. LAHIRI. Differential effects of oligomycin on carotid
chemoreceptor responses to O_2 and CO_2 in the cat. *J. Appl. Physiol.* 63:2084–2092,
1987.
30. WILSON, D. F., W. L. RUMSEY, T. J. GREEN, M. ROBIOLIO, AND J. M. VANDERKOOI. Intracellular
oxygen concentration and its role in energy metabolism. In: *Chemoreceptors and Reflexes in Breathing: Cellular and Molecular Aspects,* ed. S. Lahiri, R. E. Forster, R. O.
Davies, and A. I. Pack. New York: Oxford University Press, 1989, pp. 164–174.

10

Excitatory and Inhibitory Influences on the Ventilatory Augmentation Caused by Hypoxia

NEIL S. CHERNIACK, NANDURI PRABHAKAR,
MUSA A. HAXHIU, AND MICHAEL RUNOLD

Maintenance of an adequate supply of O_2 to tissues depends on a complex pattern of circulatory and ventilatory adjustments that are triggered by environmental perturbations, alterations in arterial O_2 levels, and changes in metabolic rate (16, 17, 66). Ventilatory responses to hypoxia are mediated by discrete neural pathways involving peripheral chemoreceptors, primary afferents, and central neurons (16, 17, 66). Hypoxia increases ventilation entirely by its effects on the peripheral chemoreceptors, mainly the carotid body (17, 18, 51, 63, 66). The characteristics of the response, however, depend on complex interactions at multiple levels of the neuraxis, including the primary afferent neurons and bulbopontine pathways through which the carotid body signals are processed and transduced to ventilation. Neurons in the nucleus of the tractus solitarius and near the ventrolateral surface of the medulla, for example, particularly in the nucleus paragigantocellularis lateralis, play a pivotal role in amplifying respiratory responses to hypercapnia and hypoxia (8, 38, 50, 62). Moreover, hypoxia can affect breathing by direct actions on the brain, including alterations in cerebral blood flow, stimulation or depression of diencephalic and cortical neurons, and possibly changes in cerebral metabolism (16–18, 54, 66).

It is likely that hypoxic responses are controlled by a complex interplay of multiple neuroactive substances. Relatively little is known about underlying neurochemical mechanisms that mediate ventilatory responses to hypoxia. An increasing number of neuroactive substances, including monoamines, peptides, and amino acids, have been implicated in the regulation of chemoreceptor afferent pathways (16, 17). Two classes of putative neurotransmitters, tachykinin peptides and catecholamines, appear to be critically involved at several levels of the neuraxis in mediating the hypoxic response (1, 2, 7, 9–11, 16, 17, 20, 21, 24, 33, 41, 48, 53, 56–58). Tachykinins, particularly substance P (SP), and neurokinin A (NKA) and catecholamines are localized to, and/or act on major cell groups in the chemoreceptor pathway, including the peripheral chemoreceptors, the primary afferent neurons, the nucleus tractus solitarius (nTS), and the nucleus paragigantocellularis (NPG) (17, 22, 23, 36, 40, 43, 57, 67). The specific roles played by these molecules, and their interactions, however, remain largely undefined.

In many physiological systems besides feedback regulation, biological processes and the maintenance of optimum levels of critical substances are controlled by both excitatory and inhibitory (push–pull) mechanisms. Stimulating drives are opposed by processes that inhibit stimulation. This allows for fine tuning of regulation and allows the physiological system to operate over a wide range without saturation of its biological elements. At the chemoreceptors, for example, SP and dopamine appear to have excitatory and inhibitory actions, respectively, and could conceivably function as elements in a push–pull regulatory system (17, 19, 47). Although a similar kind of regulation may take place at other sites, the precise interaction undoubtedly depends on the immediate biochemical environment, including the presence of multiple other transmitters, and local anatomic connections. In addition, the neurons producing the hypoxic response may exhibit a certain degree of plasticity, and the interplay between tachykinins and dopamine may vary as hypoxic stimulation is maintained (66).

MECHANISM OF PERIPHERAL CHEMORECEPTOR RESPONSES

The carotid body consists primarily of type I (glomus) cells containing norepinephrine- and dopamine-storing dense-cored vesicles, type II (sustentacular) cells, and sensory nerve terminals that are apposed mainly to type I cells (47). The complex formed between sensory terminals and glomus cells is generally believed to be the major sensing unit for hypoxia. Different subsets of type I cells have been described largely on the number and types of vesicles present (16, 17, 47). Different tachykinins (SP and NKA) have also been shown to be present in type I cells, and sometimes even in the small cell, and may provide an additional source of biochemical heterogeneity (16, 17).

Various theories of how the carotid body operates have been proposed (see Refs. 17, 36). A common element in all is that hypoxia eventually leads to the release of some excitatory neurotransmitters probably from type I cells. Acetylcholine, norepinephrine, vasoactive intestinal polypeptide (VIP), and adenosine, which are all present in the carotid body, increase nerve activity when exogenously administered (16, 17, 68). They are probably not crucial in the transduction of the hypoxic response, although they may modify its expression. For example, neither cholinergic nor beta-adrenergic antagonists consistently eliminate the carotid body response to hypoxia (39).

Recent evidence suggests that tachykinin peptides are involved in this excitatory response to hypoxia and cyanide (56, 57, 68). Antagonists to SP, for example, abolish or substantially attenuate the increase in carotid body activity produced by hypoxia. To test this idea further, we studied the effects of different doses of SP on chemoreceptor activity in artificially ventilated, anesthetized cats. Single or paucifiber preparation of the peripheral ends of the nerve to the carotid body in the cat responded to increasing doses of SP during normoxic conditions. Chemoreceptor activity significantly increased (by 4.3 ± 1.0 to 10.6 ± 1.4 impulses/second) with increasing doses of SP (from 1 to 10 µg/kg). The maximal effect occurred with 3 µg/kg of SP. Associated with the increased chemoreceptor activity, a transient decrease of about 20 mm Hg in arterial blood pressure was seen. Unlike chemosensory activity, however, this hypotensive response was not dose dependent. The effects of SP (3 μg/kg) on chemoreceptor activity were also studied at three different levels of severity of hypoxia. Substance P increased chemoreceptor activity at all levels of PaO_2 tested. The magnitude of the excitation was significantly more with the lowest PaO_2 compared with the highest PaO_2 ($P < 0.01$).

Experiments were performed on anesthetized, paralyzed, and artificially ventilated cats to evaluate the importance of SP-like peptide on the carotid body responses to combinations of hypoxia and hypercapnia (58). The effect of intracarotid infusion of an antagonist, that is, D-Pro^2-D-Trp$^{7.9}$Substance P (10 to 15 μg/kg per minute), on carotid responses was examined during (1) hyperoxic hypercapnia (7% CO_2 and 93% O_2), (2) isocapnic hypoxia (11% O_2 and N_2), and (3) hypoxic hypercapnia (11% O_2 and 7% CO_2). Anti-SP had no effect on carotid body response to hyperoxic hypercapnia but significantly attenuated the chemoreceptor excitation caused by isocapnic hypoxia, and hypoxic hypercapnia. These results indicate that the effect of SP antagonists seems to be quite specific and that endogenous SP may play an important role in carotid body responses to hypoxia but not to CO_2.

AORTIC BODY

The aortic body, like the carotid body, responds to tachykinins. We assessed aortic chemoreceptor responses to exogenous SP and, in addition, evaluated the role of endogenous SP in hypoxic stimulation by using the SP antagonist, D-Pro^2-D-Trp$^{7.9}$Substance P. Administration of SP into the aortic arch of artificially ventilated, normoxic cats in doses of 10, 50, and 100 nmol increased the chemosensory discharge of paucifiber preparations. Hypoxic excitation (PaO_2, 42 mm Hg) of chemosensory activity was significantly enhanced after infusion of SP at a rate of 1 μg/kg per minute for 3 minutes as compared with pre-SP controls (Fig. 10.1). Furthermore, intraaortic infusion of SP antagonist (15 μg/kg per minute for 10 minutes) markedly attenuated the hypoxic excitation of chemosensory discharge. Anti-SP, however, did not affect (10 μg) the chemosensory stimulation induced by nicotine, which acts directly on sensory nerve endings. These results confirm similar studies of the effects of anti-SP on the carotid body (59). They suggest that aortic chemoreceptors respond to exogenous SP in a dose-dependent manner like the carotid body, and that SP-like peptide may be important for hypoxic stimulation of both aortic and carotid chemoreceptors.

CHARACTERIZING AND LOCALIZING TACHYKININS IN THE CAROTID BODY

We examined the distribution of SP immunoreactivity (Substance P-IR) in the carotid body of the cat using immunocytochemical techniques (Fig. 10.2). Substance P-IR was present in many type I cells and in both fine and coarse nerve fibers (60). Section of the carotid sinus nerve 2 weeks before assay did not affect SP-IR in type I cells, but eliminated all of the fine nerve fibers, leaving a sparse plexus of coarse axons. Removal of the superior cervical and nodose

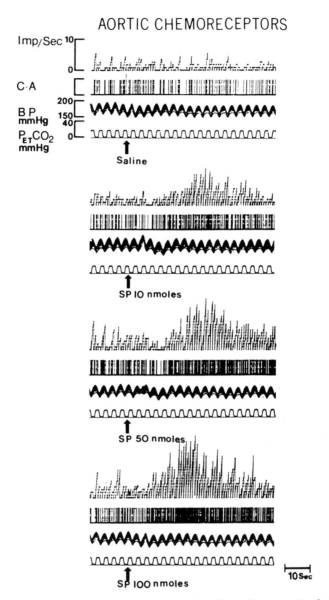

FIGURE 10.1. Example of an experiment illustrating the effect of intraaortic administration of substance P (SP) on aortic chemoreceptor discharge rate in an anesthetized, paralyzed, and mechanically ventilated cat. Imp/Sec, rate meter output; C·A, action potentials recorded from the filament of aortic nerve; BP mm Hg, systemic arterial blood pressure; $P_{ET} CO_2$ mm Hg, partial pressure of end-tidal CO_2. All three doses of SP produced a clear dose-dependent augmentation of aortic chemoreceptor activity.

ganglia had no effect on SP-IR in type I cells or in the fine terminal plexus. Neurokinin A was also found in type I cells in the carotid body and was, in some cells, co-localized with SP. When administered into the lingual artery, NKA, like SP, augmented carotid body activity.

The chemical identity of the SP-like tachykinin(s) in the carotid body has not been clearly established. The studies described indicate that both NKA and

SP are present in the carotid body, but other tachykinins may also be present. We have carried out studies to identify the nature of tachykinin(s) present in the cat carotid body and relate them to the chemoceptive function. Carotid bodies were surgically removed from artificially ventilated cats and placed in a formic acid containing dithiothreitol (DTT, 10^{-4} M) and a proteolytic enzyme inhibitor (PMSF), and constantly mixed for 24 hours at 4°C. The supernatants were collected after centrifugation. The proteins were separated by acetone precipitation. The resulting supernatant was lyophilized and subjected to analysis using a reverse phase high-performance liquid chromatography. The elutents were monitored at 225 nM for peptide absorption. The carotid body extracts showed a peptide with an elution profile corresponding to synthetic SP. In addition, distinct peaks with elution patterns identical to SP 1-4 (N-terminal fragment) and SP 5-11 (C-terminal fragment), and NKA, other tachykinins seemed to be present such as physalaemine and eledoisin. Thus, the results suggest the occurrence in the carotid body of at least four different

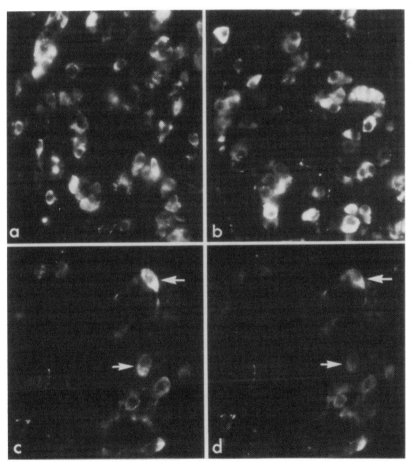

FIGURE 10.2. Immunocytochemical localization of NKA-LI and SP-LI immunoreactivities in the cat carotid body. NKA-LI (**a,c**) and SP-LI (**b,d**) are present in many glomus cells and a sparse plexus of fibers. The intensity of the glomus cell immunoreactivity is variable. The result of a double-label elution study is shown in **c** and **d**. Cells and processes that contain NKA-LI (**c**) also contain SP-LI. (**a,b**, X375; **c,d**, X525)

peptides belonging to the tachykinin family. To test the significance of these peptides for the carotid body chemoceptive function, the following experiments were performed. Afferent chemosensory activity was recorded from "single" or paucifibers of the carotid sinus nerve in 20 anesthetized, paralyzed, and artificially ventilated cats. Close carotid body injection of the peptides were made through a cannula in the lingual artery. The magnitude of the chemosensory responses to various tachykinins (Δimp/sec per nmol of peptide) were expressed as multiples of the response to the intact SP molecule (SP 1-11). The results showed that on an equimolar basis N-terminal fragment of SP 1-4 was less potent by about 50% than SP 1-11; whereas the C-terminal fragment (SP 5-11) was almost as active as SP 1-11. Physalaemine was two times more effective (1.96 $\pm$ 0.3), whereas NKA and eledoisin were both slightly less effective (0.9 $\pm$ 0.2) than SP 1-11.

SUBSTANCE P AND NEUROKININ A CONTENT OF THE CAT CAROTID BODY UNDER DIFFERENT LEVELS OF ARTERIAL P_{O_2}

Neurokinin A originates from beta-preprotachykinin, a precursor peptide that also gives rise to SP. Using radioimmunoassay techniques, we analyzed SP and NKA contents of the carotid bodies under different levels of arterial P_{O_2}.

Substance P content of the carotid bodies from the animals breathing room air averaged 57 fmol/mg, whereas NKA content averaged 85 fmol/mg. There were no significant differences in the tachykinin content of right and left carotid bodies. After 1 hour of hyperoxic ventilation, the SP and NKA content of the carotid body decreased to 51 and 29 fmol/mg. With hypoxic exposure, however, tachykinin content rose (SP to 146 fmol/mg and NKA to 98 fmol/mg). The increase in both NKA and SP levels in hypoxia versus hyperoxia was statistically significant (60).

Although tachykinins are present and can clearly influence carotid body activity, it is not clear as yet whether they are the neurotransmitters involved in the transduction of the hypoxic signal at the carotid body (25, 48). The increase in carotid body activity produced by exogenous tachykinins is delayed, therefore, it is possible that some metabolite of SP other than SP itself is released from the carotid body during hypoxia. In addition, SP antagonists have been reported to have some local anesthetic effect that may contribute to its effect in blocking the stimulation caused by hypoxia and cyanide injection. Against this contention is the finding that the increase in carotid body discharge produced by hypercapnia is not affected by anti-SP. In addition, SP antagonists do not prevent the augmented discharge caused by CO_2 or by nicotine, which acts directly on the afferent nerve ending (23, 56, 57, 68).

ENDOPEPTIDASES

It has been shown in other areas of the body that tachykinins are mainly broken down by endopeptidases (44). Biochemical analysis using high-performance liquid chromatography has revealed the presence of a neutral endopep-

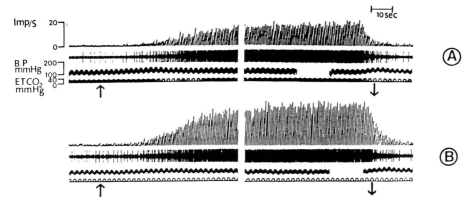

FIGURE 10.3. Example of an experiment illustrating the effect of intracarotid administration of phosphoramidon (30 μmol/ml per minute for 3 minutes) on carotid chemoreceptor responses to hypoxia in an anesthetized, paralyzed, and artificially ventilated cat. **(A)** depicts the chemoreceptor response to hypoxia after vehicle infusion and **(B)** illustrates the chemoreceptor response to low Po_2 after infusion of phosphoramidon. At arrow (↑) animal's ventilation was switched from 100% O_2 to 12% O_2 in N_2, and at the second arrow (↓) the gas mixture was switched back to 100% O_2. Imp/S, rate meter output; Action potentials from a chemoreceptor fiber; BP mm Hg, arterial blood pressure; ET CO_2 mm Hg, tidal Pco_2. Interruption in blood pressure tracing was due to collection of arterial blood sample for blood gas analysis. Note the potentiation of hypoxic response after administration of phosphoramidon.

tidaselike enzyme attached to the membrane fraction and in the cytosolic fraction of homogenized carotid body cells. Although this enzyme catabolizes SP and is inhibited by phosphoramidon, a relatively specific inhibitor of neutral endopeptidase, the identity of the endopeptidase in the carotid body is not definitely established.

Neutral endopeptidase also catabolizes enkephalins. Because enkephalins inhibit carotid body discharge, blockade of neutral endopeptidase by phosphoramidon might exaggerate the inhibitory actions on carotid body discharge of enkephalins. Intraarterial injection of phosphoramidon in cats in vivo, however, increases carotid body activity, as shown in Fig. 10.3. As might be expected, the effect of phosphoramidon on carotid body activity is enhanced if enkephalin action is prevented by the injection of naloxone (the enkephalin antagonist).

INHIBITORY MECHANISMS AT THE CAROTID BODY

Hypoxia, besides exciting the carotid body, also triggers mechanisms that may depress chemoreceptor discharge (16, 18, 47). An inhibitory efferent discharge that increases as hypoxia intensifies has been observed in nerve fibers to the carotid body (16, 17). Reciprocal synapses have been reported between type I cells and efferent nerves that would allow the response to hypoxia to be shaped and controlled by inhibitory neurotransmitters (47). Dopamine, as well as norepinephrine, are present in type I carotid body cells. Dopamine may mediate this inhibitory action by binding with D_2 receptors. Dopamine synthesis and release increases with hypoxia even if the carotid sinus nerve is severed (17). Dopamine in most species in vivo reduces carotid body activity, whereas dopamine antagonists augment carotid body responses to hypoxia (17). The carotid body responses to exogenous dopamine, however, are not entirely consistent and may depend on the amount of dopamine administered (16, 17). In some species dopamine can excite the carotid body, particularly if it is given in large doses. It should be noted, however, that other inhibitory substances may participate in carotid body regulation. For example, enkephalins have been reported to decrease, and naloxone (the opiate antagonist) to enhance carotid body responses to hypoxia (16, 17).

POSSIBLE ACTIONS OF DOPAMINE AND TACHYKININS
IN THE PETROSAL GANGLION

The petrosal ganglion contains the cell bodies of the primary afferent neurons, which link the carotid body chemoreceptors to brainstem respiratory neurons, and thereby exert critical modulatory influences on the hypoxic response. Despite widespread interest in chemoreceptor afferent transmission, relatively little is known about the expression and regulation of neurotransmitters in these cells. Specific neurochemical markers expressed by carotid body afferent neurons in the petrosal ganglion of the rat have been identified (31, 33). In particular, carotid body afferents are distinguished from all other sensory ganglion neurons by expression of catecholaminergic phenotypic traits, including functional tyrosine hydroxylase, the rate-limiting catecholamine biosynthetic enzyme, and formaldehyde-induced catecholamine fluorescence. More specifically, these cells appear to synthesize dopamine (31). These findings suggest that dopamine plays a specific role in respiratory regulation as a neurotransmitter of chemoreceptor sensory neurons. Moreover, the fact that carotid body afferents express catecholaminergic traits suggests that these cells may be the loci at which catecholamines perturb normal respiratory controls. Katz et al. (32, 34) have found that depolarizing stimuli, including SP, markedly increase the activity in the petrosal ganglion in vitro. These data suggest that tachykinin peptides, which are present in glomus cells, may normally regulate dopamine metabolism in carotid body afferents. Moreover, they also raise the possibility that prolonged carotid body stimulation may lead to long-term increases in the activity in carotid body afferents, perhaps by enzyme induction. These changes may, in turn, alter ventilatory adjustments to hypoxia, and could provide a molecular basis for long-term adaptation of chemoreceptor responses.

In addition to dopamine, some carotid body afferents contain peptides, such as SP (10, 20, 21, 25, 29, 30, 41). The precise relationship between peptidergic expression and carotid body innervation, and between peptidergic and catecholamine expression in petrosal sensory neurons, however, is unknown. It may be that catecholamine and peptidergic primary afferent neurons project to different locations in the medulla or subserve different physiological functions.

INHIBITORY AND EXCITATORY EFFECTS AT THE NUCLEUS
TRACTUS SOLITARIUS

Carotid body afferents are known to project to the nucleus tractus solitarius
(nTS), another critical locus at which tachykinins and dopamine may modulate
respiratory responses to hypoxia (3, 13–16, 28). The nTS is a heterogeneous
complex composed of multiple subnuclei that are distinguished by cytoarchitecture, afferent and efferent connections, and cytochemistry (for reviews see
Refs. 35, 39, 61, 64). Afferent fibers that innervate different peripheral targets,
for example, project to different subnuclei (27). Anatomic and physiological
techniques have been used to map chemoreceptor afferent projections to the
nTS of several species (3, 12–14, 26, 52, 55). In cats, carotid sinus nerve afferents, including chemoreceptor and baroreceptor fibers, are predominantly localized (1) dorsal and dorsolateral to the tractus solitarius, corresponding
roughly to the region of the lateral subnucleus of Loewy and Burton; (2) dor-
somedial to the tractus solitarius in the medial subnucleus; and (3) in the commissural subnuclei (3, 13, 14, 52, 55). Although still controversial, projections
to the ventrolateral subnucleus (3, 13, 14, 52, 55) and to the region of the nucleus ambiguus (13) have also been identified. Electrophysiologic studies indicate that chemoreceptor afferents alone may have a somewhat restricted distribution within the carotid sinus nerve terminal field, occupying sites medial
to baroreceptor fibers (14).

The nTS regions that receive chemoreceptor inputs are densely innervated
by SP (9, 24) and catecholamine-containing nerve terminals (1, 11, 28), which
may be derived from both peripheral afferents and intrinsic neurons. Peripheral deafferentation, for example, markedly depletes SP from the commissural
and intermediate zones of nTS (20, 21), and afferent depolarization releases
SP from a slice preparation of the nTS in vitro (22). Moreover, specific SP antagonists block the hypoxic stimulation of breathing but not the respiratory
stimulation caused by CO_2 when injected close to the nTS into the fourth ventricle of the rabbit pup, and SP injected into the nTS increases breathing even
when the pups were decerebrated (67). In rats, however, opposite effects have
been observed (7). Because some primary afferents contain SP (20, 21, 29, 41),
the peptide may regulate hypoxic responses by acting on second order neurons
after release from presynaptic sensory terminals (20–22). In addition, however,
brain neurons that project to nTS, interneurons within nTS, and circulating
SP may also participate in the peptidergic regulation of brainstem respiratory
control.

In vivo release of SP was measured in the nTS in adult cats using a microdialysis technique. A tungsten microelectrode was stereotactically implanted into the nTS for localization of respiration-related neuronal activity.
Thereafter, a microdialysis probe was stereotactically implanted in the same
position. The position of the probe was also histologically confirmed after the
experiment. Substance P in perfusates was measured with radioimmunoassay
using a specific C-terminal directed antiserum to SP.

After 90 minutes of control period, a hypoxic gas mixture (9% O_2 in N_2)
was administered. Hypoxia was given in periods of 5 minutes three times with
5 minutes of room air in between, and samples collected during these 30-min-

ute hypoxic periods as before. Phrenic nerve activity was monitored as an index of central inspiratory activity.

The results demonstrate that SP-LI was significantly increased with hypoxia increasing to 0.44 fmol from 0.24 fmol. These data strongly support the conjecture that SP is a central mediator of chemoreception of hypoxia.

The catecholamine mechanisms that regulate chemoreceptor pathways within the nTS are unknown. Catecholamines are present in many regions of the nTS. Catecholamines, released either from afferent terminals (30) or intrinsic neurons (2, 28), may modify respiratory responses to hypoxia, as has been suggested for vasomotor responses (4).

EFFECTS OF SUPERFICIAL VENTROLATERAL MEDULLARY REGIONS ON THE RESPONSE TO HYPOXIA

Superficial groups of neurons that can profoundly affect breathing and blood pressure are located near the ventral medullary surface (VMS) in the nucleus paragigantocellularis (NPG) (5, 8, 38, 45, 46, 50, 62, 65). It has been shown that microinjection of lidocaine or gamma aminobutyric acid (GABA) in this area can produce apnea, and that local cooling depresses the ventilatory responses to both hypercapnia and hypoxia (5, 8, 38). Neurons containing catecholamines and SP are also present in the same area (40). Although it seems clear that catecholamine-containing neurons near the VMS can modify vasomotor activity, it is not known whether the same neurons also affect respiration (8, 50). Interventions in this area that affect blood pressure do affect respiration, but the two responses can be separated (5, 8, 45, 46, 49, 65). It may be that respiratory neurons in the nTS communicate with spinal respiratory neurons by units in the NPG. The activity of NPG neurons can be affected by stimulation of a number of different sources, including the carotid body (51).

Studies in our laboratory indicate that application of SP or microinjection of other related tachykinins (NKA, for example) to the ventral medullary surface on the intermediate area of Schlaefke also augment ventilation even under hyperoxic situations in cats and dogs. But investigations of the effect on hypoxic responses of SP or its antagonists have not been reported.

Substance P immunoreactivity has been shown in both a rostral and caudal group of neurons in the ventrolateral medulla. The rostral group lies ventral to the facial nucleus less than 0.5 mm deep from the surface and extends 3 to 4.5 mm lateral to the midline (37). These cells seem to form a lateral extension of the NPG. The caudal group lies ventrolateral to the inferior olivary nucleus. The cells are found adjacent to the pial membrane and extend about 0.6 mm deep from the surface and extend 3.8 mm lateral to the midline.

In addition, Moracic et al. (42), using a polyclonal antibody and by staining for glial acidic protein, have been able to show the presence of neutral endopeptidase in glial cells near the VMS (Fig. 10.4), often in close proximity to tachykinin-containing fibers.

In dogs, topical application of neutral endopeptidase inhibitors, such as phosphoramidon and bestatin, to the ventral surface of the medulla potentiates both hypoxic and hypercapnic respiratory response by about 200%. Phos-

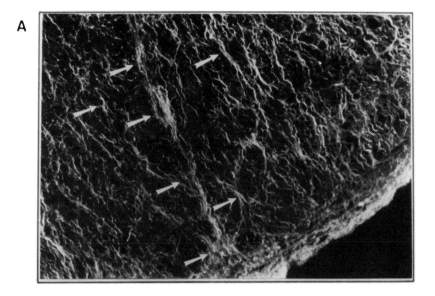

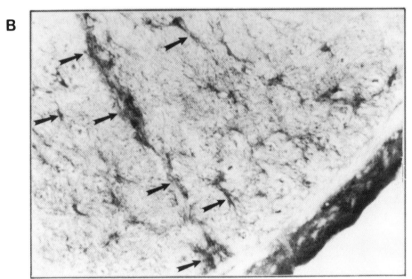

FIGURE 10.4. Immunohistochemical reactions for the co-localization of specific glial marker glial fibrillary acidic protein (GFAP) and NEP in the same section. **(A)** GFAP-like immunoreactivity. Indirect fluorescence method. **(B)** NEP-like immunoreactivity. ABC method. *Arrows* indicate the glial processes stained with both the GFAP and the NEP antibodies. (bar, 5 μM)

phoramidon injections in the carotid body, however, had no effect on chemoreceptor responses to hypercapnia.

SUMMARY

The possibility of chains of neurons containing specific chemicals (like tachykinins or catecholamines) that operate in a regulatory network by amplifying and suppressing the hypoxic actions on breathing at multiple sites is an intriguing possibility, but much work remains to be done. The complex responses to hypoxia certainly suggest the presence of equally complex control mechanisms. For example, the peripheral chemoreceptors are responsible for the ventilatory augmentation caused by hypoxia but may also have inhibitory effects. Hypoxia of the central nervous system is believed to cause respiratory depression and it is currently conjectured that central nervous system hypoxic depression is produced by the release of neuroinhibitory agents from central nervous system tissues (54). Recent studies by Schramm and Grunstein (63) and Bureau et al. (6), however, suggest that carotid body stimulations may, in fact, exaggerate hypoxic depression. Bureau et al. (6) have shown that hypoxic depression from peak levels of excitation is found in greater abundance in chemodenervated animals. Thus, the regulatory system proposed may not only shape the acute respiratory responses to hypoxia but may also be involved in producing more long-term effect of hypoxia on ventilation such as hypoxic depression and even altitude acclimatization.

REFERENCES

1. ARMSTRONG, D. M., V. M. PICKEL, T. H. JOH, D. J. REIS, AND R. J. MILLER. Immunocytochemical localization of catecholamine synthesizing enzymes and neuropeptides in area prostrema and medial nucleus tractus solitarius of rat brain. *J. Comp. Neurol.* *196*:505–517, 1981.
2. ARMSTRONG, D. M., C. A. ROSS, V. M. PICKEL, T. H. JOH, AND D. J. REIS. Distribution of dopamine-, noradrenaline-, and adrenaline-containing cell bodies in the rat medulla oblongata: demonstrated by the immunocytochemical localization of catecholamine biosynthetic enzymes. *J. Comp. Neurol.* *212*:173–187, 1982.
3. BERGER, A. J. Distribution of carotid sinus nerve afferent fibers to solitary tract nuclei of the cat using transganglionic transport of horseradish peroxidase. *Neurosci. Lett.* *14*:153–158, 1979.
4. BOLME, P., K. FUXE, T. HOKFELT, AND M. GOLDSTEIN. Studies on the role of dopamine in cardiovascular and respiratory control: central vs. peripheral mechanisms. *Adv. Biochem. Psychopharmacol.* *16*:281–290, 1977.
5. BUDZINSKA, K., C. VON EULER, F. F. KAO, T. PANTALEO, AND Y. YAMAMOTO. Effects of graded cold block in rostral areas of medulla. *Acta Physiol. Scand.* *124*:329–340, 1985.
6. BUREAU, M. A., J. LAMARCHE, P. FOULON, AND P. DALLE. The ventilatory response to hypoxia in the newborn lamb after carotid body denervation. *Respir. Physiol.* *60*:109–119, 1985.
7. CARTER, D. A., AND S. L. LIGHTMAN. Cardio-respiratory actions of substance P, TRH and 5-HT in the nucleus tractus solitarius of rats: evidence for functional interactions of neuropeptides and amine neurotransmitters. *Neuropeptides* *6*:425–436, 1985.
8. CHERNIACK, N. S., C. VON EULER, I. HOMMA, AND F. F. KAO. Graded changes in central chemoreceptor input by local temperature changes on the ventral surface of the medulla. *J. Physiol. (London)* *287*:191–211, 1979.
9. CUELLO, A. C., AND I. KANAZAWA. The distribution of substance P immunoreactive fibers in the rat central nervous system. *J. Comp. Neurol.* *178*:129–156, 1978.
10. CUELLO, A. C., AND D. S. McQUEEN. Substance P: a carotid body peptide. *Neurosci. Lett.* *17*:215–219, 1980.
11. DAHLSTROM, A., AND K. FUXE. Evidence for the existence of monamine neurons in the central nervous system. II. Experimentally induced changes in the amine levels of bulbospinal neuron systems. *Acta Physiol. Scand.* *247*:1–36, 1965.
12. DAVIES, R. O., AND M. W. EDWARDS, JR. Distribution of carotid body chemoreceptor afferents in the medulla of the cat. *Brain Res.* *64*:451–454, 1973.
13. DAVIES, R. O., AND M. KALIA. Carotid sinus nerve projections to the brain stem in the cat. *Brain Res. Bull.* *6*:531–541, 1981.
14. DONOGHUE, S., R. B. FELDER, D. JORDAN, AND K. M. SPYER. The central projections of carotid baroreceptors and chemoreceptors in the cat: a neurophysiological study. *J. Physiol. (London)* *347*:397–409, 1984.
15. EULER, C. VON. Brain stem mechanisms for generation and control of breathing pattern. In: *Handbook of Physiology,* Section 3, Vol. II, ed. N. S. Cherniack and J. G. Widdicombe. Bethesda, MD: American Physiological Society, 1986, pp. 1–68.

16. EYZAGUIRRE, C., AND P. ZAPATA. Perspectives in carotid body research. *J. Appl. Physiol.* 57:931–957, 1984.
17. FIDONE, S. J., AND C. GONZALEZ. Initiation and control of chemoreceptor activity in the carotid body. In: *Handbook of Physiology,* Section 3, Vol. II, ed. N. S. Cherniack and J. G. Widdicombe. Bethesda, MD: American Physiological Society, 1986, pp. 247–312.
18. FITZGERALD, R. S., AND S. LAHIRI. Reflex responses to chemoreceptor stimulation. In: *Handbook of Physiology,* Section 3, Vol. II, ed. N. S. Cherniack and J. G. Widdicombe. Bethesda, MD: American Physiological Society, 1986, pp. 313–362.
19. FOLGERING, H., J. PONTE, AND T. SADIG. Adrenergic mechanisms and chemoreception in the carotid body of the cat and rabbit. *J. Physiol. (London) 325*:1–21, 1982.
20. GILLIS, R. A., C. J. HELKE, B. L. HAMILTON, W. P. NORMAN, AND D. M. JACOBOWITZ. Evidence that substance P is a neurotransmitter of baro- and chemoreceptor afferents in nucleus tractus solitarius. *Brain Res. 181*:476–481, 1980.
21. HELKE, C. J., T. L. O'DONOGHUE, AND D. M. JACOBOWITZ. Substance P as a baro- and chemoreceptor afferent neurotransmitter: immunocytochemical and neurochemical evidence in the rat. *Peptides 1*:109, 1980.
22. HELKE, C. J., D. M. JACOBOWITZ, AND N. B. THOA. Capsaicin and potassium evoked substance P release from the nucleus tractus solitarius and spinal trigeminal nucleus in vitro. *Life Sci. 29*:1779–1785, 1981.
23. HELKE, C. J., J. J. NEIL, V. J. MASSARI, AND A. D. LOEWY. Substance P neurons project from the ventral medulla to the intermediolateral cell column and ventral horn in the rat. *Brain Res. 243*:147–152, 1982.
24. HOKFELT, T., J. KELLERTH, A. LJUNGDAHL, G. NILSSON, A. NYGARDS, AND B. PERNOW. Immunohistochemical localization of substance P in the central and peripheral nervous systems. In: *Neuroregulators and Psychiatric Disorders,* ed. E. Usdin, D. A. Hamburg, and J. D. Barchos. New York: Oxford University Press, 1977, pp. 299–311.
25. JACOBOWITZ, D. M., AND C. J. HELKE. Localization of substance P immunoreactive nerves in the carotid body. *Brain Res. Bull. 5*:195–197, 1980.
26. JORDAN, D. AND K. M. SPYER. Studies on the termination of sinus nerve afferents. *Pflugers Arch. 369*:65–73, 1977.
27. KALIA, M., AND M. MESULAM. Brainstem projections of the sensory and motor components of the vagus complex in the cat. II. Laryngeal, tracheobronchial, pulmonary, cardiac and GI branches. *J. Comp. Neurol. 193*:467–508, 1980.
28. KALIA, M., K. FUXE, AND M. GOLDSTEIN. Rat medulla oblongata. II. Dopaminergic, nonadrenergic (A1 and A2) and adrenergic neurons, nerve fibers, and presumptive terminal processes. *J. Comp. Neurol. 233*:308–332, 1985.
29. KATZ, D. M., AND H. J. KARTEN. Substance P in the vagal sensory ganglia: localization in cell bodies and pericellular arborizations. *J. Comp. Neurol. 193*:549–564, 1980.
30. KATZ, D. M., K. A. MARKEY, J. E. ADLER, AND I. B. BLACK. Target regulation of adult sensory neurotransmitter plasticity. *Soc. Neurosci. (Abstr) 9*:305, 1983.
31. KATZ, D. M., K. A. MARKEY, M. GOLDSTEIN, AND I. B. BLACK. Expression of catecholaminergic characteristics by primary sensory neurons in the normal adult rat in vivo. *Proc. Natl. Acad. Sci.* (USA) *80*:3526–3530, 1983.
32. KATZ, D. M., J. E. ADLER, AND I. B. BLACK. Peptide regulation of catecholaminergic transmitter metabolism in adult primary sensory neurons in vitro. *Soc. Neurosci. (Abstr) 11*:668, 1985.
33. KATZ, D. M., AND I. B. BLACK. Expression and regulation of catecholaminergic traits in primary sensory neurons: relationship to target innervation in vivo. *J. Neurosci. 6*:983–989, 1986.
34. KATZ, D. M., J. E. ADLER, AND I. B. BLACK. Expression and regulation of tyrosine hydroxylase in adult sensory neurons in culture: effects of elevated potassium and nerve growth factor. *Brain Res. 385*:68–73, 1986.
35. KING, G. W. Topology of ascending brainstem projections to nucleus parabrachialis of the cat. *J. Comp. Neurol. 191*: 615–638, 1980.
36. LANDIS, S. G., N. R. PRABHAKAR, J. MITRA, AND N. S. CHERNIACK. Localization of substance P and CGRP immunoreactivity in the cat carotid body. *Fed. Proc. 46*:824, 1987.
37. LIEBSTEIN, A. G., R. DERMIETZEL, I. M. WILLENBERG, AND J. DAUSCHERT. Mapping of different neuropeptides in the lower brainstem of the rat: with special reference to the ventral surface. *J. Auton. Nerv. Syst. 14*:299–313, 1985.
38. LOESHCKE, H. H. Central chemosensitivity and the reaction theory. *J. Physiol. (London) 332*:1–24, 1982.
39. LOEWY, A. D., AND H. BURTON. Nuclei of the solitary tract: efferent projections to the lower brain stem and spinal cord of the cat. *J. Comp. Neurol. 181*:421–450, 1978.
40. LOEWY, A. D., J. H. WALLACH, AND S. MCKELLAR. Efferent connections of the ventral medulla oblongata in the rat. *Brain Res. 3*: 63–80, 1981.

41. LUNDBERG, J. M., T. HOKFELT, H. FAHRENKRUG, G. NILSSON, AND L. TERENIUS. Peptides in the cat carotid body (glomus caroticum): VIP-, enkephalin-, and substance P-like immunoreactivity. *Acta Physiol. Scand.* 107:279–281, 1979.

42. MORACIC, V., G. K. KUMAR, E. C. DEAL, N. S. CHERNIACK, AND M. A. HAXHIU. Neutral endopeptidase (NEP) is present in the ventrolateral medulla (VLM). *Fed. Proc. (Abst)* 1027:A403, 1989.

43. MALEY, B., AND R. ELDE. Immunohistochemical localization of putative neurotransmitters within the feline nucleus tractus solitarii. *Neuroscience* 7:2469–2490, 1982.

44. MATSAS, R., A. J. KENNY, AND A. J. TURNER. The metabolism of neuropeptides: the hydrolysis of peptides including enkephalins, tachykinins and their analogues by endopeptidase 24.11. *Biochem. J.* 223:443–440, 1984.

45. MCALLEN, R. M., J. J. NEIL, AND A. D. LOEWY. Effects of kainic acid applied to the ventral surface of the medulla oblongata on vasomotor tone, the baroreceptor reflex and hypothalamic autonomic response. *Brain Res.* 238:65–76, 1982.

46. MCALLEN, R. M. Location of neurons with cardiovascular and respiratory function at the ventral surface of the cat's medulla. *Neuroscience* 18:43–49, 1986.

47. MCDONALD, D. M., AND R. A. MITCHELL. The innervation of the glomus cells, ganglion cells and blood vessels in the rat carotid body: a quantitative ultrastructural analysis. *J. Neurocytol.* 4:177–230, 1975.

48. MCQUEEN, D. S. Effects of substance P on carotid chemoreceptor activity in the cat. *J. Physiol. (London)* 302:31–47, 1980.

49. MILLHORN, D. E. Neural respiratory and circulatory interaction during chemoreceptor stimulation and cooling of ventral medulla in cat. *J. Physiol. (London)* 370:217–231, 1986.

50. MILLHORN, D. E., AND F. ELDRIDGE. Role of ventrolateral medulla in regulation of respiratory and cardiovascular system. *J. Appl. Physiol.* 61:1249–1263, 1986.

51. MITRA, J., N. R. PRABHAKAR, T. PANTALEO, M. RUNOLD, E. VAN LUNTEREN, C. VON EULER, AND N. S. CHERNIACK. Do structures in the region of nucleus paragigantocellularis (nPG) integrate and mediate ventilatory drive inputs? *Soc. Neurosci. (Abstr)* 12:304, 1986.

52. MIURA, M., AND D. J. REIS. Termination and secondary projections of carotid sinus nerve in the cat brain stem. *Am. J. Physiol.* 217:142–153, 1969.

53. MULLIGAN, E., S. LAHIRI, A. MOKASHI, S. MATSUMOTO, AND K. H. MCGREGOR. Adrenergic mechanisms in oxygen chemoreception in the cat aortic body. *Respir. Physiol.* 63: 375–382, 1986.

54. NEUBAUER, J. A., T. V. SANTIAGO, M. A. POSNER, AND N. H. EDELMAN. Ventral medullary pH and ventilatory responses to hyperperfusion and hypoxia. *J. Appl. Physiol.* 58:1659–1668, 1985.

55. PANNETON, W. M., AND A. D. LOEWY. Projections of the carotid sinus nerve to the nucleus of the solitary tract in the cat. *Brain Res.* 191:239–244, 1980.

56. PRABHAKAR, N. R., M. RUNOLD, Y. YAMAMOTO, H. LAGERCRANTZ, AND C. VON EULER. Effect of substance P antagonist on the hypoxia-induced and carotid chemoreceptor activity. *Acta Physiol. Scand.* 121:301–303, 1984.

57. PRABHAKAR, N. R., J. MITRA, E. M. ADAMS, AND N. S. CHERNIACK. Role of substance P in the hypercapnic excitation of carotid chemoreceptors. *Fed. Proc.* 45:160, 1986.

58. PRABHAKAR, N. R., J. MITRA, AND N. S. CHERNIACK. Role of substance P in hypercapnic excitation of carotid chemoreceptors. *J. Appl. Physiol.* 63:2418–2425, 1987.

59. PRABHAKAR, N. R., J. MITRA, H. LAGERCRANTZ, C. VON EULER, AND N. S. CHERNIACK. Substance P and hypoxic excitation of the carotid body. In: *Substance P and Neurokinins,* ed. J. L. Henry, R. Couture, A. C. Cuello, G. Pelletier, R. Quirion, and D. Regoli. New York: Springer-Verlag, 1988, pp. 263–265.

60. PRABHAKAR, N. R., S. C. LANDIS, G. K. KUMAR, D. MILLIKIN-KILPATRICK, N.S. CHERNIACK, AND S. E. LEEMAN. Substance P and neurokinin A in the cat carotid body: localization, exogeneous effects and changes in content in response to arterial P_{O_2}. *Brain Res.* 481:205–214, 1989.

61. RICARDO, J. A., AND E. T. KOH. Anatomical evidence of direct projections from the nucleus of the solitary tract to the hypothalamus, amygdala, and other forebrain structures in the rat. *Brain Res.* 153:1–26, 1978.

62. SCHLAEFKE, M. E. Central chemosensitivity: a respiratory drive. *Rev. Physiol. Biochem. Pharmacol.* 90:171–244, 1981.

63. SCHRAMM, C. M., AND M. GRUNSTEIN. Respiratory influence of peripheral chemoreceptor stimulation in maturing rabbits. *J. Appl. Physiol.* 63:1671–1680, 1987.

64. TABER, E. The cytoarchitecture of the brain stem of the cat. I. Brain stem nuclei of the cat. *J. Comp. Neurol.* 116:27–70, 1961.

65. VAN LUNTEREN, E., J. MITRA, N. R. PRABHAKAR, M. A. HAXHIU, AND N. S. CHERNIACK. Ventral

medullary surface inputs to cervical sympathetic respiratory oscillations. *Am. J. Physiol. 252* (Reg. Integ. Comp. Physiol. 21): R1032–1038, 1987.

66. WEIL, J. V. Ventilatory control at high altitude. In: *Handbook of Physiology,* Section 3, Vol. II, ed. N. S. Cherniack and J. G. Widdicombe. Bethesda, MD: American Physiological Society, 1986, pp. 703–727.

67. YAMAMOTO, Y., AND H. LAGERCRANTZ. Some effects of substance P on central respiratory control in rabbit pups. *Acta Physiol. Scand. 124*:449–455, 1985.

68. YAMAMOTO, Y., AND H. LAGERCRANTZ. Substance P: a putative mediator of the hypoxic drive. In: *Neurobiology of the Control of Breathing,* ed. C. von Euler and H. Lagercrantz. New York: Raven, 1986, pp. 97–100.

11

Control of Ventilation in Chronic Hypoxia
Role of Peripheral Chemoreceptors

JOHN V. WEIL

When confronted by ambient hypoxia, mammalian species are known to man-ifest a number of responses, some with potential adaptive value. These include increases in ventilation and cardiac output, a rise in circulating red blood cell concentration, and changes in the architecture of the peripheral tissue includ-ing increased density of capillaries and mitochondria. Some of these, such as the rise in ventilation and cardiac output, may be rapidly activated but are energy costly, whereas others, such as the development of polycythemia and changes in tissue architecture, are slower to evolve but may be more efficient, and, as we shall see, may be the modes of choice for species with the most successful adaptation to very high altitude. For individuals unaccustomed by prior extensive exposure to hypoxia, however, ventilation seems to be among the earliest and most important adaptive responses. In this discussion, I briefly review evidence that bears on the potential functional significance of the ventilatory response in adaptation to hypoxia and indicate that this re-sponse is altered by hypoxia itself in ways that may have important influences on ventilation and on the extent and quality of functional adaptation to high altitude (38).

VARIABILITY OF VENTILATION IN HYPOXIA

Increased ventilation evoked by hypoxia is widespread among mammalian species. This response develops rapidly, within a few seconds to a minute, is proportional to and triggered by a fall in arterial oxygen tension, and is me-diated almost entirely by peripheral chemoreceptors, largely the carotid body. The extent of this response, however, may be quite variable. Under conditions of identical ambient or arterial oxygen tension, there may be broad differences in the observed increases in ventilation. These differences may be observed either among individuals or may occur within an individual as a function of the duration of hypoxic exposure and indicate that there must be differences in the controlling stimulus–response relationship—the hypoxic ventilatory re-sponse (34). Two fundamental kinds of variation appear to be involved, that which precedes hypoxic exposure, and that which develops during, and may be attributable to hypoxia.

It is now well known that there is considerable variation in the strength of the ventilatory response to hypoxia among low altitude populations (15). In part, such variation seems attributable to familial (11, 17, 20, 24, 27, 30), genetic (6, 21), hormonal (41), and gender (40) effects. Whatever its cause, several studies suggest that the preexistent strength of the hypoxic ventilatory response may be an important determinant of ventilation and of the quality of hypoxic adaptation. As an example, individuals having a vigorous hypoxic ventilatory response measured at low altitude develop higher ventilation and maintain better oxygenation during exercise at high altitude (32). Furthermore, individuals with demonstrated capacity to climb to very high altitudes, as a class, have a greater ventilatory responsiveness to hypoxia than individuals without such an ability (23, 31). In contrast, a relatively low ventilatory response to hypoxia before altitude ascent seems to be associated with the development of syndromes of maladaptation to high altitude—acute mountain sickness (13) and high altitude pulmonary edema (18, 22). Thus, on balance, antecedent variation in hypoxic ventilatory response correlates with, and may be a determinant of, subsequent exercise capacity and symptoms that follow ascent to high altitude. As will be pointed out, however, the hypoxic ventilatory response that existed before ascent is probably modified in important ways, both negatively and positively by the hypoxia itself.

HYPOXIA AS A VENTILATORY DEPRESSANT

It has been known for some time that in addition to its well-known stimulatory effects on ventilation, hypoxia is also under certain circumstances capable of depressing ventilation or partially negating its stimulatory effects. This depressant effect on ventilation has been most clearly documented in very severe hypoxia (Pa_{O_2}, 18 to 20 mm Hg) (5, 25) and in the newborn (14). Whether moderate hypoxia of a sort commonly encountered at high altitude can also depress ventilation or offset the stimulatory effect of hypoxia has been investigated more recently. Among the early observations pointing to such an effect was the finding that ventilation, measured in humans during subacute high altitude exposure, was substantially less than that observed when hypoxia of similar severity and at comparable Pa_{CO_2} was induced in the laboratory. This suggested a smaller ventilatory response to persistent than to brief hypoxia (7) (see Fig. 11.1). Subsequent studies revealed a biphasic temporal sequence for the hypoxic response such that after the abrupt induction of hypoxia, ventilation rises promptly to a peak response within a few minutes and subsequently falls from this maximum value to a new plateau that is commonly 20 to 30% below the peak value (39). In contrast to newborns, in which ventilation falls to normoxic levels, adults show a ventilation during sustained hypoxia that consistently remains above normoxic values (14). In the newborn, this decrease or roll-off from peak values is associated with decreased metabolic rate (26), whereas in adults we have been unable to detect changes in oxygen consumption or CO_2 production during the transition from peak to lower plateau values of ventilation.

Subsequent studies have further emphasized the potential role of this hypoxic ventilatory roll-off as a determinant of the initial ventilatory response to

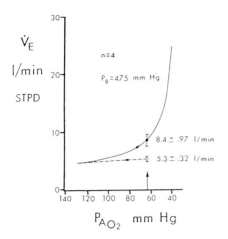

FIGURE 11.1. Ventilatory response to acute iso-capnic hypoxia measured in the laboratory (*solid line* and *filled circle*) is compared with ventilation during simulated high altitude exposure with CO_2 replacement to prevent the development of hypocapnia (*open circle*). The results indicate that during hypobaric exposure in which hypoxia is sustained, ventilation is substantially reduced below that for brief exposure to hypoxia of the same extent, and suggest that hypoxic ventilatory stimulation may be diminished during prolonged exposure. Figure reproduced from Ref. 7.

high altitude by demonstrating that on the first day after ascent, ventilation falls well below values measured during acute laboratory exposures to hypoxia under isocapnic conditions (16). This ventilatory shortfall at altitude is probably due in part to hypocapnia because when the P_{CO_2} is allowed to fall during acute laboratory hypoxia, ventilation is reduced somewhat but only to about half the extent observed at high altitude. Similarly, when the acute, isocapnic hypoxic exposure was prolonged for a few minutes, ventilation stabilized at plateau values below those seen during briefer exposure, but again not to the extent seen at altitude. When the two effects, hypocapnia and sustained exposure, were combined, measurements in the laboratory closely approached those at high altitude (Fig. 11.2). This suggested that ventilation at high altitude was substantially less than that during very brief hypoxic exposure, and that the difference may be in large part attributable to the additive effects of hypocapnia and the roll-off effect of persistent hypoxia.

To further explore the mechanism of the ventilatory roll-off in hypoxia, studies were undertaken to determine the functional locus of this phenomenon. There were several possibilities. The effect might depend on changes within the peripheral chemoreceptor reflecting either failure or rapid adaptation of the carotid body. Alternatively, it could represent a change in central nervous system integration with attenuated conversion of chemoreceptor input

FIGURE 11.2. Ventilation plotted in relation to arterial oxygen saturation for 12 subjects to show the acute ventilatory response to progressive isocapnic hypoxia (*solid line*) in comparison with values measured in those same individuals several hours after ascent to the summit of Pikes Peak (4300 m). The results indicate that for the same degree of hypoxia, ventilation is considerably lower during the altitude exposure than in acute hypoxic exposure. (**A**) During acute exposure, a decrease in ventilatory response is seen when the P_{CO_2} is allowed to fall (poikilocapnic conditions). (**B**) When isocapnia is maintained but the exposure is sustained for 30 minutes, a reduction is also seen. (**C**) When the two effects are combined as responses to sustained poikilocapnic hypoxia, substantial reductions of ventilation are found with values that closely resemble those measured on the first day of altitude exposure. The results suggest that ventilation at high altitude may reflect stimulation by hypoxia and attenuation by the combined effects of hypocapnia and time-dependent ventilatory depression. Figure reproduced from Ref. 16.

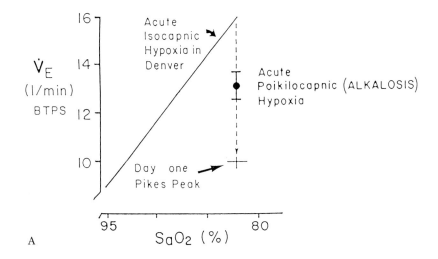

A

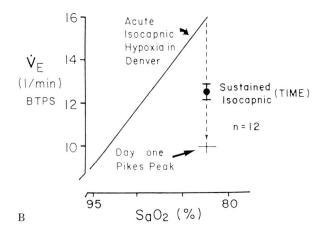

B

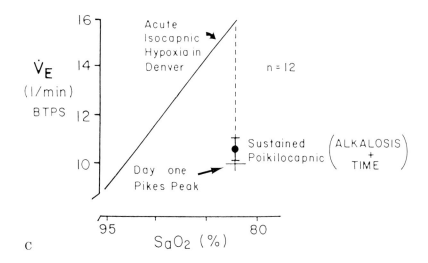

C

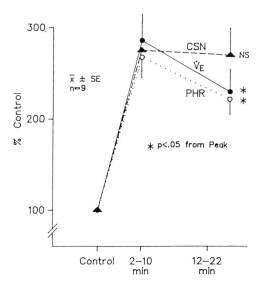

FIGURE 11.3. Responses of ventilation, phrenic, and carotid sinus neurograms to brief and more sustained hypoxia in anesthetized cats. The results demonstrate that after a rise to an early peak, there is a significant decline in both ventilation and phrenic nerve activity, but no significant decrement in carotid sinus nerve activity. The data suggest that the ventilatory roll-off during sustained hypoxia is not explained by a diminution in carotid body activity, but reflects the operation of central depressant mechanisms. Figure reproduced from Ref. 35.

into ventilatory output. Finally, it could reflect a failure of response of the peripheral respiratory apparatus to respiratory neural activation. Accordingly, studies were undertaken in cats that demonstrated that during wakefulness and anesthesia, there is a ventilatory roll-off with magnitude and time course similar to those observed in humans (35). Simultaneous recording of ventilation, carotid sinus nerve activity, and phrenic nerve activity during anesthesia revealed a parallel decline in ventilation and phrenic neural activity, but no change in carotid sinus nerve traffic. This suggested that the locus of the ventilatory roll-off lays somewhere between the carotid sinus and the phrenic nerves, that is, within the central nervous system (CNS) and that neither changes in carotid body sensitivity nor in the peripheral respiratory apparatus response to respiratory neural activation were involved (Fig. 11.3). Thus, it appears that attenuated central transduction of carotid sinus nerve input into ventilatory output is an important contributor to the hypoxic ventilatory roll-off. Although the mechanisms for this effect remain unknown, several possibilities exist. First, hypoxia could stimulate a time-dependent release of a depressant neuromodulator. Endogenous opiates would be good candidates, but are probably not involved because the hypoxic roll-off is unmodified by administration of naloxone (19). On the other hand, adenosine might be implicated as the roll-off is significantly attenuated by aminophylline, which blocks effects of adenosine; however, unexpected differences in breathing pattern confound the interpretation of the findings (10). The role of other inhibitors, such as dopamine or gamma-aminobutyric acid, in relation to the hypoxic roll-off remain largely unexplored. Alternatively, it could be that the decline in ventilation is related to an hypoxia-induced increase in cerebral blood flow with consequent accelerated removal of carbon dioxide and relative hypocapnic alkalosis in and around the central chemoreceptor as has been suggested to explain the hypoventilation of rapid eye movement sleep (29). The failure, however, of added hypercapnia to prevent the preservation of the hypoxic roll-off makes this less likely (9). Finally, it is possible that the roll-off reflects a true depression of CNS function by hypoxia. Further studies are necessary to elucidate the mechanism of this phenomenon (see Chapter 22).

PROGRESSIVE INCREASE IN VENTILATION DURING SUBACUTE HYPOXIA—
VENTILATORY ACCLIMATIZATION

Within a few hours, exposure to continued hypoxia leads to a slow, steady rise in ventilation, which progresses over several days. This ventilatory acclimatization to hypoxia has been exhaustively studied and in addition to increased ventilation, is manifested as a decrease in $Paco_2$ and in the bicarbonate concentration of arterial blood and cerebrospinal fluid (8, 37). The ventilatory response to carbon dioxide shows a steepened slope and a shift to the left, that is, to lower $Paco_2$ values. Numerous theories have been proposed to explain this phenomenon and include a progressive, general, or selective resolution of alkalosis in the cerebrospinal fluid or brain interstitium. Alternatively, it has been proposed that there may be a general increase in ventilatory responsiveness reflecting CNS sensitization to a variety of respiratory stimuli. Finally, it has been suggested that the increased ventilation of acclimatization might reflect an enhanced expression of ventilatory drive produced by improved lung mechanics. Although some evidence has been produced in support of each of these ideas, none has stood the test of repeated reexamination and the mechanism of this phenomenon remains unresolved.

Until relatively recently, little attention had been given to the possibility that acclimatization might reflect a progressive enhancement of the ventilatory sensitivity to hypoxia. This notion is suggested by one of the more obvious features of the phenomenon. During acclimatization, there seems to be a progressive increase of the response, ventilation, whereas the presumed stimulus, hypoxia, remains unchanged or decreased (Fig. 11.4). This idea is consistent with earlier findings that acclimatization is largely prevented by denervation or resection of the carotid body (1), that the magnitude and rapidity of acclimatization is correlated across species with the strength of the ventilatory re-

FIGURE 11.4. Ventilation in relation to arterial oxygenation during five days after ascent to the summit of Pikes Peak (4300 m) in 12 healthy subjects in comparison with the ventilatory response to acute isocapnic hypoxia measured in ventilation before ascent (*solid line*). The data indicate a progressive increase in ventilation during high altitude exposure despite a declining hypoxic stimulus measured as increasing arterial oxygenation. This suggests that ventilatory acclimatization to hypoxia might be associated with progressive enhancement of the ventilatory stimulus potential of hypoxia. Figure reproduced from Ref. 6.

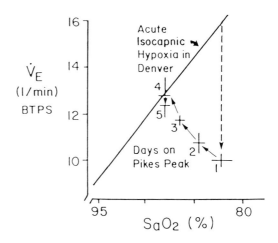

sponse to hypoxia (3), and that acclimatization is associated with augmented responsiveness to other putative stimuli to the carotid body such as very brief hypercapnia and doxapram (12). In contrast to the numerous studies of hypercapnic ventilatory response, there have been few direct sequential measurements of the hypoxic ventilatory response during acclimatization. At least two studies, however, have encompassed measurements of ventilatory response to progressive isocapnic hypoxia before and at various times during acclimatization to high altitude and both show progressive increases in the magnitude of this response (7, 39) (Fig. 11.5). This increase is especially remarkable considering that it occurs in a setting of hypocapnic alkalosis, which in acute studies profoundly attenuates the hypoxic ventilatory response. Thus, it would appear that in subacute hypoxia, there is a progressive increase in the ventilatory sensitivity to hypoxia that could be an important contributor to the progressive rise in ventilation seen during acclimatization. These studies, however, provide no clear clues as to whether this change is mediated by alterations in carotid body sensitivity, CNS translation of chemoreceptor activity into ventilation, or might even be due to changes in respiratory mechanics or muscle function.

Several recent studies suggest that changes within the carotid body may be responsible for the enhanced hypoxic ventilatory sensitivity in acclimatization. First, reports from the Madison, Wisconsin group indicate that a progressive rise in ventilation during sustained hypoxia, which closely resembles acclimatization, is induced when hypoxia is confined to the carotid body by isolated closed-loop perfusion of the carotid bifurcation in goats (2, 4). This suggests that a progressive rise in ventilation during sustained hypoxia is triggered by an action of hypoxia on the carotid body, but does not indicate whether the enhancement of sensitivity to that stimulus occurs peripherally or centrally. Subsequent studies done by the Denver group showed that in cats, 48 hours of exposure to simulated altitude produced a fall in Pa_{CO_2} and an increase in hypoxic ventilatory sensitivity that was paralleled by an increase in

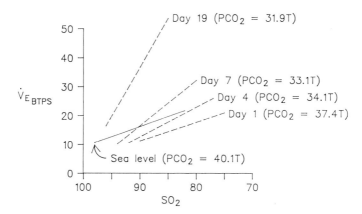

FIGURE 11.5. Ventilatory responses to acute isocapnic hypoxia in six subjects measured at low altitude (*solid line*) and at various times after ascent to the summit of Pikes Peak (4300 m). The results show substantial and progressive steepening of the slope of the response despite a progressive decline in the basal P_{CO_2} at which the responses were measured (values shown in parenthesis). The results suggest that ventilatory acclimatization to high altitude is associated with an increase in the hypoxic ventilatory response. Figure reproduced from Ref. 39.

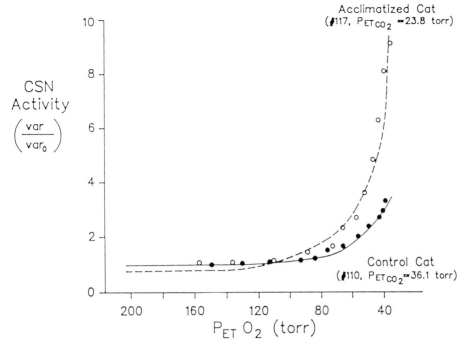

FIGURE 11.6. Carotid sinus nerve responses to progressive isocapnic hypoxia in a control cat (*solid circles* and *solid line*) compared with the response measured in another cat after 48 hours of exposure to simulated altitude, P_b = 440 mm Hg (*broken lines* and *open circles*). After altitude exposure, there is an augmentation of the carotid sinus nerve response to hypoxia despite the lower basal P_{CO_2} at which these measurements were made. The results suggest that the hypoxic sensitivity of the carotid body is enhanced during the acclimatization phase of high altitude exposure. Figure reproduced from Ref. 36.

hypoxic response of the carotid body (36) (Fig. 11.6). This augmented carotid body response persisted after section of the sinus nerve, above the point of recording, to eliminate the potential influence of efferent sinus nerve activity on the function of the carotid body. Direct comparison of carotid sinus nerve activity with simultaneous measures of ventilation produce a linear relationship describing the central translation of peripheral chemoreceptor activity into ventilation and indicate that central translation is unchanged during acclimatization. Similarly, recent studies in the goat using continuous carotid sinus nerve recordings over several hours of hypoxia show a progressive rise in nerve activity indicating progressive enhancement of hypoxic sensitivity of the carotid body (28). These findings suggest that the increase in ventilatory sensitivity to hypoxia during subacute hypoxia may reflect enhanced carotid body sensitivity.

POSTHYPOXIC RESIDUAL HYPERVENTILATION

Although this information suggests an association and perhaps a dependency of ventilatory acclimatization on enhanced carotid body sensitivity, the question arises as to how to account for the commonly observed persistence of acclimatization-induced hyperventilation after abrupt relief of hypoxia with oxygen administration when hypoxic sensitivity should have no influence on ventilation (residual hyperventilation). The answer is unclear but it may be that different factors are involved in the induction and maintenance of increased ventilation in acclimatization. In particular, hyperventilation, especially when associated with hypocapnic alkalosis, seems to possess a self-perpetuating quality that is well described but poorly understood (33) and this was recently illustrated by the work of the Madison group with isolated carotid body hypoxia. These studies showed that in animals in which systemic hypocapnic alkalosis developed as a consequence of hyperventilation induced by the action of local hypoxia on the carotid body, residual ventilation was manifested by the failure of ventilation to return to baseline levels after the discontinuation of hypoxia. In experiments in which systemic hypocapnic alkalosis was prevented by CO_2 administration, however, ventilation reverted promptly to baseline values after discontinuance of hypoxia suggesting that hypocapnic alkalosis may play a role in the development of residual hyperventilation in acclimatization (2).

SUMMARY

Thus, there is considerable variation in strength of the hypoxic ventilatory response, which may contribute to variability in the extent of adaptation to sustained hypoxia. High hypoxic ventilatory sensitivity may be associated with better function and fewer symptoms of maladaptation. Furthermore, important variation in the strength of the hypoxic response may reflect the operation of both antecedent factors that determine the basal hypoxic ventilatory response preceding hypoxic exposure, and the influence of hypoxia itself that alters the hypoxic ventilatory response. These latter effects are comprised of hypoxic ventilatory depression that can develop even in moderate hypoxia after a few minutes, and based on studies in experimental animals, may largely involve a decrease in the CNS translation of peripheral chemoreceptor activity into ventilation. On the other hand, more sustained hypoxic exposure leads to a progressive augmentation of ventilation (ventilatory acclimatization) associated with, and perhaps due to, progressive augmentation in ventilatory sensitivity to hypoxia that may predominantly reflect enhanced hypoxic sensitivity of the carotid body. Future studies might be profitably directed toward better delineation of the mechanism of the central depressant actions of intermediate duration hypoxia and the peripheral chemoreceptor sensitizing effects of more sustained hypoxic exposure.

REFERENCES

1. BISGARD, G. E., AND J. H. K. VOGEL. Hypoventilation and pulmonary hypertension in calves after carotid body excision. *J. Appl. Physiol.* 31:431–437, 1971.
2. BISGARD, G. E., M. A. BUSCH, AND H. V. FORSTER. Ventilatory acclimatization to hypoxia is not dependent on cerebral hypocapnic alkalosis. *J. Appl. Physiol.* 60:1011–1015, 1986.
3. BOUVEROT, P. Rate of ventilatory acclimatization to altitude and strength of the O_2-chemoreflex drive. In: *Les Colloques de l'Institut National de la Santé et de la Recherche Médicale.* ed. B. Duron. Paris: INSERM, 1976, vol. 59, pp. 213–219.

4. Busch, M. A., G. E. Bisgard, and H. V. Forster. Ventilatory acclimatization to hypoxia is not dependent on arterial hypoxemia. *J. Appl. Physiol. 58*:1874–1880, 1985.
5. Cherniack, N. S., N. H. Edelman, and S. Lahiri. Hypoxia and hypercapnia as respiratory stimulants and depressants. *Respir. Physiol. 11*:113–126, 1970.
6. Collins, D. D., C. H. Scoggin, C. W. Zwillich, and J. V. Weil. Hereditary aspects of decreased hypoxic response. *J. Clin. Invest. 21*:105–110, 1978.
7. Cruz, J. C., J. T. Reeves, R. F. Grover, J. T. Maher, R. E. McCullough, A. Cymerman, and J. C. Denniston. Ventilatory acclimatization to high altitude is prevented by CO_2 breathing. *Respiration 39*:121–130, 1980.
8. Dempsey, J. A., and H. V. Forster. Mediation of ventilatory adaptations. *Physiol. Rev. 62*:262–346, 1982.
9. Easton, P. A., and N. R. Anthonisen. Carbon dioxide effects on the ventilatory response to sustained hypoxia. *J. Appl. Physiol. 64*:1451–1456, 1988.
10. Easton, P. A., and N. R. Anthonisen. Ventilatory response to sustained hypoxia after pretreatment with aminophylline. *J. Appl. Physiol. 64*:1445–1450, 1988.
11. Fleetham, J. A., M. E. Arnup, and N. R. Anthonisen. Familial aspects of ventilatory control in patients with chronic obstructive pulmonary disease. *Am. Rev. Respir. Dis. 129*:3–7, 1984.
12. Forster, H. V., J. A. Dempsey, E. Vidruk, and G. DoPico. Evidence of altered regulation of ventilation during exposure to hypoxia. *Respir. Physiol. 20*:379–392, 1974.
13. Hackett, P. H., J. T. Reeves, R. F. Grover, and J. V. Weil. Ventilation in human populations native to high altitude. In: *High Altitude and Man*, ed. J. West and S. Lahiri. Bethesda, MD: American Physiological Society, pp. 179–191, 1984.
14. Haddad, G. G., and R. B. Mellins. Hypoxia and respiratory control in early life. *Ann. Rev. Physiol. 46*:629–643, 1984.
15. Hirshman C. A., R. E. McCullough, and J. V. Weil. Normal values for hypoxic and hypercapnic drives in man. *J. Appl. Physiol. 38*:463–471, 1975.
16. Huang, S. Y., J. K. Alexander, R. F. Grover, J. T. Maher, R. E. McCullough, R. G. McCullough, L. G. Moore, J. B. Sampson, J. V. Weil, and J. T. Reeves. Hypocapnia and sustained hypoxia blunt ventilation on arrival at high altitude. *J. Appl. Physiol. 56*:602–607, 1984.
17. Hudgel, D. W., and J. V. Weil. Asthma associated with decreased hypoxic ventilatory drive: A family study. *Ann. Int. Med. 80*:622–625, 1974.
18. Kafer, E. R., and J. Leigh. Recurrent respiratory failure associated with the absence of ventilatory response to hypercapnia and hypoxemia. *Am. Rev. Respir. Dis. 106*:100–108, 1972.
19. Kagawa, S., M. J. Stafford, T. B. Waggener, and J. W. Severinghaus. No effect of naloxone on hypoxia-induced ventilatory depression in adults. *J. Appl. Physiol. 52*:1031–1034, 1982.
20. Kawakami, Y., I. Tadashi, A. Shida, and T. Yoshikawa. Control of breathing in young twins. *J. Appl. Physiol. 52*:537–542, 1982.
21. Kawakami, Y., T. Yoshikawa, A. Shida, and Y. Asanuma. Control of breathing in young twins. *J. Appl. Physiol. 52*:537–542, 1982.
22. Lakshminarayan, S., and D. J. Pierson. Recurrent high altitude pulmonary edema with blunted chemosensitivity. *Am. Rev. Respir. Dis. 111*:869–872, 1975.
23. Masuyama, S., H. Kimura, T. Sugita, T. Kuriyama, K. Tatsumi, F. Kunitomo, S. Okita, H. Tojima, Y. Yuguchi, S. Watanabe, and Y. Honda. Control of ventilation in extreme-altitude climbers. *J. Appl. Physiol. 61*:500–506, 1986.
24. Moore, G. C., C. W. Zwillich, J. O. Battaglia, E. K. Cotton, and J. V. Weil. Respiratory failure associated with familial depression of ventilatory response to hypoxia and hypercapnia. *N. Engl. J. Med. 295*:861–865, 1976.
25. Morrill, C. G., J. R. Meyer, and J. V. Weil. Hypoxic ventilatory depression in dogs. *J. Physiol. (London) 38*:143–146, 1975.
26. Mortola, J. P., and R. Rezzonico. Metabolic and ventilatory rates in newborn kittens during acute hypoxia. *Respir. Physiol. 73*:55–68, 1988.
27. Mountain, R., C. W. Zwillich, and J. V. Weil. Hypoventilation in obstructive lung disease: The role of familial factors. *N. Engl. J. Med. 298*:521–525, 1978.
28. Nielsen, A. M., G. E. Bisgard, and E. H. Vidruk. Carotid chemoreceptor activity during acute and sustained hypoxia in goats. *J. Appl. Physiol. 65*:1796–1802, 1988.
29. Parisi, R. A., J. A. Neubauer, M. M. Frank, T. V. Santiago, and N. H. Edelman. Linkage between brain blood flow and respiratory drive during rapid-eye-movement sleep. *J. Appl. Physiol. 64*:1457–1465, 1988.
30. Saunders, N. A., S. R. Leeder, and A. R. Rebuck. Ventilatory response to carbon dioxide in young athletes. A family study. *Am. Rev. Respir. Dis. 113*:497–502, 1976.

31. SCHOENE, R. B. Control of ventilation in climbers to extreme altitude. *J. Appl. Physiol.* 53:836–891, 1982.
32. SCHOENE, R. B., S. LAHIRI, P. H. HACKET, R. M. PETERS, JR., J. S. MILLEDGE, C. J. PIZZO, F. H. SARNQUIST, S. J. BOYER, D. J. GRABER, K. H. MARET, AND J. B. WEST. Relationship of hypoxic ventilatory response to exercise performance on Mount Everest. *J. Appl. Physiol.* 56:1478–1483, 1984.
33. SMITH, A. C., M. K. SPALDING, AND W. E. WATSON. CO_2 as stimulus to spontaneous ventilation after prolonged artificial ventilation. *J. Physiol. (London)* 160:32–39, 1962.
34. SORENSON, S. C., AND J. C. CRUZ. Ventilatory response to a single breath of CO_2 and O_2 in normal man at sea level and high altitude. *J. Appl. Physiol.* 27:186–190, 1969.
35. VIZEK, M., C. K. PICKETT, AND J. V. WEIL. Biphasic ventilatory responses of adult cats to sustained hypoxia has central origin. *J. Appl. Physiol.* 63:1658–1664, 1987.
36. VIZEK, M., C. K. PICKETT, AND J. V. WEIL. Increased carotid body hypoxic sensitivity during acclimatization to hypobaric hypoxia. *J. Appl. Physiol.* 63:2403–2410, 1987.
37. WEIL, J. V. Ventilatory control at high altitude. In: *Handbook of Physiology. Section 3: The Respiratory System. Vol II Control of Breathing. Part 2*, ed. N. S. Cherniack and J. G. Widdicombe. Bethesda, MD: American Physiological Society, 1986, pp. 703.
38. WEIL, J. V., AND C. W. ZWILLICH. Assessment of ventilatory response to hypoxia: methods and interpretation. *Chest* 70:124S–128S, 1976.
39. WHITE, D. P., K. GLEESON, C. K. PICKETT, A. M. RANNELS, A. CYMERMAN, AND J. V. WEIL. Altitude acclimatization: influence on periodic breathing and chemoresponsiveness during sleep. *J. Appl. Physiol.* 63:401–412, 1987.
40. WHITE, D. P., N. J. DOUGLAS, C. K. PICKETT, J. V. WEIL, AND C. W. ZWILLICH. Sexual influence on the control of breathing. *J. Appl. Physiol.* 54:874–879, 1983.
41. ZWILLICH, C. W., M. R. NATALINO, F. D. SUTTON, AND J. V. WEIL. Effects of progesterone on ventilation in normal man. *J. Lab. Clin. Med.* 92:262–269, 1978.

12

Molecular Mechanisms of Carotid Body Afferent Neuron Development

DAVID M. KATZ

Peripheral chemoreflexes undergo marked developmental changes in the perinatal period (11, 16, 21, 22, 26, 27, 45). In the fetus, for example, it is generally agreed that the carotid chemoreceptors are relatively ineffective in increasing respiration during hypoxia (11, 14, 27, 45). In neonates, on the other hand, hypoxia produces a transient hyperventilation, followed by a return to normal or below normal levels of ventilation (11, 14, 16, 21, 22, 44, 45). In adults, however, hypoxia evokes a relatively sustained increase in ventilation, primarily by acting on the carotid bodies (17). Although physiologic studies have delineated how chemoreflexes change with development, the underlying cellular and molecular mechanisms remain undefined. What, for example, triggers the emergence of peripheral chemoreflexes after birth? What regulates the transition from a transient to a sustained ventilatory response to hypoxia? Moreover, what can these developmental changes tell us about the underlying plasticity of the neural pathways that mediate peripheral chemoreflexes?

One way to approach these questions is to identify components of the chemoreflex pathway that undergo significant developmental changes during the perinatal period. Many cell groups may be involved in regulating the development of chemoresponsiveness, including the peripheral chemoreceptors themselves, primary afferent neurons, and brain and spinal cord respiratory neurons. In addition, mechanical and metabolic influences may also be important (11, 16, 21, 22, 26, 27, 45).

This chapter focuses on the biochemical maturation of one subset of respiratory-related neurons, namely, primary sensory neurons that innervate the carotid body (Fig. 12.1). These cells, located in the petrosal ganglion (PG) of the glossopharyngeal nerve, project peripherally in the carotid sinus nerve (CSN) to innervate glomus cells within the carotid body. In addition, carotid body afferents extend a central process that terminates in the brainstem nucleus tractus solitarius, thereby forming the afferent link between the carotid body chemoreceptors and the central nervous system. Activation of second-order neurons in the brainstem is believed to be mediated by the release of neuroactive substances from primary afferent terminals. Therefore, transmission of carotid body stimulation to the central nervous system is critically dependent on the maturity of neurochemical properties expressed by carotid body afferent neurons. The potential role of afferent development in postnatal chemoreflex maturation is underscored by our recent finding that these cells are

133

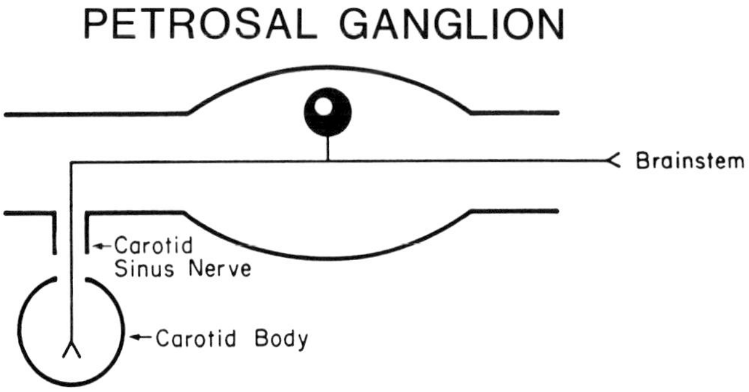

PETROSAL GANGLION

FIGURE 12.1. Schematic diagram illustrating the carotid body afferent pathway. Primary sensory neurons with cell bodies in the petrosal ganglion project peripherally, by the carotid sinus nerve, to the carotid body and centrally to the brainstem nucleus tractus solitarius.

relatively immature at birth and undergo marked biochemical development in the perinatal period (29). Before discussing these data, however, the following sections briefly review background studies on (1) chemoreflex development and (2) transmitter expression in adult carotid body afferent neurons.

CHEMOREFLEX DEVELOPMENT

Considerable experimental evidence indicates that the carotid body afferent pathway is either functional, or capable of being stimulated, in the fetus and the neonate (6, 14, 15, 40–43). The carotid chemoreceptors, however, appear to be relatively ineffective in increasing ventilatory responses during hypoxia in the fetus, possibly due to inhibition by central mechanisms (14, 15). The transition from a fetal to a neonatal response is accompanied by a marked shift in the sensitivity of the chemoreceptors to arterial Po_2 (10). Mechanisms underlying resetting of the chemoreceptors are unknown, although changes in carotid body blood flow may contribute to this shift (1). Similarly, it is unknown what mechanisms mediate the transition from transient to sustained increases in ventilation in response to hypoxia, although neurologic, mechanical, and metabolic factors may all play a role (21, 22). It is thought that in neonates a sustained hyperventilation with hypoxia is inhibited primarily by a depressive effect of low oxygen on central respiratory activity (14). Alternatively, Bureau et al. (12) suggest that the hypoxic sensitivity of neonatal peripheral chemoreceptors is blunted due to their relative immaturity, and functionally unable to sustain hyperventilation in the face of counteracting inhibitory drives. Another possibility is that the carotid chemoreceptors themselves are fully active (see Ref. 40), but transmission between carotid body afferents and the brainstem is functionally immature. This is similar to the proposal by Saetta and Mortola (44) that chemoreceptor inputs in newborns may not be sufficiently powerful to oppose the central depressive effects of hypoxia (see Ref. 33). Moreover, recent studies by Eden and Hanson (16) indicate that chemoreflex development may be modulated by the increase in inspired O_2 that occurs after birth, and suggest that environmental signals may regulate maturational changes by altering the balance between peripheral and central factors. Cellular mechanisms by which environmental factors may influence chemoreflex maturation, however, remain undefined.

TRANSMITTER PROPERTIES EXPRESSED BY CAROTID BODY AFFERENT NEURONS

The expression and regulation of transmitter properties are critical processes through which developmental events can regulate neuronal maturation (7, 39). Until recently, however, relatively little was known about the neurochemistry of carotid body afferents, hampering investigation of developmental mechanisms. Recently, immunocytochemical and biochemical studies have begun to identify neurochemical properties expressed by carotid body afferents in adult animals, thereby laying the foundation for investigations of development at the molecular level.

Visceral afferent neurons in general exhibit a wide diversity of transmitter phenotypes, similar to those found in peripheral ganglia of the somatosensory system. For example, cells in the nodose ganglion of the vagus nerve are now known to exhibit a variety of peptidergic properties, including substance P (SP; 4, 24, 31, 35), calcitonin gene-related peptide (CGRP; 13, 20, 35), vasoactive intestinal peptide (24, 35), somatostatin (24, 35), and cholycystokinin (24, 35). Substance P (4) and CGRP have also been localized to cells in the rat PG (24, Katz, D.M., unpublished observations).

In addition to these peptidergic phenotypes, some nodose and petrosal ganglion cells are distinguished by expression of monoaminergic transmitter properties not previously associated with sensory neurons. In the nodose and petrosal ganglia of adult rats, for example, a subpopulation of sensory neurons express catecholaminergic transmitter traits, including catalytically active tyrosine hydroxylase (TH), the rate-limiting enzyme in catecholamine biosynthesis, formaldehyde-induced catecholamine fluorescence (FIF), and a monoamine-oxidase-like pathway for catecholamine metabolism (32) (Fig. 12.2). These cells exhibit morphologic features typical of primary sensory neurons, such as an initial axon glomerulus and a single primary neurite that branches into a central and peripheral process (32). Tyrosine hydroxylase-containing petrosal neurons are readily distinguished from sympathetic and small intensely fluorescent (SIF) cells by cytochemical, morphometric, and pharmacologic criteria (32). For example, catecholaminergic sensory neurons are insensitive to neonatal treatment with the neurotoxin 6-hydroxydopamine, thereby distinguishing them from sympathetic neurons (32). The catecholaminergic neurons in the nodose and petrosal ganglia appear to synthesize dopamine, as they do not express immunoreactivity for dopamine-beta-hydroxylase, the enzyme that converts dopamine to norepinephrine (32).

Some visceral afferents express other monoaminergic properties, distinct from the catecholaminergic phenotype. Gaudin-Chazal and colleagues, for example, found serotoninlike immunoreactivity (18) and uptake of exogenous radiolabeled serotonin (19) in subpopulations of nodose ganglion cells in the cat. It is not yet known, however, if nodose ganglion cells that contain serotonin

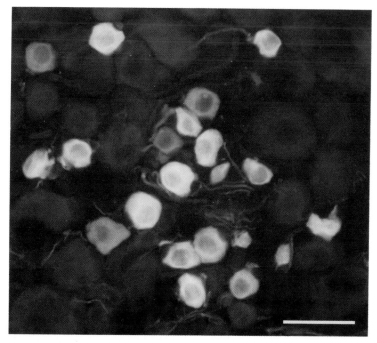

FIGURE 12.2. Fluorescence micrograph showing tyrosine hydroxylase immunoreactivity in petrosal ganglion sensory neurons from an adult rat. Section thickness is 10 μm and scale bar equals 50 μm.

actually synthesize the amine or simply take it up from exogenous stores. In addition, studies of nodose ganglion cells in culture indicate that, under experimental conditions, some visceral afferents are capable of synthesizing acetylcholine (5).

Of the many transmitter properties expressed by visceral sensory neurons, only one phenotype has been shown to be selectively associated with carotid body afferent neurons. By combining immunocytochemical staining with retrograde tracing methods, Katz and Black (30) found that expression of catecholaminergic properties by PG afferents is highly correlated with innervation of the carotid body. In these experiments, carotid body afferent neurons in the PG were labeled by retrograde transport of fluorescent tracers applied either to the carotid sinus nerve or selectively infused into the carotid body (30). Cryostat sections of the PG were then stained with a highly specific antiserum against rat TH (36) and examined for co-localization of the retrograde marker and antibody labeling. These studies demonstrated that 93% of the TH-containing cells in the PG project peripherally in the CSN and 84% innervate the carotid body (30). Tyrosine hydroxylase is, therefore, a highly selective marker for carotid body afferents in the rat PG. This contrasts, for example, with the peptide SP, which is found in sensory neurons innervating a wide variety of diverse target tissues (see Ref. 31). Potential targets of the small number of TH neurons that do not terminate in the carotid body include extracarotid glomus tissue and the carotid sinus, although such projections have not yet been demonstrated.

The fact that some carotid body afferents exhibit biochemical properties typical of dopaminergic neurons raises the possibility that dopamine is used as a neurotransmitter or neuromodulator by these cells. Recent studies, for example, raise the possibility that dopamine can be released from both the central and peripheral terminals of carotid body afferents. Thus, Yamamoto and co-workers found that stimulation of the rabbit carotid body by hypoxia, or electrical stimulation of the carotid sinus nerve, evokes dopamine release from primary afferent terminal fields in the brainstem nucleus tractus solitarius (Yamamoto, Y., Lagercrantz, H., and von Euler, C., personal communication). It remains to be established, however, whether the dopamine was released from the afferent endings themselves, or from surrounding brain structures. Similarly, Almaraz and Fidone (2) have shown that electrical stimulation of the cut peripheral end of the cat sinus nerve evokes dopamine release from the carotid body in vitro. Here, too, however, it is unknown whether the dopamine was released directly from sinus nerve terminals in the carotid body or from glomus cells activated transsynaptically after CSN stimulation. It must also be pointed out that catecholaminergic afferents have thus far only been described in the PG of rats (32), and postulated to exist in the nodose ganglion of dogs (46); similar findings in cat and rabbit have not yet been reported.

It is tempting to speculate that dopaminergic afferents could provide an anatomic substrate for the so-called efferent pathway for chemosensory inhibition in the carotid body. As described by numerous investigators, electrical stimulation of the cut peripheral end of the CSN in cats inhibits chemsosensory discharge (see Ref. 17). This pathway, which is now believed to originate in the PG (38), is thought to be mediated by dopamine release in the carotid body (34). We hypothesize that during peripheral CSN stimulation, antidromic activation of dopaminergic sensory fibers could depress chemosensitivity by causing a local release of dopamine from afferent nerve terminals. A role for afferent endings in this phenomenon was first suggested by McDonald and Mitchell (38), and is supported by the abundance of transmitter storage vesicles within afferent terminals apposed to carotid body glomus cells (37). Much further work is required, however, to elucidate the physiological role of dopaminergic afferents in chemoreception, as well as their possible involvement in "efferent" inhibition.

DEVELOPMENT OF CATECHOLAMINERGIC PROPERTIES IN CAROTID BODY
AFFERENT NEURONS

The highly selective localization of catecholaminergic properties within the rat PG provided us with sensitive markers for defining the biochemical development of carotid body afferent neurons in this species. To begin investigating the ontogeny of transmitter properties, immunocytochemical and biochemical methods were used to define the appearance and maturation of catecholaminergic traits in the rat PG (28). Immunocytochemical studies demonstrated that the TH cells found in the adult PG first become detectable around embryonic day (E) 16.5 (birth = E22.5). The number of TH cells subsequently rises to 70% of adult levels by E22.5, the day before birth, and then an additional 50% to reach adult values by postnatal day one (P1). As cell division has ceased in the PG by E14.5 (3), these increases in TH cell number most likely reflect a rise in TH levels per cell, above the threshold for immunostaining. This is further supported by the observation that the sharp increase in the number of detectable TH cells between E22.5 and P1 was accompanied by an increase in the staining intensity of individual neurons.

The marked rise in TH expression between E22.5 and P1 also suggested that a rapid induction of TH protein per cell occurs around birth. To quantify the magnitude of this induction, the relative amount of TH protein in E21.5 and P1 ganglion homogenates was compared on Western blots (28). Samples containing equal numbers of ganglia per volume were probed with a mouse monoclonal TH antibody and compared by densitometric scanning of the stained blots. These studies revealed a 4- to 10-fold increase, depending on the experiment, in the amount of immunoreactive TH protein per ganglion (Fig. 12.3). As the number of immunoreactive neurons rose by 50% during this period, these data indicate that on average, TH levels per cell rose approximately 3.5-fold between E21.5 and P1. Thus, the development of this specific catecholaminergic trait in carotid body afferents appears to be highly regulated around birth.

Although adult numbers of TH neurons are present by P1, the amount of TH protein per cell continues to increase during the first few postnatal weeks. In preliminary experiments, Western blot analysis demonstrated an approximate fourfold rise in TH levels per ganglion between P1 and 3 to 4 weeks of age (Fig. 12.3; Katz, D.M., Moracic-Piperski, V., and Siegel, R., unpublished observations). In view of the role of TH in catecholamine biosynthesis, these obervations suggested that catecholamine levels per cell also rise during the perinatal period. To address this issue, histochemical methods were used to compare catecholamine levels in P1 and adult PG neurons. Whereas P1 neurons exhibited relatively faint catecholamine fluorescence, intensely labeled sensory perikarya and fibers were detected by 1 month of age. These findings demonstrate, therefore, that catecholamine levels in PG neurons rise substantially during postnatal development. As TH levels also rise during this period, the increase in catecholamine fluorescence most likely reflects increased amine synthesis. A possible contribution, however, from decreased amine turnover cannot be ruled out at this time.

These data indicate that carotid body afferent neurons in the PG are biochemically immature at birth, raising the possibility that they are functionally immature as well. Although the role of dopamine in these cells has not yet been defined, we can speculate on the potential implications of biochemical immaturity in the perinatal period. For example, if transmitter synthesizing mechanisms are not fully developed at birth, neonatal ganglion cells may be unable to sustain effective synaptic transmission at high rates of stimulation. Much additional work on this point is required, however, including studies of evoked transmitter release from carotid body afferents in neonatal animals.

The time course of catecholaminergic development in the PG parallels, in many respects, the development of peripheral chemoreflexes. For example, the

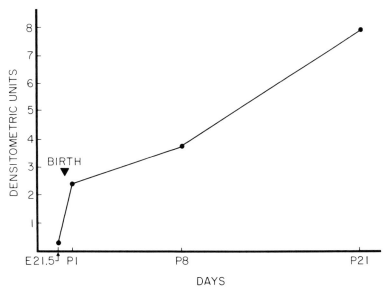

FIGURE 12.3. Comparison of TH protein levels in the petrosal ganglion at different stages of development; embryonic day (E) 21.5, postnatal day (P) 1, postnatal day 8, and postnatal day 21. Homogenates of equal numbers of ganglia of each age were run simultaneously in different lanes of an SDS–polyacrylamide gel. The separated proteins were then transferred to nitrocellose and the filter probed with a monoclonal antibody against rat tyrosine hydroxylase (Boehringer-Manheim). The density of tyrosine hydroxylase immunoreactivity in each lane, corresponding to the amount of tyrosine hydroxylase protein per homogenate, was then quantified by scanning densitometry; these values are displayed as densitometric units along the ordinate.

rapid perinatal accretion of TH coincides with the appearance of peripheral chemoreflexes on P1 in the rat (25). Moreover, TH and catecholamine levels continue to increase postnatally, at a time when peripheral drives to respiration are also increasing (25, 26). It is too early to know whether any causal relationship exists between these biochemical events and the development of peripheral chemoreflexes. For example, the development of catecholaminergic properties in carotid body afferents may be a prerequisite for mature synaptic transmission. This could explain the absence of a significant peripheral drive to respiration before birth, when TH and catecholamine levels in the PG are relatively low. Similarly, the failure of neonatal animals to sustain hyperventilation during hypoxia could result from a rapid depletion of still immature transmitter stores. Alternatively, the perinatal maturation of catecholaminergic properties in the PG could be a consequence, rather than a cause, of chemoreflex development during this period. Nonetheless, these findings illustrate the biochemical immaturity of carotid body afferents in the fetus and the newborn. This population of cells may consequently be a locus at which developmental changes influence the maturation of neural respiratory controls. Therefore, elucidating factors that regulate catecholaminergic development in the PG may reveal cellular and molecular mechanisms that underlie the development of peripheral chemoreflex controls.

MOLECULAR MECHANISMS OF CATECHOLAMINERGIC DEVELOPMENT

In most catecholaminergic populations, including sympathoadrenal cells, extracellular factors are known to play a major role in regulating transmitter development. In sympathetic neurons, for example, TH development is regulated by both anterograde and retrograde transsynaptic factors, including depolarizing stimuli and nerve growth factor, respectively (7). As shown by Black and co-workers (see Ref. 7), ganglionic blockade, or surgical deafferentation of postganglionic neurons, prevents the normal postnatal maturation of catecholaminergic properties in the sympathetic superior cervical ganglion. Conversely, exposure of neonatal sympathetic neurons to depolarizing stimuli in tissue culture increases levels of TH activity (23), suggesting that impulse activity may normally regulate catecholaminergic development in vivo (7).

At present it is unknown whether similar mechanisms regulate catecholaminergic development in primary sensory neurons. Is it possible, for example, that the postnatal accretion of TH and catecholamines in carotid body afferents is stimulated by changes in the level of afferent activity? Studies of TH regulation in adult PG neurons suggest that such mechanisms may indeed be important. For example, exposure of ganglion cells to depolarizing stimuli in tissue culture significantly increased levels of TH activity (28). These findings indicate that TH expressed by sensory neurons can be regulated by extracellular factors in vitro. Studies in progress are aimed at determining whether depolarizing influences might similarly regulate the perinatal increase in TH levels observed in the PG in vivo.

The mutability of TH activity in response to extracellular factors indicates that this enzyme may also be a site at which nerve stimulation leads to long-term changes in neuronal function (8, 47). As previously shown for sympathetic neurons, for example, even short periods of impulse activity can lead to prolonged changes in enzyme induction, which may last for days (47). Moreover, some long-term changes clearly involve altered expression of the TH gene (9). Therefore, regulation of catecholaminergic synthesizing enzymes provides a mechanism by which altered neural activity can lead to relatively stable changes in neuronal function (8, 47). It will be of great interest to determine whether stimulation of peripheral chemoreceptors might similarly alter catecholaminergic enzyme expression in carotid body afferent neurons. Such long-term changes could provide a molecular substrate for adaptive responses to chronic environmental perturbations, including hypoxia. Investigating such possibilities remains an exciting area for further research.

ACKNOWLEDGMENTS

The author gratefully acknowledges the outstanding technical assistance of Melissa Erb and the secretarial skills of Vicky Maloy. Supported by American Heart Association grant PL 653 (Ohio Affilliate) and the Dysautonomia Foundation.

REFERENCES

1. ACKER, H., D. W. LUBBERS, M. J. PURVES, AND E. D. TAN. Measurements of the partial pressure of oxygen in the carotid body of fetal sheep and newborn lambs. *J. Devel. Physiol.* 2:323–338, 1980.

2. ALMARAZ, L. AND S. FIDONE. Carotid sinus nerve C-fibers release catecholamines from the cat carotid body. *Neurosci. Letts.* 67:153–158, 1986.

3. ALTMAN, J., AND S. BAYER. Development of the cranial nerve ganglia and related nuclei in the rat. *Adv. Anat. Embryol. Cell Biol.* 74:1–90, 1982.

4. AYER-LELIEVRE, C. S., AND A. SEIGER. Development of substance P-immunoreactive neurons in cranial sensory ganglia of the rat. *Int. J. Devel. Neurosci.* 2:451–463, 1984.

5. BACCAGLINI, P. I., AND E. COOPER. Influences on the expression of acetylcholine receptors on rat nodose neurons in cell culture. *J. Physiol.* 324:429–439, 1981.

6. BISCOE, T. J., M. J. PURVES, AND S. R. SAMPSON. Types of nervous activity which may be recorded from the carotid sinus nerve in the sheep fetus. *J. Physiol.* 202:1–23, 1969.

7. BLACK, I. B. Regulation of autonomic development. *Ann. Rev. Neurosci.* 1:183–214, 1978.

8. BLACK, I. B., J. E. ADLER, C. F. DREYFUS, W. F. FRIEDMAN, E. F. LAGAMMA, AND A. H. ROACH. Biochemistry of information storage in the nervous system. *Science* 236:1263–1268, 1987.

9. BLACK, I. B., D. M. CHIKARAISHI, AND E. J. LEWIS. Transsynaptic increase in RNA coding for tyrosine hydroxylase in a rat sympathetic ganglion. *Br. Res.* 339:151–153, 1985.

10. BLANCO, C. E., G. S. DAWES, M. A. HANSON, AND H. B. MCCOOKE. The response to hypoxia of arterial chemoreceptors in fetal sheep and new-born lambs. *J. Physiol. (London)* 351:25–37, 1984.

11. BRYAN, A. C., G. BOWES, AND J. E. MALONEY. Control of breathing in the fetus and the newborn. In: *Handbook of Physiology,* Vol. II, eds. Cherniack, N. S. and Widdicombe, J. G. Bethesda, MD: American Physiological Society, 1986, pp. 621–647.

12. BUREAU M. A., J. LAMARCHE, P. FOULON, AND D. DALLE. The ventilatory response to hypoxia in the newborn lamb after carotid body denervation. *Respir. Physiol.* 60:109–119, 1985.

13. CADIEUX, A., D. R. SPRINGALL, P. K. MULDERRY, J. RODRIGO, M. A. GHATEI, G. TERENGHI, S. R. BLOOM, AND J. M. POLAK. Occurrence, distribution and ontogeny of CGRP immunoreactivity in the rat lower respiratory tract: Effect of capsaicin treatment and surgical denervations. *Neurosci.* 19:605–627, 1986.

14. DAWES, G. S. The central control of fetal breathing and skeletal movements. *J. Physiol.* 346:1–18, 1982.

15. DAWES, G. S., L. B. DUNCAN, B. V. LEWIS, C. L. MERLET, J. B. OWEN-THOMAS, AND J. T. REEVES. Cyanide stimulation of the systemic arterial chemoreceptors in foetal lambs. *J. Physiol.* 201:117–128, 1968.

16. EDEN, G. J., AND M. A. HANSON. The effect of hypoxia from birth on the biphasic respiratory response of the newborn rat to acute hypoxia. *J. Physiol.* 366:59P, 1985.

17. FIDONE, S. J., AND C. GONZALES. Initiation and control of chemoreceptor activity in the carotid body. In: *Handbook of Physiology,* Vol. II, eds. Cherniack, N. S. and Widdicombe, J. G. Bethesda, MD: American Physiological Society, 1986, pp. 247–312.

18. GAUDIN-CHAZAL, G., P. PORTALIER, M. C. BARRIT, AND J. J. PUIZILLOUT. Serotonin-like immunoreactivity in paraffin-sections of the nodose ganglia of the cat. *Neurosci. Letts.* 33:169–172, 1982.

19. GAUDIN-CHAZAL, G., L. SEGU, N. SEYFRITZ, AND J. J. PUIZILLOUT. Visualization of serotonin neurons in the nodose ganglia of the cat. An autoradiographic study. *Neuroscience* 6:1127–1137, 1981.

20. GREEN, T., AND G. J. DOCKRAY. Calcitonin gene-related peptide and substance P in afferents to the upper gastrointestinal tract in the rat. *Neurosci. Letts.* 76:151–156, 1987.

21. HADDAD, G. G., AND R. B. MELLINS. Hypoxia and respiratory control in early life. *Ann. Rev. Physiol.* 46:629–643, 1984.

22. HANSON, M. A. Maturation of the peripheral chemoreceptor and CNS components of respiratory control in perinatal life. In: *Neurobiology of the Control of Breathing,* eds. Euler, C. von and Lagercrantz, H. New York: Raven Press, 1986, pp. 59–65.

23. HEFTI, F., H. GNAHN, M. E. SCHWAB, AND H. THOENEN. Induction of tyrosine hydroxylase by nerve growth factor and by elevated K^+ concentrations in cultures of dissociated sympathetic neurons. *J. Neurosci.* 2:1554–1566, 1982.

24. HELKE, C. J., AND K .M. HILL. Immunohistochemical study of neuropeptides in vagal and glossopharyngeal afferent neurons in the rat. *Neuroscience* 26:539–551, 1988.

25. HERTZBERG, T., S. HELLSTROM, J.-M. PEQUIGNOT, AND H. LAGERCRANTZ. Carotid body catecholamines and the development of the arterial chemoreflex in newborn rats. Salt Lake City; Faredrag, August, 1988.

26. HERTZBERG, T., AND H. LAGERCRANTZ. Postnatal sensitivity of the peripheral chemoreceptors in newborn infants. *Arch. Dis. Child.* 62:1238–1241, 1987.

27. JANSEN, A. M., AND V. CHERNICK. Development of respiratory control. *Physiol. Rev.* 63:437–483, 1983.

28. KATZ, D. M. Expression and regulation of tyrosine hydroxylase in adult sensory neurons in

culture: Effects of elevated potassium and nerve growth factor. *Brain Res. 385:*68–73, 1986.

29. KATZ, D. M., AND M. J. ERB Developmental regulation of tyrosine hydroxylase expression in primary sensory neurons of the rat. *Dev. Biol. 137:*233–242, 1990.

30. KATZ, D. M., AND I. B. BLACK. Expression and regulation of catecholaminergic traits in primary sensory neurons: relationship to target innervation in vivo. *J. Neurosci.* 6:983–989, 1986.

31. KATZ, D. M., AND H. J. KARTEN. Substance P in the vagal sensory ganglia: localization in cell bodies and pericellular arborizations. *J. Comp. Neurol. 193:*549–564, 1980.

32. KATZ, D. M., K. A. MARKEY, M. GOLDSTEIN, AND I. B. BLACK. Expression of catecholaminergic characteristics by primary sensory neurons in the normal adult rat in vivo. *Proc. Natl. Acad. Sci. USA 80:*3526–3530, 1983.

33. LAHIRI, S., J. S. BRODY, E. K. MOTOYAMA, AND T. M. VELASQUES. Regulation of breathing in newborns at high altitude. *J. Appl. Physiol. 44:*673–678, 1978.

34. LAHIRI, S., N. SMATRESK, M. POKORSKI, P. BARNARD, A. MOKASHI, AND K. H. McGREGOR. Dopaminergic efferent inhibition of carotid body chemoreceptors in chronically hypoxic cats. *Am. J. Physiol., 247:*R24–R28, 1984.

35. LUNDBERG, J. M., T. HOKFELT, G. NILSSON, L. TERENIUS, J. REHFELD, R. ELDE, AND S. SAID. Peptide neurons in the vagus, splanchnic and sciatic nerves. *Acta Physiol. Scand.* 104:499–501, 1978.

36. MARKEY, K. A., S. KONDO, AND M. GOLDSTEIN. Purification and characterization of tyrosine hydroxylase from a clonal pheochromocytoma cell line. *Mol. Pharmacol. 17:*79–85, 1980.

37. McDONALD, D. M., AND R. A. MITCHELL. The innervation of glomus cells, ganglion cells and blood vessels in the rat carotid body: a quantitative ultrastructural analysis. *J. Neurocytol. 4:*177–230, 1975.

38. McDONALD, D. M., AND R. A. MITCHELL. The neural pathway involved in "efferent inhibition" of chemoreceptors in the cat carotid body. *J. Comp. Neurol. 201:*457–476, 1981.

39. PATTERSON, P. H. Environmental determination of autonomic neurotransmitter functions. *Ann. Rev. Neurosci. 1:*1–18, 1978.

40. PURVES, M. J. The effect of a single breath of oxygen on respiration in the newborn lamb. *Respir. Physiol. 1:*297–307, 1966.

41. PURVES, M. J. The effects of hypoxia in the newborn lamb before and after denervation of the carotid chemoreceptors. *J. Physiol. 185:*60–77, 1966.

42. PURVES, M. J. Respiratory and circulatory effects of breathing 100% oxygen in the newborn lamb before and after denervation of the carotid chemoreceptors. *J. Physiol. 185:*42–59, 1966.

43. RIGATTO, H., J. P. BRADY, B. CHIR, AND R. DE LA TORRE VERDUZCO. Chemoreceptor reflexes in preterm infants. *Pediatrics 55:*604–613, 1974.

44. SAETTA, M., AND J. P. MORTOLA. Interaction of hypoxic and hypercapnic stimuli on breathing patterns in the newborn rat. *J. Appl. Physiol. 62:*506–512, 1987.

45. WALKER, D. Peripheral and central chemoreceptors in the fetus and newborn. *Ann. Rev. Physiol. 46:*687–703, 1984.

46. YOSHIDA, M., Y. KONDO, N. KARASAWA, K. YAMADA, I. TAKAGI, AND I. NAGATSU. Immunohistocytochemical localization of catecholamine-synthesizing enzymes in suprarenal, superior cervical and nodose ganglia of dogs. *Acta Histochem. Cytochem. 14:*588–595, 1981.

47. ZIGMOND, R. E., AND Y. BEN-ARI. Electrical stimulation of preganglionic nerve increases tyrosine hydroxylase activity in sympathetic ganglia. *Proc. Natl. Acad. Sci. (USA)* 74:3078–3080, 1977.

13

Relationship Between Erythropoiesis and Ventilation in High Altitude Natives

ROBERT M. WINSLOW

Erythrocytosis, an increased rate of red blood cell production, is one of the main physiologic adjustments to hypoxia (18). The response is mediated by the glycoprotein hormone, erythropoietin, which is synthesized in the kidney (9). Upon exposure to hypoxia, the erythropoietin concentration increases in the blood of sojourners within about 6 hours (10). Peak concentrations are reached in about 48 hours, and significant elevations can still be measured after 9 days (1). After that, the serum erythropoietin concentration is indistinguishable from sea-level normal. It is not known whether variation in the erythropoietin response can explain the variation in hematocrit observed in sojourners to altitude, but based on a few subjects (14), there seems to be no striking correlation.

In contrast to sojourners, highland natives of Peru clearly have elevated steady-state erythropoietin concentrations (13, 15). Faura and co-workers (10) demonstrated elevated urine erythropoietin in residents of Morococha, Peru (4500 m), but these early studies failed to show a correlation between the erythropoietin production and the degree of erythrocytosis. Since the recent availability of sensitive radioimmunoassays for erythropoietin, systematic studies of the erythropoietic regulation in high-altitude natives have not been performed, and a quantitative description of the regulation of erythropoiesis in high-altitude natives has not been provided.

Of particular interest is the clinical entity, chronic mountain sickness (Monge's disease), which is the occurrence of symptomatic, excessive polycythemia in long-term residents of high altitude (23). Symptoms result from a severe expansion of the blood volume and a consequent burden on the circulatory system. The cure for the syndrome is descent to sea level or phlebotomy. Whittembury and Monge (20) suggested that chronic mountain sickness results from the normal age-dependent loss of ventilation with arterial hypoxemia. This point has been difficult to prove, however, because in large surveys, no striking relationship between ventilation, age, and erythrocytosis could be demonstrated (23).

The degree of hypoxia-induced erythrocytosis is dependent on geographical location (see Ref. 23). High hematocrits and hemoglobin concentrations traditionally have been observed in northern Peru, Bolivia, Chile, the North American Rocky Mountains, and on the Tibetan plateau. Lower, almost sea-level normal values have been observed in southern Peru and Nepal. Moreover, in some instances, the same authors have reported different values depending on the site of their studies, and significant differences seem to occur between Peruvian sites separated by only a few hundred meters in altitude (8).

Lifelong natives of high altitudes and sojourners, even with nearly equal exposure to hypoxia, may have different ventilatory drives. Hackett and co-workers (11) pointed out that hypoxia should be viewed as the product of years of exposure and altitude. The observation that chronic mountain sickness is more common in Tibetan sojourners than in high-altitude natives (12) has special significance if one believes in the hypoventilatory etiology of chronic mountain sickness.

It is often stated that chronic mountain sickness does not occur in Sherpas, whereas it is relatively common in Quechua Indians. Such differences between two populations could have many possible explanations. Some of them are not of genetic or physiologic interest, such as nutritional deficiencies or endemic diseases that cause anemia. Nutritional causes for lower hematocrits found in the Himalayas have not been identified (2, 3). Differences in the mean altitude of exposure for the two populations could also occur. If such explanations cannot be established, however, then differences in O_2 transport or the erythropoietic response to hypoxia remains. If genetic adaptation to hypoxia occurred in humans it will provide a unique opportunity to observe evolution in progress. We undertook to study comparable populations of male natives in the Andes and Himalayas to attempt to resolve some of these questions.

METHODS

Location

The Andean studies were done in Ollagüe, Chile (21.12° south, 70.29° west, 3700 m altitude, barometric pressure 493 mm Hg), located on the Andean altiplano, near the Chile–Bolivia border. The subjects were either employees of the railway or were farmers or other types of laborers.

The Himalayan studies were done in Khunde, Nepal (27.49° north, 86.43° east, 3700 m altitude, barometric pressure 481 mm Hg), located in the Khumbu region. The work pattern of the residents of Khunde is typical of Sherpas, and follows the seasons: in the premonsoon and postmonsoon season, they work as porters and guides. During the monsoon, they remain in their native villages.

Subjects

Experimental subjects in Chile were recruited from the local residents of Ollagüe and surrounding villages. We chose only nonsmoking men between 20 and 30 years of age for the complete set of studies. We did not accept subjects who had visited lower altitudes in recent months, who used tobacco or drugs, or who reported or demonstrated evidence of significant illness of any kind. Blood was also obtained from four residents of Amincha (5400 m). These subjects worked in the sulfur mine at the summit of Aucanquilcha (6300 m).

In Nepal, we used the same criteria for acceptance of subjects into the studies. This phase of the work was carried out at the beginning of the monsoon, which ensured that the maximum number of potential subjects would be in their native villages. It was virtually impossible to obtain detailed information about the altitude exposure in the months just before the studies. As the subjects worked as porters, however, they had been intermittently exposed to altitudes slightly higher than their altitude of residence.

Protocols

In most of the cases, the studies were performed over 2 days. On the first, we obtained histories and performed physical examinations. Also on the first day we obtained venous blood for routine hematologic measurements. We performed exercise and tests of ventilatory sensitivity to hypoxia in the afternoon of the first day. Samples of blood or separated plasma were frozen in liquid nitrogen to return to the United States for special measurements such as erythropoietin concentration.

General Evaluation

Native physicians took histories in the subjects' native language. They paid special attention to questions relating to symptoms of polycythemia, intolerance to altitude, recent descent to lower altitude, therapeutic phlebotomy, or respiratory symptoms. We selected for study only subjects who did not work underground. Native physicians also performed physical examinations; they had extensive experience with high-altitude medical problems.

Hematology

Methods for the hematologic measurements, erythropoietin concentrations, and blood O_2 affinity measurements have been published elsewhere (21, 24).

Ventilatory Measurements

The methods and apparatus used for gas exchange measurements were as previously described (22). In addition, an ear oximeter (Ohmeda) was used to monitor arterial saturation. Analysis of gas exchange data was carried out on-line and the data were recorded also on FM tape for later, more extensive, evaluation (22).

In the hypoxic ventilatory response tests, the subjects were judged to be in the steady state when the gas exchange ratio (R) was constant and usually not greater than 1. A valve was then turned that introduced N_2 into the inspired side of the breathing valve. This was done in such a way that the subject could not see when the valve was turned. The response to the inspired N_2 was estimated from the saturation measured by the ear oximeter and by the pattern of ventilation. If the saturation did not fall below 80% and there was no apparent increase in ventilatory rate, maximum expired flow, or tidal volume, then after reestablishing the steady state a second stimulus was provided, larger than the first.

Subjective Analysis of Gas Exchange Signals

A subjective assessment of the response to N_2 was made by visual inspection of the analog recording. The largest response was in one of the Westerners. He was given a score of 4. If no response occurred after either stimulus, a value of 0 was assigned. The values 1 to 3 were used for intermediate responses. The patterns of response allowed the subjects to be divided into two groups, responders and nonresponders. The nonresponders were those subjects who had no discernible response to either N_2 stimulus.

Statistical Methods

Normalcy of distributions was evaluated using the Wilk–Shapiro test. After analysis of variances, group means were compared using either a pooled variance *t*-test (equal variances) or unpooled *t*-test (unequal variances). Differences were accepted as significant when $P<0.05$.

RESULTS

Subjects

Table 13.1 presents some characteristics of the study populations. The Chile subjects were slightly older ($P=0.05$), shorter ($P=0.03$), and heavier ($P=0.003$). The detailed anthropometric data for these subjects were reported elsewhere (7), but it is worthy of note that the two populations could not be distinguished with regard to vital capacity or FEV_1, whereas the chest volumes in Chile were significantly larger.

TABLE 13.1. Characteristics of the Study Subjects

		Chile	Nepal	P
Age	n	29	30	
(yr)	mean	27.3	24.7	
	SD	±5.9	±3.8	0.05
Height	n	28	30	
(cm)	mean	162.2	165.0	
	SD	±4.4	±5.1	0.03
Weight	n	28	30	
(kg)	mean	60.4	54.5	
	SD	±8.8	±4.5	0.003
FVC	n	28	30	
(1,BTPS)	mean	5.111	5.248	
	SD	±.472	±.715	NS
FEV_1	n	28	30	
(% VC)	mean	86.4	82.9	
	SD	±6.0	±7.3	NS
Chest volume	n	23	30	
(1,BTPS)	mean	10.22	8.94	
	SD	±1.65	±1.47	0.004

FVC, forced vital capacity; FEV_1, forced expiratory volume in 1 second.

TABLE 13.2. Hematology (Summary)

		Chile	Nepal	P
Hct	n	24	30	
(%)	mean	52.2	48.4	
	SD	±4.6	±4.5	0.003
Hb	n	24	30	
(g/dl)	mean	18.0	16.9	
	SD	±1.8	±1.2	0.012
RBC	n	21	30	
($\times 10^6$/mm^3)	mean	6.14	5.84	
	SD	±1.29	±1.01	NS
plat	n	23	39	
($\times 10^3$/mm^3)	mean	253	265	
	SD	±85	±68	NS
WBC	n	24	39	
($\times 10^3$/mm^3)	mean	6.40	6.53	
	SD	±2.4	±2.1	NS
Epo	n	21	30	
(mu/ml)	mean	9.6	8.4	
	SD	±4.3	±7.1	NS

Hct, hematocrit; Hb, hemoglobin; RBC, red blood cell count; MCHC, mean cell hemoglobin concentration; MCV, mean cell volume; MCH, mean cell hemoglobin; Retic, reticulocytes; plat, platelet count; WBC, white blood cell count; Epo, erythropoietin.

Hematology

Table 13.2 summarizes the hematologic results. The most significant difference between the two groups is in hematocrit ($P = 0.003$), the values in Nepal being lower. Hemoglobins are also lower in Nepal ($P = 0.012$). There is no statistical difference in red blood cell counts between the two groups, suggesting that the red cells in Sherpas are smaller and contain less hemoglobin than those in Quechuas. Differences in other red blood cell parameters calculated from these primary measurements are not statistically significant.

Figure 13.1 shows the hematocrit distributions. Except for one case, the hematocrits in Nepal are distributed normally around a mean of 48.4%. The single exception was a Sherpa whose hematocrit was 63.5%. He had recently worked as a high-altitude porter and had no symptoms to suggest chronic mountain sickness. In contrast, the hematocrit values in Chile are skewed toward higher values with a mean of 52.2%. Nevertheless, the medians (50.8% in Chile, 47.7% in Nepal) are still significantly different ($P < 0.05$).

In Chile, one subject who volunteered for our studies had typical symptoms of chronic mountain sickness, although his hematocrit was only 57.5%. These symptoms included headache, confusion, and sleeplessness. On physical examination he appeared cyanotic and his conjunctivae were markedly erythremic, as is commonly seen in subjects with chronic mountain sickness. In Nepal, no subject reported symptoms of chronic mountain sickness, regardless of hematocrit. Furthermore, a physician who had worked in Khunde for 2 years had not encountered any case of chronic mountain sickness in his practice there.

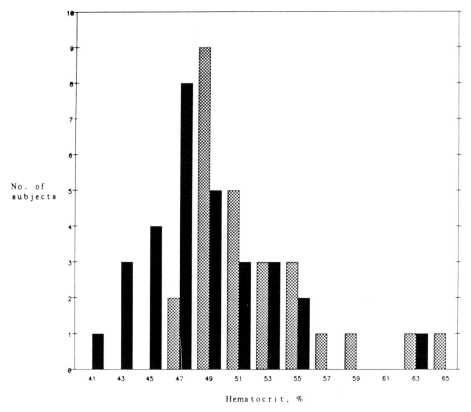

FIGURE 13.1. Hematocrit distributions in Nepal and Chile. *Filled bars,* Nepal; *crosshatched bars,* Chile.

Erythropoietin

The erthropoietin values ranged from almost undetectable, 0.6 mU/ml in Nepal, to 45 mU/ml in the subject with chronic mountain sickness in Chile. All of the values are plotted against hematocrit in Fig. 13.2. The points for two expedition members measured after arrival at altitude in Nepal and again about 2 weeks later are shown as connected points. These values show an appropriate decline in erythropoietin as red blood cell production increases. The two exceptions indicated in Fig. 13.2, are the Chilean subject with chronic mountain sickness and subjects who resided at Amincha (altitude, 5400 m) and worked at the summit of Aucanquilcha (altitude 6300 m). In these subjects, the erythropoietin concentrations are significantly elevated, suggesting that the observed hematocrit does not compensate for hypoxia.

In 13 cases, hematocrits could be matched in Chile and Nepal to within 1%. The difference in erythropoietin concentration in the two groups (Chile 10.5 ± 4.8 mU/ml, Nepal 6.1 ± 5.6 mU/ml) is still significant ($P = 0.02$) using a paired t-test.

Other Hematologic Comparisons

No differences between the osmotic fragility of red blood cells of Sherpas and Quechua Indians could be demonstrated. We have previously demonstrated that the whole blood oxygen affinity of Quechua Indians is subject to the same control mechanisms as that in lowlanders (21). The various parameters of the oxygen equilibrium curves for Sherpas and Westerners are equivalent (24). These findings confirm the earlier conclusions of Samaja et al. (16) that there are no unusual factors controlling oxygen affinity of Sherpa blood. Taken together with our similar data in Quechuas (21), these results exclude the possibility that differences in red cell O_2 transport mechanisms, such as mutant hemoglobins, or other effectors of hemoglobin function might explain hematocrit differences between Sherpas and Quechua Indians.

Hypoxic Ventilatory Response

A wide range of ventilatory response to inspired N_2 was observed. In general, the Westerners demonstrated greater responses than Sherpas, but this was not uniformly true; some Westerners had modest responses, whereas some

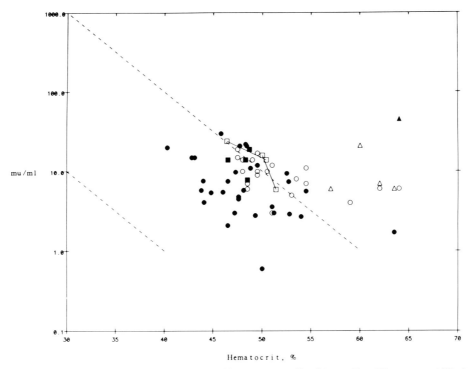

FIGURE 13.2. Erythropoietin as a function of hematocrit, all subjects. Two Westerners (*filled squares*) were studied immediately after arrival at 3700-m altitude and again 2 weeks later. They showed an appropriate suppression of erythropoietin as hematocrits rose. *Dashed lines* indicate the sea level range of normal (17). *Filled circles,* Nepal study subjects; *open circles,* Chile study subjects; *open triangles,* residents of Amincha (altitude, 6300 m); *open square,* low altitude Sherpa, Nepal.

Sherpas had brisk ones. Two Sherpas and one Westerner suppressed at low N_2. One Sherpa stimulated after minimal N_2 administration and suppressed after a more severe stimulation.

No significant correlations were found between either hematocrit or erythropoietin and baseline maximum expired flow, tidal volume, minute ventilation, end tidal O_2 or CO_2, saturation, or anthropometric parameters. Weak (but significant) correlations were found between erythropoietin and the response to N_2 (r = 0.44, $P < 0.04$).

The difference between the hematocrit values of responders and nonresponders is significant ($P < 0.02$), the hematocrits being higher in the nonresponders. Because hematocrit and erythropoietin have an inverse relationship at sea level, this difference is consistent with the higher erythropoietin values in the responders ($P < 0.002$).

The degree of arterial blood desaturation (as judged by ear oximetry) produced by the N_2 breathing appeared to be slightly greater in the responders compared with the nonresponders, but the difference was not statistically significant. Moreover, the ratio of the volume of N_2 breathed to the drop in saturation was not different. Thus, we conclude that, within the limits of the small numbers of subjects we studied, an approximately equal volume of N_2 produced about the same drop in arterial saturation in the two groups of subjects. This conclusion seems to indicate that the lower ventilatory response in the nonresponders was due to insensitivity to hypoxia, rather than to a difference in gas transport.

Exercise Tests

Breath-by-breath analysis of incremental exercise tests allowed correlation of the ventilatory response to exercise with the response to N_2, and between both ventilatory responses and the hematologic values. A wide range of initial $\dot{V}_E/\dot{V}_{CO_2}$ slopes was observed, but there was no significant correlation between the response to N_2 and the $\dot{V}_E/\dot{V}_{CO_2}$ slope for the incremental exercise tests.

The two groups, responders and nonresponders, could not be distinguished on the basis of maximum work performed in an incremental exercise test, the anaerobic threshold, the ventilatory response to exercise, or the maximum heart rate during exercise.

DISCUSSION

Geographic and cultural differences restrict the selection of strictly comparable population samples in the Andes and Himalayas. The climatic conditions in the Andean altiplano are extremely arid and constant over the year; the Himalayas are more vertical, with a marked seasonality. Therefore, although the study subjects were native to the same altitude, it is impossible to know the exact mean exposure to hypoxia. Our subjective impression was that native residents in Nepal are more likely to move vertically than those in the Andes, and their exposure to altitude may be more intermittent.

Our results generally support the previous findings of Beall (4, 5, 6) that hematocrits tend to be lower in Sherpas than in Quechua Indians in spite of the slightly lower barometric pressure in Khunde compared with Ollagüe. Beall has interpreted this difference as showing a greater degree of adaptation in Sherpas. Although a clear demonstration of the advantage of a 4% lower hematocrit value is lacking, we have argued, on the basis of hemodilution studies, that even mild polycythemia may serve no useful physiologic purpose (23). We also have the clinical impression that Sherpas suffer less from the stress of altitude than do Quechua Indians.

A clear explanation for the lower hematocrit and hemoglobin values in Nepal compared with Chile cannot be determined from our data. Simple nutritional differences might be expected to be apparent in the mean cell hemoglobin concentration, mean cell hemoglobin, or mean cell volume, in the case of iron deficiency. Our data provide only a suggestion (without statistical significance) that the red blood cells in Sherpas contain slightly less hemoglobin than those in the Quechua Indians we studied. Two possible causes for reduced red blood cell hemoglobin are iron deficiency and alpha thalassemia. We have no evidence for either, but previous surveys in the Khumbu region of Nepal (2, 3, 5) and in the Peruvian Andes (23) have failed to reveal iron deficiency.

It is possible that the red cell lifespan is slightly longer in the Andes, accounting for the higher hematocrits there. This explanation would require a slightly younger population of red cells in Sherpas, with higher 2,3-DPG concentrations, larger red cell volumes, and lower hemoglobin concentrations. We have no evidence to support this hypothesis, and the equivalent osmotic fragility and red cell indices seem to be against it (24). Careful measurements of red blood cell survival, however, would be needed to settle the issue.

If the hematopoietic response to hypoxia is different in Sherpas and Quechuas, there are several possible control points. First, the stimulus to erythropoiesis could be less (higher PaO_2) in the population with lower hematocrit (Sherpas). This could occur because of a higher alveolar PO_2 due to differences in ventilation, higher PaO_2 because of differences in pulmonary diffusion, or differences in the ventilatory response to hypoxia or exercise. Second, the production of erythropoietin in response to a given level of hypoxic stimulation could be different. Finally, the effect of erythropoietin on the stimulation of red blood cell production could be different, either because of structural alterations in erythropoietin, or in sensitivity of the erythropoietic tissue to it.

The high erythropoietin in our single case of chronic mountain sickness in Chile is particularly interesting. This case is neither like sea-level secondary polycythemia nor polycythemia vera (low erythropoietin). In our case, the red blood cell response is apparently less than that demanded and is consistent with the "vicious cycle" hypothesis: excessive red cell production diminishes O_2 supply to the kidney (23).

Our data cannot establish a "normal" erythropoietin concentration in either of these populations, but they do suggest that above a hematocrit of 55% the erythropoietin concentration is stable, around a mean of about 4 to 5 mU/ml. For most subjects, therefore, a hematocrit of between 50% and 55% seems to be normal for the altitude (3700 m). This agrees quite well with our previous observations at Cerro de Pasco (4200 m) where the median hematocrit is about 52% (23).

The data also show that many subjects in Nepal who have hematocrits below about 47% have elevated erythropoietin and, therefore, their red cell production does not compensate for hypoxia. What limits the red cell production in these subjects? Further attention should be directed at the ability of the bone marrow to produce red blood cells at high altitude, including nutritional factors necessary for hemoglobin and red blood cell production.

Weil and co-workers (19) showed lower saturation of ear lobe blood during sleep in subjects with excessive polycythemia in Leadville, Colorado. They interpreted their finding as indicating a ventilatory etiology for chronic mountain sickness. Nevertheless, a direct relationship between PaO_2 and hematocrit was not found in approximately 150 Quechua Indians residing between 4200 and 4500 m in Peru (23). This negative result could have been caused by sampling errors, as PaO_2 probably varies enough during wakefulness to mask mean differences in these subjects. Thus, studies during sleep are more likely to reflect the control of ventilation than are awake measurements.

Our studies of hypoxic sensitivity indicate that Sherpas who are most sensitive to inspired N_2 have the lowest hematocrits and the highest erythropoietin concentrations. In this regard, they are similar to sea-level sojourners to high-altitude. This greater hypoxic sensitivity would imply a higher mean PaO_2 and, therefore, a lower hematocrit. These data provide a link between ventilatory sensitivity and red blood cell production in Sherpas. The studies need to be extended to Quechua Indians and, especially, to subjects with chronic mountain sickness.

ACKNOWLEDGMENTS

Supported, in part, by grant PCM 84-16125 from the National Science Foundation, and by a grant from the National Geographic Society.

The views presented herein are the private opinions of the authors and not of the U.S. Army or the Department of Defense.

REFERENCES

1. ABBRECHT, P. H., AND J. K. LITTEL. Plasma erythropoietin in men and mice during acclimatization to different altitudes. *J. Appl. Physiol.* 32(1):54–58, 1972.
2. ADAMS, W. H., AND S. M. SHRESTA. Hemoglobin levels, vitamin B_{12}, and folate status in a Himalayan village. *Am. J. Physiol.* 27:217–219, 1974.
3. ADAMS, W. H., AND L. STRANG. Hemoglobin levels in persons of Tibetan ancestry living at high altitude. *Proc. Soc. Exp. Biol. Med.* 149:1036–1039, 1975.
4. BEALL, C. M. Reappraisal of Andean high altitude erythrocytosis from a Himalayan perspective. *Semin. Respir. Med.* 5(2):195–201, 1983.
5. BEALL, C. M., AND A. B. REICHSMAN. Hemoglobin levels in a Himalayan high altitude population. *Am. J. Physiol.* 63:301–306, 1984.
6. BEALL, C. M. Hemoglobin concentration of pastural nomad permanent residents of 4850–5450 m in Tibet. *Am. J. Phys. Anthrop.* 73:433–438, 1987.
7. BLUME, F. D., R. SANTOLAYA, M. G. SHERPA, AND C. C. MONGE. Anthropometric and lung volume measurements in Himalayan and Andean natives. *FASEB J.* 2(5):A1281, 1988.
8. COSIO, G. Trabajo minero a gran altura y los valores hematicos. *Boletin Instituto de Salud Occupacional, Lima* 10:5–12, 1965.
9. ERSLEV, A. J., J. WILSON, AND J. CARO. Erythropoeitin titers in anemic, nonuremic patients. *J. Lab. Clin. Med.* 109:429–433, 1987.
10. FAURA, J., J. RAMOS, C. REYNAFARJE, E. ENGLISH, P. FINNE, AND C. FINCH. Effect of altitude on erythropoiesis. *Blood* 33(5):668–676, 1969.
11. HACKETT, P. H., J. T. REEVES, R. F. GROVER, AND J. V. WEIL. Ventilation in human popula-

tions native to high altitude. In: *Man at High Altitude,* eds. J. B. West and S. Lahiri. Bethesda, MD: American Physiological Society, 1984, pp. 179–191.

12. HUANG, S. Y., X. H. NING, Z. N. ZHOU, Z. Z. GU, AND S. T. HU. Ventilatory function in adaptation to high altitude: studies in Tibet. In: *Man at High Altitude,* eds. J. B. West and S. Lahiri. Bethesda, MD: American Physiological Society, 1984, pp. 173–177.

13. MERINO, C. F. The plasma erythropoietic factor in the polycythemia of high altitudes. Report 56-103 to the Air University, School of Aviation Medicine, USAF, Randolph AFB, Texas, 1956, p. 103.

14. MILLEDGE, J. S., AND P. M. COTES. Serum erythropoietin in humans at high altitude and its relation to plasma renin. *J. Appl. Physiol. 59:*360–364. 1985.

15. REYNAFARJE, C., J. RAMOS, J. FAURA, AND D. VILLAVICENCIO. Humoral control of erythropoietic activity in man during and after altitude exposure. *Proc. Soc. Exp. Biol. Med. 116:*649–650, 1964.

16. SAMAJA, M., A. VEICSTEINAS, AND P. CERRETELLI. Oxygen affinity of blood in altitude Sherpas. *J. Appl. Physiol. 47(2):*337–341, 1979.

17. SHERWOOD, J. B., AND E. GOLDWASSER. A radioimmunoassay for erythropoietin. *Blood 54(4):*885–893, 1979.

18. VIAULT, F. Sur l'augmentation considerable du nombres des globules rouges dans le sang chez les habitants des hautes plateaux de l'Amerique du Sud. *Compt. Rend. Soc. Biol. (Paris) 30:*917–918, 1890.

19. WEIL, J. V., E. BRYNE-QUINN, I. E. SOLAL, G. F. FILLY, AND R. F. GROVER. Acquired attenuation of chemoreceptor function in chronically hypoxic man at high altitude. *J. Clin. Invest. 50:*186–195, 1972.

20. WHITTEMBURY, J., AND C. MONGE C. High altitude, hematocrit, and age. *Nature(London) 238:*278–279, 1976.

21. WINSLOW, R. M., C. C. MONGE, N. J. STATHAM, C. G. GIBSON, S. CHARACHE, J. WHITTEMBURY, O. MORAN, AND R. L. BERGER. Variability of oxygen affinity of blood: human subjects native to high altitude. *J. Appl. Physiol. 51:*1411–1416, 1981.

22. WINSLOW, R. M., AND S. S. MCKNEALLY. Analysis of breath-by-breath exercise data from field studies. *Int. J. Clin. Monit. Comput. 2:*167–190, 1986.

23. WINSLOW, R. M., AND C. MONGE. *Hypoxia, Polycythemia, and Chronic Mountain Sickness.* Baltimore, Johns Hopkins University Press, 1987.

24. WINSLOW, R. M., K. W. CHAPMAN, C. C. GIBSON, M. SAMAJA, C. C. MONGE, E. GOLDWASSER, M. SHERPA, F. D. BLUME, AND R. SANTOLAYA. Different hematologic responses to hypoxia in Sherpas and Quechua Indians. *J. Appl. Physiol. 66:*1561–1569, 1989.

IV

OXYGEN BIOLOGY OF ADAPTATION

14

Geometrical Relationship Between Capillaries and Muscle Fibers in Chronic Hypoxia

ODILE MATHIEU-COSTELLO

Capillary-to-fiber geometrical relationships are important for several aspects of blood–tissue transfer in skeletal muscles. Fiber size determines maximal diffusion distances within the muscle fiber. Transmembrane flux depends on the amount of capillary and fiber surfaces. From the Fick law of diffusion, the increased capillary surface area found after endurance training indicates a reduction of the pressure drop necessary for a given O_2 flux (23). Ellis et al. (7) stressed the importance of capillary geometry for the efficiency of blood–tissue transfer. The dramatic change in capillary configuration with muscle shortening (22, 25) tends to create a more uniform circumferential O_2 supply around the muscle fibers. At the extreme (circumferentially homogeneous O_2 supply), the Hill model (8) predicts that the muscle fiber can achieve a five-fold increase in O_2 flux for the same drop in PO_2 from capillary to the center of a 50-μm fiber compared with the Krogh geometry (7, 11). This chapter reviews our morphometric data on capillary-to-fiber geometry in skeletal muscles in response to hypoxia. We addressed the question of whether or not systematic difference(s) are found in the arrangement of capillaries relative to the muscle fibers after chronic exposure or adaptation, or both, to hypoxia. Specifically, we examined fiber size, capillary amount, and configuration in muscles of deer mice native to 3800 m compared with sea-level deer mice, in rats and pigeons kept at 3800 m for 5 months with sea-level controls, and in animals tolerant to prolonged periods of anoxia (harbor seal) compared with dogs. These animal models were selected to provide a wide range of functional demands or constraints.

MATERIAL AND METHODS

Skeletal muscles were perfusion fixed in situ in the following animals: deer mice (*Peromyscus maniculatus*) native to Barcroft, California (3800 m; inspired PO_2, 91 mm Hg), Sprague-Dawley rats and White King pigeons kept at UC station at White Mountain (Barcroft) for 5 months, sea level mice, rats, and pigeons, harbor seal (*Phoca vitulina*), and mongrel dogs (*Canis familiaris*). There was no difference in body mass, M_b, between altitude and sea-level animals in either mice or rats [M_b, 21 to 27 g and 244 to 305 g respectively; (21)].

Altitude pigeons were slightly larger (M_b, 647 ± 6 g) than sea-level animals (M_b, 598 ± 22 g). The body mass of the other animals was 14 kg and 22 kg (yearling seals), 41 kg (2-year-old female seal), 14, 20, and 29.5 kg (dogs). The average body mass of adult male and female seals was 87 and 65 kg, respectively (6).

Before perfusion fixation, the position of the wings (pigeon), knee, or ankle joints (limb muscles) was controlled so as to obtain muscles fixed at different degrees of extension or shortening. Samples were taken from calf and thigh muscles (mice), soleus (rat), pectoralis (pigeon), gastrocnemius, semitendinosus, and vasti (dog and seal), rectus femoris and sartorius (dog), diaphragm, subcutaneous, latissimus, and longissimus dorsi (seal). All tissues were prepared following a procedure described elsewhere in detail (15). They were fixed with a 6.25% solution of glutaraldehyde in sodium cacodylate buffer, postfixed in 1% osmium tetroxide solution, and embedded in plastic. Four to eight blocks were cut from each muscle, yielding four transverse and four longitudinal sections (1 μm thick). The angle of each section was carefully controlled as described previously (15).

Sarcomere length, l_o, was measured at magnification X 630 (10 measurements of 10 consecutive sarcomeres per longitudinal section). Fiber cross-sectional area, $\bar{a}(f)$, was obtained by one of two methods: standard point counting using 50 to 200 fibers measured at magnification X 2060 (15) or tracing the contours of a total of 30 to 180 fibers per muscle at magnification X 1050, with a Videometric 150 image analyzer (American Innovision Inc.). Fiber cross-sectional area was normalized to l_o 2.1 μm using the equation.

$$\bar{a}(f)_{2.1} = \bar{a}(f) * l_o / 2.1 \tag{1}$$

Capillary density at 2.1 μm was calculated from capillary number per fiber cross-sectional area, $Q_A(0)$, using the equation

$$Q_A(0)_{2.1} = Q_A(0) * 2.1 / l_o \tag{2}$$

Capillary-to-fiber ratio, $N_N(c,f)$ was computed as

$$N_N(c,f) = Q_A(0) * \bar{a}(f) \tag{3}$$

Capillary diameter, $\bar{d}(c)$, was measured with the image analyzer, using circular capillary profiles (difference between smaller and larger diameters less than 15 percent; average of 25 to 150 profiles measured per sample), based on our previous findings of capillary cross-section circularity in perfusion-fixed rat muscles (15).

The method used to estimate capillary anisotropy in each muscle has been described elsewhere in detail (13). Briefly, the ratio between the number of capillaries per sectional area of muscle fibers in transverse and longitudinal sections of muscle fibers, $Q_A(0)$ and $Q_A(\pi/2)$, respectively, was used to calculate, by a table of known coefficients, (1) the capillary orientation concentration parameter, K, (2) the coefficient $c(K,0)$ relating capillary counts per unit area of fiber in transverse sections, $Q_A(0)$, and (3) capillary length/volume muscle fiber, $J_v(c,f)$. Knowing $c(K,0)$, an estimate of $J_v(c,f)$ can be obtained by using the following equation:

$$J_V(c,f) = c(K,0) * Q_A(0) \qquad (4)$$

For straight and unbranched capillaries, all parallel to the muscle fiber axis (perfect anisotropy), $K = \infty$ and $c(K,0)=1$. For capillaries with no preferred orientation (isotropy), $K=0$ and $c(K,0)=2$ (ref. 28).

Capillary-to-fiber perimeter ratio, $B_B(c,f)$ was obtained using the following equation (19):

$$B_B(c,f) = c(K,0) * Q_A(0) * \pi * \bar{d}(c) * \bar{d})(f) / [4 * c'(K',0)] \qquad (5)$$

where $c'(K',0)$ is an anisotropy coefficient relating capillary perimeter per fiber cross-sectional area and capillary surface per volume of fiber. Except for muscles with large degree of capillary tortuosity (coefficient $c(K,0)>1.53$), the value of $c'(K',0)$ is 1. The maximal value of $c'(K',0)$ is 1.27 (for $c(K,0)=2$).

RESULTS AND DISCUSSION

Fiber Size

Light micrographs of transverse sections of muscles from each animal are shown in Fig. 14.1. The size of the muscle fibers was approximately the same in muscles of rat (Fig. 14.1A), pigeon (glycolytic fibers; Fig. 14.1C), 41-kg seal (Fig. 14.1E), and dog (Fig. 14.1F). The aerobic fibers of pigeon pectoralis muscle (Fig. 14.1C) were small, as were those of mice (Fig. 14.1B) and yearling seals (Fig. 14.1D). It is known that considerable variation exists in fiber size in muscles of mammals (10). Except for very small fibers in very small animals (bat and mice), no relationship was found between fiber size and body weight (rat to cattle) (26).

We have stressed the importance of considering sarcomere length when comparing fiber size among muscles and/or after different experimental conditions. Unless sarcomere length is known, it is difficult if not impossible to demonstrate relatively small changes (i.e.,<30%) in fiber size and related variables (e.g., capillary number per fiber cross-sectional area) in skeletal muscles (21). The expected inverse relationship between $\bar{a}(f)$ and l_o was found in each species, with no systematic difference in fiber size with chronic exposure to altitude. Fiber cross-sectional area normalized to sarcomere length, $\bar{a}(f)_{2.1}$, was not different between muscles of altitude (A) mice and rats (21) or pigeons (16) compared with sea-level (SL) animals. The range of sarcomere lengths at which muscles were examined in seal (1.84 to 3.13 μm) and dog (1.57 to 2.69 μm) indicates that about 40% to 70% of the variation in fiber cross-sectional area was related to sarcomere length rather than intrinsic differences between samples or animals (Fig. 14.2). The correlation of the linear transform, $\bar{a}(f)$ versus $1/l_o$ was r = 0.85 (P<0.01) in yearling seals and r = 0.80 (P<0.01) in dogs.

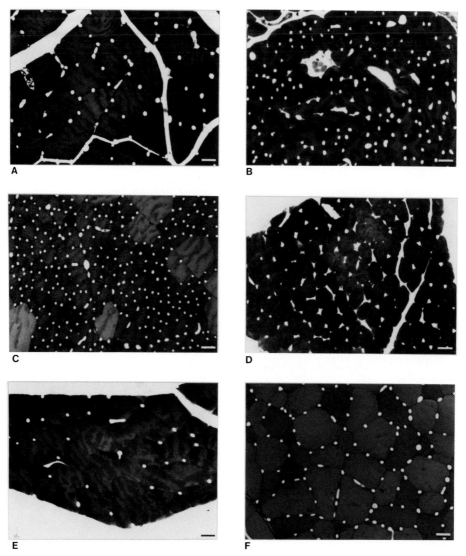

FIGURE 14.1. Light micrographs of portions of muscle bundles in 1-μm thick transverse sections from each species. Note that capillaries are empty after the vascular perfusion fixation.
(A) Rat soleus at intermediate sarcomere length (1.99 μm). **(B)** Calf muscle of deer mice in an
extended position (sarcomere length, 2.35 μm). **(C)** Pigeon pectoralis muscle at 2.2 μm sarcomere length. Note narrow aerobic (fast-twitch red) and broad glycolytic fibers (fast-twitch
white), easily distinguishable by light microscopy. **(D)** Latissimus dorsi of yearling seal (M_b, 22
kg) extended (sarcomere length, 2.43 μm). **(E)** Vastus profundus of young seal (M_b, 41 kg), at
2.15 μm sarcomere length. **(F)** Dog semitendinosus at intermediate sarcomere length (1.95
μm). (Bar = 20 μm)

Capillary Density

Because of its effect on fiber cross-sectional area, sarcomere length has a direct
effect on capillary number per fiber cross-sectional area, $Q_A(0)$. The number of
capillaries per fiber mm^2 normalized to sarcomere length, $Q_A(0)_{2.1}$, was unchanged by chronic hypoxia in both native mice (A, 3399 ± 281; SL, 3168 ±

396 mm^{-2}) (17) and chronically exposed rats (A, 1292 ± 79; SL, 1282 ± 43 mm^{-2}) (24). In pigeon pectoralis muscle, capillary number per fiber cross-sectional area depends both on sarcomere length and the relative proportion of aerobic fibers (16). For a given relative area of aerobic fibers, there was no systematic difference in capillary number per fiber cross-sectional area normalized to sarcomere length, $Q_A(0)_{2.1}$, in A compared with SL pigeons (Fig. 14.3). Although fiber size was much smaller in yearling seals than in dogs (Fig. 14.1 D to F), the range of values obtained for $Q_A(0)_{2.1}$ was approximately the same in seals (883 to 1811 mm^{-2}) and in dogs (1207 to 2028 mm^{-2}). This was because of the substantially lower capillary-to-fiber ratio, $N_N(c,f)$, in seals (M_b, 14 to 41 kg) compared with dogs (Table 14.1). We found no difference in capillary-to-fiber ratio in A and SL mice (range, 1.2 to 3.1) (17), or in rats (range, 2.1 to 3.1) (24). As for capillary density, comparing capillary-to-fiber ratio in pigeon pectoralis muscle can be misleading because of the difference in the relative proportion of aerobic fibers among samples (Fig. 14.3). There was no systematic difference in capillary-to-fiber ratio normalized to the relative area of the aerobic fibers in A and SL pigeons (unpublished observation).

Capillary Tortuosity

We have reported the substantial increase in capillary tortuosity with fiber shortening within physiological sarcomere lengths in skeletal muscles of mammals (15, 17, 20, 22). In muscles of Japanese Waltzing mice kept at a simulated altitude of 3000 m for 2 weeks, Appell (1) found "no evidence for the development of new capillaries," but qualitative evidence of increased capillary tor-

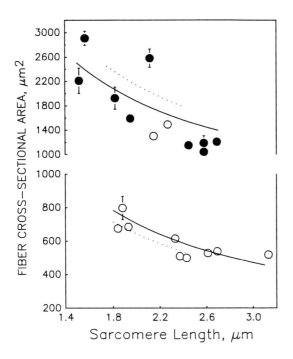

FIGURE 14.2. Relationship between fiber cross-sectional area and sarcomere length. **Upper panel**: Dog (*filled circles; solid line,* predicted change assuming constant fiber volume); *broken line,* predicted change in rats (21); data from 41-kg seal (*open circles*) shown for comparison. **Lower panel**: Yearling seals (*open circles; solid line,* predicted change); *broken line,* predicted change in HA and SL mice (21); Note that practically similar fiber size was found in muscles in yearling seals and mice (lower panel), and in muscles of dog, rat, and 41-kg seal (upper panel).

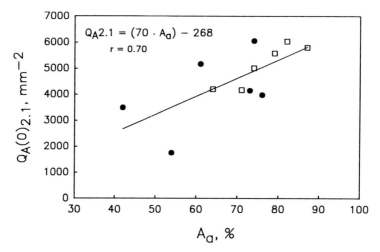

FIGURE 14.3. Relationship between capillary density per fiber cross-sectional area normalized to 2.1 μm sarcomere length, $Q_A(0)_{2.1}$, and the relative area of aerobic fibers, A_a, in the pectoralis muscle of altitude (*open squares*) and sea-level White King pigeons (*filled circles*; data from Ref. 18).

TABLE 14.1. Fiber Cross-Sectional Area Normalized to $l_0 = 2.1$ μm, $\bar{a}(f)_{2.1}$; Capillary Number Per Fiber Cross-Sectional Area at $l_0 = 2.1$ μm, $Q_A(0)_{2.1}$; Capillary To-Fiber Ratio, $N_N(c,f)$; and Capillary to Fiber Perimeter Ratio, $B_B(c,f)$, in Seal and Dog Muscles.

#	Muscle Site	M_b (kg)	$\bar{a}(f)_{2.1}$ (μm²)	$Q_A(0)_{2.1}$ (mm⁻²)	$N_N(c,f)$	$B_B(c,f)$
Seal[a]						
1	vastus profundus	14	714 ± 63	1400 ± 73	1.0 ± 0.1	0.27
2	vastus lateralis	14	591 ± 27	1811 ± 80	1.1 ± 0.1	0.24
3	semitendinosus	14	576 ± 38	1571 ± 52	0.9 ± 0.1	0.20
4	subcutaneous	14	682 ± 35	1369 ± 89	0.9 ± 0.1	0.15
5	latissimus dorsi	14	630 ± 31	1448 ± 96	0.9 ± 0.1	0.19
6	longissimus dorsi	22	690 ± 35	1054 ± 43	0.7 ± 0.0	0.14
7	latissimus dorsi	22	579 ± 48	1355 ± 128	0.8 ± 0.1	0.13
8	diaphragm	22	774 ± 35	883 ± 86	0.7 ± 0.1	0.11
9	gastrocnemius	22	657 ± 39	1370 ± 85	0.9 ± 0.1	0.18
10	vastus profundus	41	1332 ± 127	882 ± 74	1.2 ± 0.1	0.19
11	latissimus dorsi	41	1612 ± 139	954 ± 65	1.5 ± 0.2	0.27
Dog						
12	sartorius (mid)	14	1281 ± 87	2028 ± 95	2.6 ± 0.2	0.37
13	rectus femoris (sup)	14	1343 ± 92	1456 ± 96	2.0 ± 0.1	0.27
14	vastus intermedius (sup)	14	1547 ± 77	1354 ± 65	2.1 ± 0.1	0.27
15	vastus intermedius (deep)	14	1460 ± 146	1820 ± 76	2.7 ± 0.3	0.36
16	gastrocnemius (sup)	20	1599 ± 152	1499 ± 59	2.4 ± 0.2	0.32
17	gastrocnemius (deep)	20	1667 ± 159	1544 ± 97	2.6 ± 0.3	0.40
18	vastus medialis (mid)	29.5	2604 ± 197	1207 ± 72	3.1 ± 0.2	0.34
19	gastrocnemius (mid)	29.5	2173 ± 91	1505 ± 59	3.3 ± 0.2	0.43
20	semitendinosus (mid)	29.5	1476 ± 96	1579 ± 79	2.3 ± 0.2	0.34

[a]All samples were taken midportion of midbelly.
Data calculated from Ref. 20 (dog).

tuosity and density of capillary anastomoses. Unfortunately, the sarcomere length of the muscles compared was not reported (17).

Figure 14.4 shows the substantial degree of capillary tortuosity in muscle of a sea-level rat. Had chronic exposure to altitude increased capillary tortuosity (1), this would have resulted in a larger blood volume and improved O_2 supply of the muscle fibers. When sarcomere length was taken into account, however, we found no systematic difference in muscle capillary tortuosity between A and SL animals in either mice or rats (Fig. 14.5). Hypoxia at this moderate altitude (e.g., 3800 m) may not be severe enough to induce changes in muscle fiber size and capillary density (3). It remains to be determined whether or not muscle capillary configuration (tortuosity and/or branching) at a given sarcomere length is increased after training at high altitude. In soleus muscle of rats at sea-level, endurance training produced a 35% increase in citrate synthase activity and a 30% increase in capillary-to-fiber ratio, but no change in capillary tortuosity at measured sarcomere length (23).

A different capillary-to-fiber geometry is found in pigeon pectoralis muscle compared with muscles of mammals. A large number of capillary branches running perpendicular to the muscle fiber axis are found in the bird flight muscle (16). In pigeons kept at altitude for 5 months, we found no change in capillary tortuosity but an increase in the number of capillary branches, perpendicular to the muscle fiber axis, compared with sea-level animals (14).

The effect of growth on the geometry of blood–tissue transfer in seal muscles is not known. An increased capillary tortuosity with maturation has been reported in dogs (2). At a given sarcomere length, capillary tortuosity was similar in juvenile seals (M_b, 14 to 41 kg) and in adult mammals (including dogs) (5).

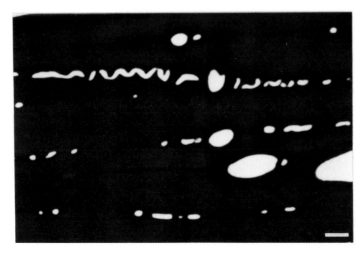

FIGURE 14.4. Light micrograph of a portion of muscle bundle in a 1-μm thick longitudinal section of sea-level rat soleus fixed at intermediate sarcomere length (1.99 μm). Note the sinuous capillaries. (Bar = 20 μm)

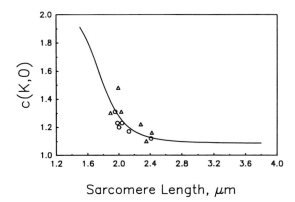

FIGURE 14.5. Relationship between the coefficient c(K,0), [relating $Q_A(0)$ to $J_V(c,f)$, Equation 4], and sarcomere length in muscles of altitude mice (*triangles*; 17) and rats (*circles*; 24). *Solid line*, curve for sea-level mammals (deer mouse to pony, including rats; 16).

Capillary-to-Fiber Perimeter Ratio

Muscle capillary diameter was not affected by chronic exposure to altitude [mice, (17); rats, (24); pigeon, unpublished observation], nor was it different in seal compared with dog muscles (4.6 ± 0.3 and 4.9 ± 0.1 μm, respectively). Because altitude exposure had no effect on fiber size or on indices of capillarity (density, diameter, and anisotropy) in either mice and rats, one can predict Equation 5) unchanged capillary-to-fiber perimeter ratios in A compared with SL muscles fixed at similar sarcomere length. In pigeon pectoralis muscle only capillary anisotropy (coefficient c(K,0) in Equation 5) was changed after altitude exposure. Therefore, a change in capillary-to-fiber perimeter ratio proportional to that of capillary anisotropy is expected (e.g., an increase of about 10% in muscles fixed at 2 μm sarcomere length) (14). In the various seal muscles, the value of capillary-to-fiber perimeter ratio was systematically smaller (range, 0.11 to 0.27) compared with both dog (0.27 to 0.43) (Table 14.1) and mice muscles (0.27 to 0.53; unpublished observation). With fiber extension (or shortening) capillary-to-fiber perimeter ratio changes less than 20% over the full range of physiological sarcomere lengths (19). Within the ranges of sarcomere lengths considered (1.84 to 3.13 μm in seals; 1.59 to 2.69 μm in dogs; 1.87 to 2.43 μm in mice), less than 10% (seal), 15% (dogs), and 9% (mice) variation in capillary to fiber perimeter ratio is attributable to the difference in sarcomere length among samples.

For similar capillary length per volume in seal (range, 1200 to 2100 mm^{-2}) and dog muscles (range, 1500 to 2600 mm^{-2}), capillary-to-fiber perimeter ratio was smaller in the seals. In yearling seals (M_b, 14 to 22 kg), muscle fibers were as small as in deer mice muscle but yet, capillary-to-fiber (and perimeter) ratio was considerably smaller. Clearly, the effect of maturation on capillary-to-fiber geometrical arrangement at measured sarcomere length in muscles of seals needs to be examined. In contrast to rodents, capillary-to-fiber ratio was found to increase linearly with fiber cross-sectional area in skeletal muscles of growing dogs, with no change in capillary density and pattern, and, therefore, unaltered diffusion distances during growth (4). In the limited number of samples considered in this study, we found a decrease in capillary density with growth in juvenile seals (M_b, 14 to 41 kg; Table 14.1). Seal pups (M_b, 10 kg) swim at birth, and they can already dive for up to 8 minutes at 10 days (6). Myoglobin concentration in muscles of 18 to 41-kg harbor seals averaged 5.5 g/ 100 g of tissue wet weight (12), a value about eight-fold larger than in dog muscles (27). The tissue O_2 stores provide energy fuel for only part of the dives. There is increasing evidence that free dives, especially those of short-term duration are fueled by aerobic metabolism, and that the muscles used in swimming remain preferentially perfused (9). Obviously, dog limb muscles can sustain considerable levels of exercise, with high $\dot{V}O_2$ and high muscle blood flow, whereas the seals sustain substantially lower levels of metabolism and must rely on the O_2 on board during the dive. Even if there is preferential perfusion of the working muscles during the dive, this perfusion as well as lactate washout and replenishment of the O_2 stores during recovery occur by a smaller capillary-to-fiber surface area available for transmembrane flux. It remains to be determined whether or not correlations exist between capillary-to-fiber geometrical arrangement in locomotor muscles and the increasing diving capacity of seals with maturation.

CONCLUSIONS

1. When account was taken of sarcomere length, we found no evidence of an increased circumferential concentration of capillaries around the muscle fibers in skeletal muscles of mammals after chronic exposure or adaptation, or both, to hypoxia.
2. The data from mice and rat muscles provided no support for increased capillary tortuosity with chronic exposure to an altitude of 3800 m.
3. In the pectoralis muscle of A pigeons, we found no change in fiber size or capillary number per fiber cross-sectional area, but an increase in blood volume by an increased number of capillary branches.
4. In seal muscles, there was no increase in blood volume or efficiency of blood–tissue transfer by an increased capillary tortuosity at measured sarcomere length compared with muscles of terrestrial mammals.

ACKNOWLEDGMENTS

This work was supported by grants 5P01-HL-17731 and HL-01534 from the National Institutes of Health.

REFERENCES

1. APPELL, H. J. Morphological studies on skeletal muscle capillaries under conditions of high altitude training. *Int. J. Sports Med.* 1:103–109, 1980.
2. AQUIN, L., AND N. BANCHERO. The cytoarchitecture and capillary supply in the skeletal muscle of growing dogs. *J. Anat.* 132: 341–356, 1981.
3. BANCHERO, N. Cardiovascular responses to chronic hypoxia. *Ann. Rev. Physiol.* 49:465–476, 1987.
4. BANCHERO, N. Long-term adaptation of skeletal muscle capillarity. *Physiologist* 25:385–389, 1982.
5. BEBOUT, D. E., AND O. MATHIEU-COSTELLO. Capillary anisotropy in skeletal muscles of Harbor seals (Abstr). *Fed. Proc. 46*:352. 1987.
6. BIGG, M. A. Harbour seal—*Phoca vitulina* and *P. larga*. In: *Handbook of Marine Mammals*, vol. 2, eds. S. H. Ridgway and R. J. Harrison. New York: Academic, 1981, pp. 1–27.

7. ELLIS, C. G., R. F. POTTER, AND A. C. GROOM. The Krogh cylinder geometry is not appropriate for modelling O_2 transport in contracted skeletal muscle. *Adv. Exp. Med. Biol.* 159:253–268, 1983.

8. HILL, A. V. The diffusion of oxygen and lactic acid through tissues. *Proc. Roy. Soc. B 104:* 39–96, 1928.

9. HOCHACHKA, P. W. Balancing conflicting metabolic demands of exercise and diving. *Fed. Proc. 45:*2948–2952, 1986.

10. HOPPELER, H., O. MATHIEU, R. KRAUER, H. CLAASSEN, R. ARMSTRONG, AND E. WEIBEL. Design of the mammalian respiratory system. VI. Distribution of mitochondria and capillaries in various muscles. *Respir. Physiol.* 44:87–111, 1981.

11. KROGH, A. The number and distribution of capillaries in muscles with calculations of the oxygen pressure head necessary for supplying the tissue. *J. Physiol. (London)* 52:409–415, 1918/19.

12. LENFANT, C., K. JOHANSEN, AND J. D. TORRANCE. Gas transport and oxygen storage capacity in some pinnipeds and the sea otter. *Respir. Physiol.* 9:277–286, 1970.

13. MATHIEU, O., L. M. CRUZ-ORIVE, H. HOPPELER, AND E. R. WEIBEL. Estimating length density and quantifying anisotropy in skeletal muscle capillaries. *J. Microsc.* 131:131–146, 1983.

14. MATHIEU-COSTELLO, O. Effect of chronic exposure to hypoxia on capillarity in avian flight muscle (Abst). *Fed. Proc. 45:*1157,1986.

15. MATHIEU-COSTELLO, O. Capillary tortuosity and degree of contraction or extension of skeletal muscles. *Microvasc. Res.* 33:98–117, 1987.

16. MATHIEU-COSTELLO, O. Histology of flight: tissue and muscle gas exchange. In: *Hypoxia: The Adaptations,* eds. J. R. Sutton, G. Coates, and J. E. Remmers. Toronto: B. C. Decker, 1990, 13–19.

17. MATHIEU-COSTELLO, O. Muscle capillary tortuosity in high altitude mice depends on sarcomere length. *Resp. Physiol.* 76:289–302, 1989.

18. MATHIEU-COSTELLO, O. Morphometric analysis of the size and geometry of the capillary network in pigeon pectoralis muscle. *Microvasc. Res.* (submitted).

19. MATHIEU-COSTELLO, O., C. G. ELLIS, R. F. POTTER, I. C. MACDONALD, AND A. C. GROOM. Muscle capillary to fiber perimeter ratio: morphometry. *J. Appl. Physiol.* (submitted).

20. MATHIEU-COSTELLO, O., H. HOPPELER, AND E. R. WEIBEL. Capillary tortuosity in skeletal muscles of mammals depends on muscle contraction. *J. Appl. Physiol.* 66:1436–1442, 1989.

21. MATHIEU-COSTELLO, O., D. C. POOLE, AND R. B. LOGEMANN. Muscle fiber size and chronic exposure to hypoxia. *Adv. Exp. Med. Biol.* 248:305–311, 1989.

22. MATHIEU-COSTELLO, O., R. F. POTTER, C. G. ELLIS, AND A. C. GROOM. Capillary configuration and fiber shortening in muscles of the rat hindlimb: correlation between corrosion casts and stereological measurements. *Microvasc. Res.* 36:40–55, 1988.

23. POOLE, D. C., O. MATHIEU-COSTELLO, AND J. B. WEST. Capillary tortuosity in rat M. soleus is not affected by endurance training. *Am. J. Physiol.* 256:H1110–H1116, 1989.

24. POOLE, D. C., AND O. MATHIEU-COSTELLO. Skeletal muscle capillary geometry: adaptation to chronic hypoxia. *Respir. Physiol.* 77:21–30, 1989.

25. POTTER, R. F., AND A. C. GROOM. Capillary diameter and geometry in cardiac and skeletal muscle studied by means of corrosion casts. *Microvasc. Res.* 25:68–84, 1983.

26. SCHMIDT-NIELSEN, K., AND P. PENNYCUIK. Capillary density in mammals in relation to body size and oxygen consumption. *Am. J. Physiol.* 200:746–750, 1961.

27. SNYDER, G. K. Respiratory adaptations in diving mammals. *Respir. Physiol.* 54:269–294, 1983.

28. WEIBEL, E. R. *Stereological Methods. Theoretical Foundations.* New York: Academic, 1980, vol. 2.

15

Muscle Function at Altitude

P. CERRETELLI, B. KAYSER, H. HOPPELER, AND D. PETTE

Exposure to chronic hypoxia exceeding 4 to 6 weeks results in a loss of body mass (1) almost equally partitioned between fat and muscle tissue (2). A reduction of muscle mass, particularly in the lower limbs, has been reported anecdotally in the past by many climbers. This has been documented by Boutellier et al. (3) who found an average of 12 percent decrease of muscle mass post- versus pre-expedition in a group of climbers of the 1981 Swiss Mt. Lhotse Shar (8398 m) expedition.

To our knowledge, until recently, there has been a lack of ultrastructural data on the adaptation of human skeletal muscle to chronic hypoxia in a natural environment. Recent data have been published concerning the changes of muscle enzymes in the course of hypoxia. Young et al. (18) reported no effects on oxidative and glycolytic enzyme activities in the vastus lateralis muscle of five subjects exposed for 18 days to 4300 m. Green et al. (8), on the other hand, have found during acclimatization to progressive hypobaria over a 40-day period (Operation Everest II) a pronounced reduction in muscle lactate concentration at 282 mm Hg as compared with sea level. These findings have been interpreted by the authors to be the consequence of a reduced ability to activate fully the contractile apparatus of the muscle, as after prolonged hypoxia resting glycogen appears to be increased (8). Alternatively, the observed reduction in maximal accumulation of muscle lactate may also be attributed to the blunting of some enzymatic steps along the glycolytic pathway with a consequent depression of the energy flow as proposed by Cerretelli et al. (5).

With regard to the functional adaptation of muscles to high altitude by natives, the only published data are those of Reynafarje (14) who reported an average of 14% higher myoglobin concentration and a 20% increase in oxidative enzyme activity in the sartorius muscle of Andean natives as compared with sea-level controls.

Himalayan natives (e.g., Sherpas), according to anthropological studies, have the longest history of high-altitude exposure. This, and the fact that the Sherpas are famous for their outstanding work performance at high altitude, recently prompted us to compare their muscle ultrastructure with that of acclimatized lowlanders.

RESULTS

The present report summarizes data on muscle ultrastructure and/or enzyme activity in the following four groups of subjects: (1) the members of the 1981 Swiss Mt. Lhotse Shar (8398 m) expedition (referred to as group A), (2) the participants in the 1986 Swiss Mt. Everest (8848 m) expedition (group B), (3) elite altitude climbers (group C) (13), and (4) five Sherpas from Nepal living permanently in the Khumbu region at altitudes between 3000 and 5000 m (group D).

The physical and physiological characteristics of the subjects participating in the various studies are given in Table 15.1.

Groups A (Lhotse) and B (Everest)

As stated in Table 15.2, the thigh muscle cross-sectional area was reduced by about 10% post- versus preexpedition in both groups. In the Lhotse group (group A), which included four nonprofessional mountaineers, a significant decrease in fat tissue cross-sectional area was also found. The mean fiber cross-sectional area (vastus lateralis muscle) was reduced in both groups by about 20%. Also the capillary-to-fiber ratio (C/F) was lower. In group B, the capillary density was significantly increased and, because of both the decreased fiber size and the increased capillary density, the fiber area supplied by one capillary was significantly reduced, with consequently a potential improvement in O_2 delivery.

As shown in Table 15.3, the volume density of total mitochondria $V_v(mt,f)$ in the analyzed muscle samples was reduced, with the greater decrease (26%) occurring in group B. The decrease was both at the expense of the interfibrillar and the subsarcolemmal mitochondria. No significant changes of the volume density of the intracellular lipids was found, whereas the volume density of the myofibrils was slightly but significantly greater, a direct consequence of the decrease in $V_v(mt,f)$. The loss of mitochondria occurred mainly at the outermost edges of the fibers (10).

The results of the enzymatic assay of both groups A and B pre- and postexpedition, appear in Tables 15.4 and 15.5, respectively. As can be seen in Table 15.4, the activity of succinate dehydrogenase (SDH), a key enzyme of the tricarboxylic acid (TCA) cycle reflecting the adaptations of the respiratory status of the muscles to physiological and pathological stress, was found in three subjects to be lower 10 to 12 days after return from altitude. Also the activities

TABLE 15.1. Physical and Physiological Characteristics of Subjects

			Body Weight (kg)		$\dot{V}O_2max$ (L/min)	
Group/Subjects		Age (yr)	pre-	post-	pre-	post-
A	Lhotse (1981)	31.6 ± 7.1	69.7 ± 7.2	67.4 ± 8.1	3.62 ± 0.45	3.26 ± 0.42
B	Everest (1986)	38.3 ± 8.7	73.6 ± 5.7	70.1 ± 6.0	4.67 ± 0.38	4.57 ± 0.43
C	Elite climbers (1986)	40.7 ± 4.9	71.2 ± 7.7		4.15 ± 0.43	
D	Sherpas (1989)	$28 \quad \pm 2.8$	54.9 ± 3.2		2.29 ± 0.40	

(Mean ± SD; pre- and postexpedition.)

TABLE 15.2. Muscle and Fat Cross-Sectional Area of the Thigh by Computerized Tomography

Group/ Subjects	Muscle Tissue Cross Sectional Area (cm^2)		Fat Tissue Cross Sectional Area (cm^2)		C/F Ratio (unitless)		Capillary Density $N_A(c,f)$ (mm^{-2})		Mean Fiber Area a(f) (μm^2)		Fiber Area Supplied by One Capillary $a_N(f,c)$ (μm^2)	
	pre-	post-	pre-	post-	pre-	post-	pre-	post-	pre-	post-	pre-	post-
A ($n = 7$)	155 ± 11	140 ± 12	30.8 ± 9.1	23.5 ± 5.6	1.94 ± 0.32	1.66 ± 0.21	499 ± 98	478 ± 77	3980 ± 870	3540 ± 620	2080 ± 430	2140 ± 350
B ($n = 7$)	184 ± 23	163 ± 23	39.3 ± 22	38.7 ± 18	2.03 ± 0.32	1.92 ± 0.45	468 ± 36	599 ± 53	4350 ± 510	3170 ± 520	2150 ± 150	1680 ± 150

Capillary to fiber ratio (C/F), capillary density ($N_A(c,f)$), mean fiber area (a(f)), and fiber area supplied by one capillary ($A_N(f,c)$) in the vastus lateralis muscle. (mean ± SD)

TABLE 15.3. Ultrastructural Composition of the Vastus Lateralis Muscle

Group/ Subject	Volume Density Total Mitochondria V_V(mt,f) (%)		Volume Density Intracellular Lipid (%)		Volume Density Myofibrils (%)	
	pre-	post-	pre-	post-	pre-	post-
A (n = 7)	5.41 ± 1.0	4.86 ± 0.57	0.680 + 0.39	1.03 ± 0.59	78.7 ± 2.2	82.3 ± 2.
B (n = 7)	6.28 ± 1.2	4.65 ± 0.73	0.944 ± 0.64	0.820 ± 0.22	76.9 ± 3.1	78.9 ± 1.

of phosphofructokinase (PFK) and of lactate dehydrogenase (LDH) were significantly reduced. The data of Table 15.5 indicate that 2 to 3 weeks after
leaving altitude, the activities of some key enzymes of the TCA cycle were still
reduced by about the same percentage as the mitochondrial volume density
(see Table 15.3, group B). At variance with the data of Table 15.4, PFK and
LDH were unchanged in this group of particularly well-trained professional
mountaineers. A positive correlation was found between individual V_V(mt,f)
values and citrate synthase (r = 0.83; P < 0.001; Fig. 15.1), cytochrome oxidase (r = 0.63; P < 0.05), 3-hydroxyacyl-CoA dehydrogenase (r = 0.84; P <
0.001; Fig. 15.2), and hydroxybutyrate dehydrogenase (r = 0.50; N.S.; Fig.
15.3) activities pre- and post-expedition.

Group C (elite climbers)

The mean cross-sectional area of the fibers of the vastus lateralis muscle was
significantly smaller in this group of outstanding climbers than in sedentary
control subjects (3108 ± 303 μm² vs. 3640 ± 260; P < 0.05; Fig. 15.4). The
number of capillaries supplying one fiber is slightly greater than the average
for sedentary subjects, but significantly smaller than for long distance run-
ners. Because the muscle fibers of the climbers are much smaller than those
of the other two groups (13), this still leads to favorable conditions for tissue
oxygenation due to reduction of the diffusion distances (Fig. 15.4, A_N (f,c)). The
volume density of total mitochondria (V_V(mt,f) = 4.95 ± 0.46) of elite climbers
is similar to that found in untrained individuals of the same age (4.74 ± 0.30)
(9) and in mountaineers (groups A and B) post-expedition (average groups A
and B = 4.76 ± 0.64; Table 15.3). The figure for the elite climbers is considerably lower than that found for endurance athletes (7.32 ± 0.89) (9, 11) and

TABLE 15.4. Muscle Enzyme Activities (mM/min/kg muscle) After Exposure to High Altitude
(10 to 12 days after return, group A)

Enzymes	pre-	post-	% change	n
SDH	7 ± 2.2	4.5 ± 0.5	− 35	3
PFK	70 ± 14	50 ± 20	− 29	7
LDH	460 ± 118	230 ± 128	− 50	7

SDH, succinate dehydrazenase; PFK, phosphofructokinase; LDH, lactate dehydrogenase.

TABLE 15.5. Enzyme Activities (U/g wet weight)

Enzymes	pre-	post-	change %
HK	1.02 ± 0.29	0.94 ± 0.28	-7.8
AMP-DA	36.0 ± 7.9	39.3 ± 11.8	$+9.2$
PFK	48.3 ± 7.9	52.6 ± 9.6	$+8.9$
LDH	161 ± 36	162 ± 53	± 0.6
GAPDH	344 ± 66	325 ± 69	-5.5
CK	370 ± 39	336 ± 70	-2.3
MDH	535 ± 66	432 ± 115^a	-19.3^b
CS	16.5 ± 3.2	12.7 ± 2.1^a	-23.0^b
HADH	24.5 ± 6.0	18.0 ± 3.9^a	-26.5^b
Cyt-Ox	10.3 ± 2.6	7.9 ± 2.7	-23.3^a
NADH-DH	2.8 ± 0.5	2.7 ± 0.6	-3.6
HBDH	0.049 ± 0.011	0.036 ± 0.012	-26.5^a

Mean $\pm$ SD; $^aP < 0.06$; $^aP < 0.05$; group B, $n = 7$.

HK, hexokinase; AMP-DA, adenine monophosphate deaminase; PFK, phosphofructokinase; LDH, lactate dehydrogenase; GAPDH, glyceraldehyde phosphate dehydrogenase; CK, creatine kinase; MDH, malate dehydrogenase; CS, citrate synthase; HADH, hydroxyacyl dehydrogenase; Cyt-Ox, cytochrome oxidase; NADH-DH, nicotinamide adenine dinucleotide dehydrogenase; HBDH, hydroxybutyrate dehydrogenase.

for unacclimatized mountaineers such as the members of groups A and B preexpedition (average groups A and B = 5.85 ± 1.2; Table 15.3).

Group D (Sherpas of Nepal)

In a group of five Sherpas analyzed after 3 months of reduced climbing activity, the mean cross-sectional area of the vastus lateralis muscle fibers was found to be 3186 ± 582 μm^2, that is, equal to that of elite Caucasian climbers (group C, 3108 ± 303). This value is lower than that of unacclimatized alpine mountaineers, but similar to that of the latter after a 6 to 8 week sojourn at 5000 to 8600 m (groups A and B; Table 15.2, Fig. 15.4). The number of capillaries per tissue area was 467 ± 25/mm^2, lower than that of elite climbers (542 ± 36; Fig. 15.4), but greater than that of sedentary subjects (387 ± 25). The volume density of total mitochondria was 3.96 ± 0.60, less than that of elite climbers (4.95 ± 0.46), of alpine mountaineers before (average groups A and B = 5.85 ± 1.2), and after exposure to 5000 to 8600 m (4.76 ± 0.64), and of sedentary subjects (4.74 ± 0.30).

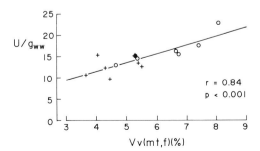

CITRATE SYNTHETASE

FIGURE 15.1. Citrate synthase activity as a function of percent volume density of mitochondria V_v(mt,f) seen in group B: 0, preexpedition; +, postexpedition (12).

HYDROXYACYL CoA DEHYDROGENASE

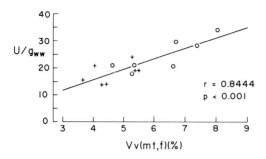

FIGURE 15.2. Hydroxyacyl CoA dehydrogenase activity as a function of $V_v(mt,f)$ (see Fig. 15.1 for symbols; 12).

DISCUSSION

The results obtained from groups A and B confirm the previous finding that a considerable weight loss follows exposure to chronic hypoxia. Such a loss is due both to a loss of muscle mass and of fat and is still significant 10 to 15 days after return to sea level. The reduction of muscle mass is particularly well documented for the vastus lateralis muscle and as the leg muscles of high altitude climbers are active even at very high altitude, the loss cannot be attributed to a lack of exercise. The reduction of fiber cross-sectional area, a confirmed finding in humans, is at variance with the results obtained in guinea pigs (15) and in rats (16) exposed to simulated altitude of 5100 and 6100 m, for 5 to 14 weeks, respectively. It is noteworthy that the fiber cross-sectional area of elite Caucasian high altitude climbers (group C) with a long personal history of exposure to hypoxia as well as that of the investigated Sherpas of Nepal (group D) is similar to that of acclimatized lowlanders. Whether this is the result of deterioration due to hypoxia (altered protein absorption and/or metabolism) or of an adaptation aimed at shortening the diffusion path between the capillary and the mitochondria is a matter for further investigation.

The increase in capillary density, due to the loss of fiber cross-sectional area, is a general feature in unacclimatized and acclimatized alpine mountaineers, in elite high altitude climbers, and in the Sherpas. The shortened O_2 diffusion distance is advantageous, particularly in hypoxia.

HYDROXYBUTYRATE DEHYDROGENASE

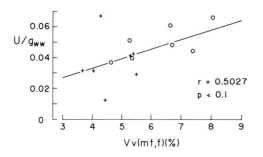

FIGURE 15.3. Hydroxybutyrate dehydrogenase activity as a function of $V_v(mt,f)$ (see Fig. 15.1 for symbols; 12).

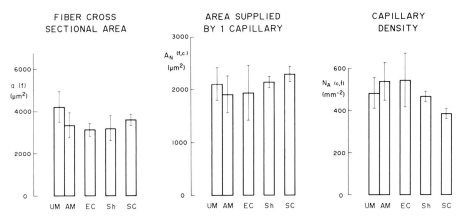

FIGURE 15.4. Fiber cross-sectional area, area of fiber cross section supplied by one capillary, and capillary density in different groups of subjects: UM, unacclimatized mountaineers (group A); AM, acclimatized mountaineers (group B); EC, elite high altitude climbers (group C); Sh, Sherpas (group D); SC, sedentary Caucasians (10).

The muscle oxidative potential estimated from $V_V(mt,f)$ appears to be closely related to the individual maximal aerobic power ($\dot{V}O_2max$) (Fig. 15.5). The correlation coefficient among the three investigated groups (A, B, and D) is 0.84 ($P < 0.001$). As appears from Fig. 15.6, the corresponding points for groups of differently trained sedentary subjects and of endurance athletes also appear to fit the line satisfactorily. This correlation can be taken as evidence for a proportional development (or deterioration) of the machinery controlling O_2 delivery and assuring the production of oxidative energy. In this context it is of note $V_v(mt,f)$ and some key enzymes of the TCA cycle and of the respiratory chain undergo a similar reduction in the course of acclimatization. Chronic hypoxia hampers not only the glycolytic pathway but also the rate of utilization of lipids and ketone bodies as indicated by the reduced activity of

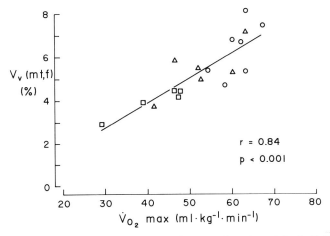

FIGURE 15.5. Percent volume density of mitochondria as a function of the individual maximal aerobic power ($\dot{V}O_2max$): Δ, group A; $\circ$, group B; $\square$, Sherpas (10).

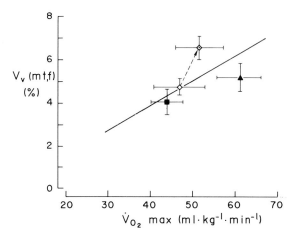

FIGURE 15.6. The same parameters as for Fig. 15.5. The regression line is also that of Fig. 15.5: ■ ▲, groups of differently trained individuals (7,9); ◇, groups after 6 weeks of training (9).

hydroxyacyl dehydrogenase and hydroxybutyrate dehydrogenase (Table 15.6, 12). This observation allows one to draw the conclusion that the observed functional impairment of the oxidative machinery is due to a loss of mitochondrial structure rather than to qualitative deterioration of specific enzymatic activities. This is also compatible with the observed unchanged efficiency of aerobic exercise in unacclimatized and acclimatized lowlanders as well as for acclimatized Sherpas (4). Although the trend is the one depicted in Fig. 15.5, V_v(mt,f) and oxidative enzyme activities in groups A and B appear to be more closely matched before than after high-altitude exposure. The latter finding seems to indicate that other factors besides the ones analyzed in the present study play a role in hypoxic deterioration of muscle function.

    The relatively high volume density of intracellular lipid droplets probably reflecting the muscle fiber's capacity to oxidize fat is particularly high in untrained and trained mountaineers, in elite climbers, and in endurance athletes compared with sedentary subjects. Such changes are probably not only adaptive but may also have a nutritional origin as in the investigated group of Sherpas not only was the increase of lipids not confirmed, but the volume density of lipid droplets was particularly low (50 % of that of acclimatized mountaineers).

TABLE 15.6. Changes of Mitochondrial Volume Density V_v(mt,f) and of the Enzymes (U/gww) Controlling the Aerobic Pathway (group B)

Variable	pre-	post-	change %
$V_v$mt	6.28 ± 1.2	4.65 ± 0.73	− 26.0
HADH	24.5 ± 6.0	18.0 ± 3.9	− 26.5
HBDH	0.049 ± 0.01	0.036 ± 0.012	− 26.5
CS	16.5 ± 3.2	12.7 ± 2.1	− 23.0
MDH	535 ± 66	432 ± 115	− 19.0
Cyt-Ox	10.3 ± 2.6	7.9 ± 2.7	− 23.0

For abbreviations, see Table 15.5.

CONCLUSION

Both indirect (reduced $\dot{V}o_2$ max) and direct (reduced $V_v(mt,f)$ and enzyme activity) evidence of hypoxia-induced muscle deterioration have been presented. This applies both to acclimatized lowlanders and Himalayan natives.

Such decreased function also affects anaerobic metabolism, particularly its glycolytic component, as shown by reduced blood (5) and muscle (8) lactate accumulation. This limitation of anaerobic metabolism as evidenced by the reduced blood lactate accumulation is not only a feature of acclimatized lowlanders but is also found in Peruvian Indians as well as in Himalayan Sherpas. Another interesting observation, pointing to some defective steps in the anaerobic glycolysis occurring in altitude residents, is the delayed onset of anaerobic glycolytic energy release during supramaximal exercise (7). Also of interest here are West's observations (17).

After a long sojourn at altitude, the peak anaerobic power has also been found to decrease (6), a finding that could be likely attributed to the loss of muscle mass.

Although there is experimental evidence pointing to an altered absorption of carbohydrates and fat from the gastrointestinal tract, the mechanisms underlying the functional impairment of the muscles at high altitude are still unknown. An additional difficulty in the search for an explanation of this problem is represented by the controversial results obtained from animal models.

REFERENCES

1. BOYER S. J., AND F. D. BLUME. Weight loss and changes in body composition at high altitude. *J. Appl. Physiol. 57*:1580–1585, 1984.
2. BRADWELL A. R., P. W. DYKES, J. H. COOTE, P. J. FORSTER, J. J. MILLES, I. CHESNER, AND N. V. RICHARDSON. Effect of acetazolamide on exercise performance and muscle mass at high altitude. *Lancet i*:1001–1005, 1986.
3. BOUTELLIER, U., H. HOWALD, P. E. DI PRAMPERO, D. GIEZENDANNER, AND P. CERRETELLI. Human muscle adaptation to chronic hypoxia. In: *Hypoxia, Exercise, and Altitude*, ed. J. R. Sutton, C. S. Houston, and H. L. Jones. New York: A. R. Liss, 1983, pp. 273–281.
4. CERRETELLI P. Gas exchange at high altitude. In: *Pulmonary Gas Exchange. Vol. II, Organism and Environment*, ed. J. B. West. New York: Academic Press, 1980, pp. 97–147.
5. CERRETELLI P., A., VEICSTEINAS, AND C. MARCONI. Anaerobic metabolism at high altitude: the lactacid mechanism. In: *High Altitude Physiology and Medicine*, ed. W. Brendel and R. A. Zink. New York: Springer, 1982, pp. 95–102.
6. CERRETELLI P., AND P. E. DI PRAMPERO. Aerobic and anaerobic metabolism during exercise at altitude. In: *Medicine Sport Science*, E. Jokl, and M. Hebbelinck. Basel: Karger, 1985, 19:1–19.
7. CERRETELLI P., P. E. DI PRAMPERO, AND H. HOWALD. Adjustments to exercise at altitude. *Prog. Resp. Res. 21*:256–261, 1986.
8. GREEN H. J., J. SUTTON, P. YOUNG, A. CYMERMAN, AND C. S. HOUSTON. Operation Everest II: muscle energetics during maximal exhaustive exercise. *J. Appl. Physiol. 66*:142–150, 1989.
9. HOPPELER H., P. LÜTHI, H. CLAASSEN, E. R. WEIBEL, AND H. HOWALD. The ultrastructure of the normal human skeletal muscle. A morphometric analysis of untrained man, woman and well-trained orienteers. *Pflüger's Archiv 344*:217–238, 1973.
10. HOPPELER H., E. KLEINERT, C. SCHLEGEL, H. CLAASSEN, H. HOWALD, S. R. KAYAR, AND P. CERRETELLI. Muscular exercise at high altitude: II. Morphological adaptations of human skeletal muscle to chronic hypoxia. *Int. J. Sports Med.* (in press).
11. HOPPELER H., H. HOWALD, K. CONLEY, S. L. LINSTEDT, H. CLAASSEN, P. VOCK, AND E. R. WEIBEL. Endurance training in humans: aerobic capacity and structure of skeletal muscle. *J. Appl. Physiol. 59*:320–327, 1985.

12. HOWALD, H., D. PETTE, J. A. SIMONEAU, A. UBER, H. HOPPELER, AND P. CERRETELLI. Muscular exercise at high altitude: III. Effects of chronic hypoxia on muscle enzymes. *Int. J. Sports Med.* (in press).
13. OELZ, O., H. HOWALD, P. E. DI PRAMPERO, H. HOPPELER, H. CLAASSEN, R. JENNI, A. BUHL-MANN, G. FERRETTI, J. CL. BRÜCKNER, A. VEICSTEINAS, M. GUSSONI, AND P. CERRETELLI. Physiological profile of world-class high-altitude climbers. *J. Appl. Physiol.* 60:1734–1742, 1986.
14. REYNAFARJE B. Myoglobin content and enzymatic activity of muscle and altitude adaptation. *J. Appl. Physiol.* 17:301–305, 1962.
15. SILLAU A. H., L. AQUIN, M. V. BUI, AND N. BANCHERO. Chronic hypoxia does not affect guinea pig skeletal muscle capillarity. *Pflüger's Arch.* 386:39–45, 1980.
16. SNYDER G. K., E. E. WILCOX, AND E. W. BURNHAM. Effects of hypoxia on muscle capillarity in rats. *Resp. Physiol.* 62:135–140, 1985.
17. WEST J. B. Lactate during exercise at extreme altitude. *Fed. Proc.* 45:2953–2957, 1986.
18. YOUNG A. J., W. J. EVANS, E. C. FISHER, R. L. SHARP, D. L. COSTILL, AND J. T. MAHER. Skeletal muscle metabolism of sea-level natives following short-term high-altitude residence. *Eur. J. Appl. Physiol.* 52:463–466, 1984.

16

Acclimatization and Adaptation:
Organ to Cell

JOHN B. WEST

The physiological responses to chronic hypoxia are many and varied. This chapter reviews acclimatization and adaptation to high altitude with an emphasis on the cellular and metabolic changes. This is an area where data in humans have become available only recently, but there is increasing evidence of its great importance.

ACCLIMATIZATION TO HIGH ALTITUDE.

Figure 16.1 reminds us that the most obvious features of high-altitude acclimatization are hyperventilation, polycythemia, and respiratory alkalosis. The topic of hyperventilation in response to chronic hypoxia was addressed in some detail in earlier chapters. The physiological advantage of hyperventilation at extreme altitude can hardly be overemphasized. For example, it can be shown that if a climber on the summit of Mt. Everest had the same alveolar ventilation as he does at sea level, his alveolar and, therefore, arterial Po_2 would be essentially zero. In the event, by increasing his alveolar ventilation some five- to sixfold, he maintains an alveolar Po_2 of about 35 mm Hg in spite of an inspired Po_2 of only 42 mm Hg (47, 48). Even so the arterial Po_2 is considerably lower than the alveolar value because of diffusion limitation across the blood–gas barrier and the value of the arterial Po_2 is about 28 mm Hg (47, 36). One of the consequences of this extreme hyperventilation is an astonishingly low alveolar Pco_2 of about 7.5 mm Hg.

The occurrence of polycythemia at high altitude is also well known and the regulation of red blood cell production through the erythropoietin mechanism in response to tissue hypoxia was also discussed in earlier chapters. Substantial degrees of polycythemia are frequently seen in lowlanders acclimatized to high altitude. For example, Pugh (31) reviewed results from five expeditions (51 observations in 40 subjects) and concluded that the hemoglobin concentration after about 6 weeks at high altitude averaged 20.5 g/dl and was independent of altitude above 5500 m. This corresponds to a mean hematocrit of about 60% to 62%. Permanent residents of the South American Andes have similar degrees of polycythemia for the same altitude as acclimatized lowlanders. Sherpas and Tibetans, however, apparently have lower hemoglobin levels for a given altitude as discussed by Winslow in Chapter 13.

Iceberg of Physiology of High Altitude

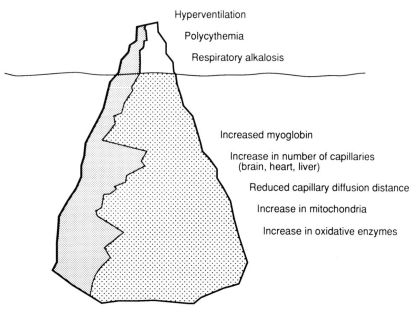

FIGURE 16.1. Physiological changes resulting from exposure to high altitude. The most obvious are hyperventilation, polycythemia, and respiratory alkalosis, but the cellular and metabolic changes may be more important.

Although at first sight the polycythemia of high altitude appears to be a useful response because it increases the oxygen-carrying capacity of the blood in the face of a low arterial Po_2, some physiologists believe that the high levels of polycythemia at extreme altitude may be counterproductive. The reason is that very high hematocrits are associated with uneven blood flow in peripheral capillaries as a result of rouleaux formation and sludging, and these phenomena may interfere with efficient oxygen unloading. Indeed some physicians, especially in Europe, have advocated hemodilution of climbers at extreme altitude claiming that this reduces the incidence of illnesses such as frostbite. This disease is believed to be caused by a combination of cold and tissue hypoxia.

In this context the results of a pilot study of hemodilution on four climbers during the 1981 American Medical Research Expedition to Everest are of interest. These subjects had the highest hematocrits seen on the expedition (mean 58%), and hemodilution was carried out by removing approximately 15% of their blood volume and replacing this with the same volume of human serum albumin. The results showed that returning the hematocrit to near normal level did not decrease exercise tolerance (33). This preliminary result certainly suggests that the polycythemia conferred little advantage. Along similar lines, Winslow and Monge (50) have actually shown improvement of exercise tolerance in high altitude Andean natives whose very high hematocrits were reduced by the removal of blood over several weeks.

These results raise the issue of whether the polycythemia of high altitude is really beneficial, at least at extreme altitudes. It should be remembered that the evolutionary pressure for the erythropoietin control of red blood cell production in response to tissue hypoxia was developed over thousands of years at sea level where it performs an important role in replacing red cells if these are lost as the result of trauma, malnutrition, or parasitic infection. The tissue hypoxia of extreme altitude, however, is caused by an entirely different mechanism and it may well be that the severe polycythemia of very high altitude actually confers no advantage.

The occurrence of respiratory alkalosis referred to in Fig. 16.1 has received relatively little attention. There is increasing evidence, however, that it plays a major role at extreme altitude by greatly increasing the oxygen affinity of the hemoglobin and thus accelerating oxygen loading in the pulmonary capillary. Although there is ample time for oxygen loading by the pulmonary capillary at sea level (Fig. 16.2A), this is not the case at extreme altitude because the rate of rise of the Po_2 of the capillary blood is so slow (Fig. 16.2B). This slow rate can be explained by two factors. First, the loading is occurring very low on the oxygen dissociation curve where the curve is very steep, and second, there is considerable polycythemia. Both factors increase the change in blood oxygen concentration per unit change of Po_2, and, therefore, delay the loading process (29).

It could be argued that the advantage that the lung gains in loading oxygen as a result of the increased hemoglobin affinity, is lost in the peripheral tissues where unloading is impeded. Modeling studies, however, show that the advantage in loading offsets the loss during unloading (6). Indeed, as will be pointed out later, an increased oxygen affinity for hemoglobin is very commonly seen in animals who live in an oxygen-deprived environment.

The alkalosis that increases the oxygen affinity of the hemoglobin is brought about by the fall in alveolar and, therefore, arterial Pco_2 as a result of the extreme hyperventilation. The degree of respiratory alkalosis is extraordinary; measurements from the 1981 American Medical Research Expedition to Everest (AMREE) indicate an arterial pH of a climber at rest on the Everest summit of between 7.7 and 7.8 (47). This calculated value is based on the measured alveolar Pco_2 of 7.5 mm Hg and a measured base excess of -7.2 mEq/L, this being the mean value of two climbers from blood taken during the morning after their successful summit climb. Measurements made during a simulated ascent of Mt. Everest during which subjects spent 40 days in a low pressure chamber (Operation Everest II, OEII) gave lower values of arterial pH on the "summit" (36). The different result, however, can be explained by the higher arterial Pco_2 values in OE II than in AMREE probably resulting from the shorter period available for acclimatization (45).

It is interesting that many members of the animal kingdom that are exposed to oxyen deprivation increase the oxygen affinity of their hemoglobin by a variety of different strategies. Perhaps the best known example is the human fetus where the oxygen affinity is enormously increased by the presence of fetal hemoglobin with an oxygen half-saturation pressure (P_{50}) of about 19 mm Hg at pH 7.4. It is remarkable that the P_{50} of a climber on the Everest summit has about the same value at his prevailing high blood pH (52). Other strategies employed include decreasing the level of 2,3-diphosphoglycerate in the red

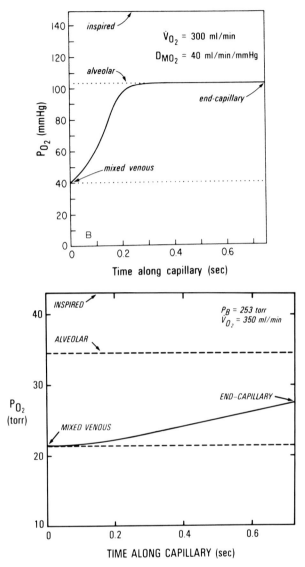

FIGURE 16.2. **(A)** Calculated time course for P_{O_2} in the pulmonary capillary at sea level in a resting human. Note that there is ample time for equilibration of the P_{O_2} between alveolar gas and end-capillary blood. From West and Wagner (49). **(B)** Similar calculation for a climber at rest on the summit of Mt. Everest. Note that there is considerable diffusion-limitation of oxygen uptake with a large alveolar end-capillary P_{O_2} difference. From West et al. (46).

blood cell (fetus of dog, horse, pig), decreasing the level of ATP in the red cell (trout, eel), and reducing the Bohr effect (tadpole). It is fascinating that the climber at extreme altitude accomplishes the same end by severe respiratory alkalosis.

Although the advantage of respiratory alkalosis is best seen at extreme altitude, there is evidence that alkalosis occurs at more moderate altitudes. For example, members of the 1981 AMREE who were living at an altitude of

6300 m at Advanced Base Camp had a mean arterial pH of 7.47 (52). Indeed, even permanent residents of Morococha in Peru (4540 m, P_B 432 mm Hg) have a mean plasma pH of 7.439 $\pm$ 0.065 according to Winslow et al. (51), indicating that they apparently have a mild degree of respiratory alkalosis as a permanent condition.

CELLULAR AND METABOLIC RESPONSES

Figure 16.1 indicates that although hyperventilation, polycythemia, and to a lesser extent respiratory alkalosis, are the traditionally recognized responses to high altitude, they may only be the tip of the iceberg. It is possible that the cellular and metabolic changes are far more important, although much less is known about these, especially in humans. This is not surprising because their investigation requires tissue samples such as muscle biopsies.

On a historical note, Paul Bert in his monumental "La Pression Barométrique" raised the question of whether the metabolism of high altitude natives is different from that of lowlanders: ". . . just as a Basque mountaineer furnished with a piece of bread and a few onions makes expeditions which require of a member of the *Alpine Club* who accompanies him the absorption of a pound of meat, so it may be that the dwellers in high places finally lessen the consumption of oxygen in their organism, while keeping at their disposal the same quantity of vital force, either for the equilibrium of temperature, or the production of work. Thus we could explain the acclimatization of individuals, of generations, of races" (7). Incidentally we now know that the oxygen requirements of a given amount of work are no different at high altitude than at sea level, or in high-altitude natives than in lowlanders. There is evidence, however, for increases in intracellular oxidative enzymes, for example, as a result of acclimatization to high altitude, supporting Bert's general thesis of metabolic adaptation.

Increased Myoglobin

Just as the concentration of hemoglobin in the blood increases at high altitude, so does the concentration of myoglobin in skeletal muscle. An early study was carried out by Hurtado et al. (16) when they showed that dogs born and raised in Morococha (4540 m) had increased concentrations of myoglobin in the diaphragm, adductor muscles of the leg, pectoral muscles of the chest, and the myocardium compared with control dogs in Lima at sea level. More recently, Reynafarje (32) showed that myoglobin concentrations in the sartorius muscle of high-altitude natives of Cerro de Pasco (4400 m) were higher (7.03 mg/g tissue) than in sea-level controls (6.07 mg/g tissue). Additional measurements of the nitrogen content of the muscle, lean body mass, and body water content confirmed that the increase in myoglobin concentration was a true high-altitude effect and not the result of dehydration. This latter factor could have explained the apparent increase in myoglobin in skeletal muscle of rats in another study (1). Other authors have also shown increases in myoglobin in skeletal muscle, myocardium, and diaphragm (10, 38, 42).

Myoglobin confers several advantages for oxygen transport in skeletal muscle including facilitating oxygen diffusion, buffering regional differences of Po_2, and providing an oxygen store for short periods of very severe oxygen deprivation. It is known that increasing oxygen demand, for example, by exercise training, raises the myoglobin content of muscles in experimental animals (22, 28). Also it is known that some animals, such as seals, that require large oxygen uptakes under conditions of reduced oxygen availability have very large amounts of myoglobin (9). Two studies of the effects of training in humans, however, have failed to show any increase in muscle myoglobin concentrations (17, 37).

Number and Density of Capillaries

Other things being equal, a reduction in intercapillary distance in peripheral tissues would enhance oxygenation, and this would be particularly valuable at high altitude where the arterial Po_2, and therefore, the diffusion head of pressure is reduced. The extent to which intercapillary distance is reduced as a result of acclimatization is not entirely clear, however, and there is evidence, for example, that if the distance is reduced in skeletal muscle, this result is brought about by a decrease in the size of the individual muscle fibers rather than an increase in the number of capillaries.

Increased vascularization of the brain, retina, skeletal muscle, and liver of experimental animals exposed to low barometric pressures over several weeks was reported in a number of early studies (8, 23, 26, 41). In addition, it was shown that the rate of loss of carbon monoxide from subcutaneous gas pockets in rats was increased by 3 weeks of simulated exposure to a 5600-m altitude in a low pressure chamber. This implied an increase in capillary number of 50% (39).

In skeletal muscle, however, the consensus now seems to be that although capillary density (number of capillaries per unit volume of tissue) is increased by exposure to high altitude, this is not caused by the formation of new capillaries, but by a reduction in size of the muscle fibers. For example, Fig. 16.3 shows data obtained by Banchero (5) in four groups of guinea pigs. Two groups were studied at sea level and Denver (1610 m), and in addition there were animals native to the Andes (3900 m), and animals exposed to a simulated altitude of 5100 m. The top panel shows that any increase in capillary density was accompanied by a reduction of fiber cross-sectional area, whereas the lower panel shows that, during normal growth, the capillary-to-fiber ratio was linearly related to the fiber cross-sectional area, and this relationship is not disturbed by exposure to hypoxia. There were no significant differences between the four groups of animals. Thus, these data are consistent with the increase in capillary density being caused by a decrease in cross-sectional area of the muscle fibers.

Recent data indicate the same result in acclimatized humans at very high altitude. As described in Chapter 15, Cerretelli and his co-workers obtained muscle biopsies on climbers after they had returned to Switzerland after attempts to climb Lhotse Shar (8398 m). These investigators found that capillary density was somewhat raised but that the increase could be wholly accounted for by a reduction of muscle fiber size.

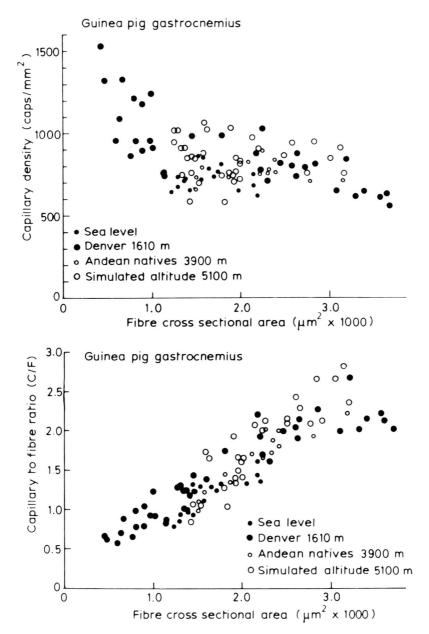

FIGURE 16.3. Capillary density (number of capillaries per mm[2] of cross section) and capillary-to-fiber ratio (number of capillaries per muscle fiber) in gastrocnemius muscle of four groups of guinea pigs. These were studied at sea level, in Denver at 1610 m, at 3900 m (Andean natives), and at a simulated altitude of 5100 m. The data are consistent with the increase in capillary-to-fiber ratio being explained by a decrease in cross-sectional area of the muscle fibers. From Banchero (5).

Similar results were obtained in Operation Everest II. In this study, eight volunteers were gradually decompressed to the simulated altitude of Mt. Everest over a period of 40 days. Capillary density increased by approximately 13% when expressed as capillaries per mm[2]. The corresponding total muscle area (as determined by CT scan), however, was reduced by approximately 11%.

Thus, the changes in capillary density reflected atrophy of the muscle and not an increase in the number of capillaries per se (MacDougall, personal communication).

A related issue is whether the configuration of the capillaries in skeletal muscle changes as a result of exposure to prolonged hypoxia. Claims that this occurs have been made (2) and it has been suggested that the increased tortuosity effectively increases capillary surface area and enhances gas diffusion. This result, however, has not been confirmed by Mathieu-Costello as described in Chapter 14. She found no change in the tortuosity of skeletal muscle capillaries in the high-altitude deer mouse *Peromyscus maniculatus* at an altitude of 3800 m, and she believes that the previous result can be explained by failure to control the state of contraction of the muscle. It should also be pointed out, however, that Mathieu-Costello did not show a decrease in muscle fiber size at 3800 m, and this may mean that the changes observed by Cerretelli and MacDougall and their colleagues only occur at high altitudes. In a recent study, Poole and Mathieu-Costello (30) showed that these results were not due to genetic factors because the same finding was seen in sea-level rats taken to 3800 m for 5 months.

The reduction of fiber size in skeletal muscle is part of the general pattern of muscle atrophy that occurs at very high altitude. The reasons for this are not fully understood. Possible factors include the reduced level of physical activity (discussed later), reduction of appetite, and impaired gastrointestinal absorption. This cannot be the whole story, however, as evidenced by experience obtained on the 1960–1961 Himalayan Scientific and Mountaineering Expedition. During several months at an altitude of 5800 m, the level of physical activity was well maintained with opportunities for daily skiing, and yet all expedition members suffered a relentless and progressive loss of weight that averaged 0.5 to 1.5 kg/week (31). Measurements of calorie intake showed that these were more than adequate for the level of physical activity. Thus, it seems very likely that there is some change in protein metabolism during severe hypoxia that results in extensive breakdown of muscle protein. Muscle biopsies taken during Operation Everest II show that the atrophy was particularly evident in type 1 compared with type 2 fibers (MacDougall, personal communication).

Volume of Mitochondria

Ou and Tenney (27) reported that the number of mitochondria in samples of myocardium was 40% greater in cattle born and raised at 4250 m compared with cattle at sea level (Fig. 16.4). They showed that the size of individual mitochondria was the same, and they argued that the increase in mitochondrial number was advantageous because it reduced the diffusion distance of the intracellular oxygen. These interesting results, however, may not apply to all species. Another study of the mitochondrial density of myocardium of rabbits and guinea pigs from Cerro de Pasco (4330 m) compared with sea level showed no increase in density (18).

Recent work shows that mitochondrial volume in human skeletal muscle decreases with exposure to very high altitude. As described in Chapter 15,

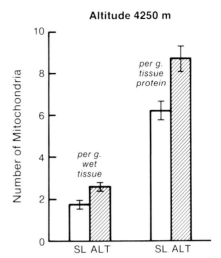

FIGURE 16.4. Increase in number of mitochondria in myocardium of cattle born and raised at 4250 m (ALT) compared with another group and raised at sea level (SL). The left hand columns show the number of mitochondria (× 10¹¹) per gram of wet tissue, and the right hand columns show the number (× 10¹¹) per gram of tissue protein. Data from Ou and Tenney (27).

Cerretelli et al. studied muscle biopsies of seven climbers shortly after they returned from the Swiss 1986 Everest Expedition and found that mitochondrial volume density decreased by 25%. This was associated with a decrease of 10% in muscle mass and a fall of 15% in muscle fiber diameter. There was also a tendency for a decrease in mitochondrial volume in leg muscle biopsies in the subjects of Operation Everest II (MacDougall, personal communication).

It should be emphasized that the level of physical activity affects mitochondrial volume. For example, physical training in humans increases mitochondrial volume density (14), and highly aerobic animals, such as the horse, have greater myochondrial densities than animals such as the cow (15). This factor should be borne in mind in interpreting the results at very high altitude (discussed later).

Intracellular Enzymes

An early study of enzymatic activity of human muscle at high altitude was carried out by Reynafarje (32). Biopsies were taken from the sartorius muscle of high altitude natives in Cerro de Pasco (4400 m), and these were compared with biopsies from residents of Lima at sea level. It was found that the activities of three of the enzymes in the electron transport chain were significantly increased in the altitude residents (NADH-oxidase, cytochrome c-reductase, and NAD[P]$^+$ transhydrogenase).

Other studies have confirmed increases in enzymes of the electron transport chain and also those of the Krebs cycle. For example, Harris et al. (13) found an increase in the activity of succinate dehydrogenase in myocardial homogenates of various species indigenous to an altitude of 4380 m, and Ou and Tenney (27) also reported increased levels of succinate dehydrogenase and several enzymes of the electron transport chain in myocardium of high-altitude cattle at 4250 m.

In contrast to the effects of moderately high altitude (3500 to 5000 m), recent measurements show that extreme altitude (above 6000 m) apparently causes a reduction in the activity of certain enzymes. As described in Chapter 15, measurements made by Cerretelli and his associates showed a reduction of enzymes of both the Krebs cycle and the electron transport chain in climbers returning from exposure to over 8000 m. Similar results were apparently found in the subjects of Operation Everest II (12).

Effect of Level of Physical Activity

Several of the cellular and metabolic variables referred to previously are altered by repeated physical exercise, such as endurance training, and this may be a factor in some of the studies at high altitude. For example, an expedition to medium altitude is very likely to be associated with an increased degree of physical activity. On the other hand, periods spent at extreme altitude (over 6000 m) are often characterized by substantial reductions of physical activity because of the difficult living conditions and the general depressive effect of severe hypoxia. Indeed the eminent mountaineer H.W. Tilman once remarked that one of the hazards of a Himalayan expedition was bed sores! (40)

Table 16.1 shows a comparison of tissue changes caused by endurance training and associated with exposure to high altitude. It shows that the fiber diameter of skeletal muscle may be increased by endurance training. By the same token, however, muscle fiber size may be decreased by inactivity (an extreme example is the muscle atrophy caused by placing a limb in a plaster cast) and this may contribute to the reduction in fiber size at extreme altitude.

Several aspects of cellular and subcellular responses to chronic hypoxia and physical training are further discussed in Chapter 2 by Wilson and Rumsey.

Medium Versus Very High Altitudes

It is probably misleading to consider medium altitudes (3500 to 5000 m) and very high altitudes (say above 6000 m) as similar environmental stresses. For example, it is known that acclimatized lowlanders can tolerate altitudes up to 5000 m with relatively few problems, and that they can live indefinitely at

TABLE 16.1. Comparison of Tissue Changes Caused by Training and Associated with Exposure to High Altitude

Tissue Changes	Endurance Training	High Altitude
Capillary density in skeletal muscle	Increase due to new capillaries	Increase due to reduction in diameter of muscle fibers
Fiber diameter of skeletal muscle	May be increased	Decreased
Myoglobin concentration	No change in humans	Increased in skeletal and heart muscle
Muscle enzymes	No change in glycolytic, increase in oxidative	Similar changes at moderate altitude? decreased at extreme altitudes

From Ward et al. (43).

such altitudes. Residence at altitudes over 6000 m, however, is generally accompanied by a substantial decrease in the level of physical activity, and a relentless loss of weight, and it is not possible for humans to live at these altitudes for more than a few months. Thus, exposure to very high altitudes inevitably causes physical deterioration, and does not result in acclimatization in the sense that the body adapts successfully to the hostile conditions.

These differences between medium and very high altitudes should be borne in mind in assessing the cellular and metabolic changes described earlier. For example, the decrease in intercapillary distance seen in humans at extreme altitudes may not reflect an improvement in oxygen delivery so much as the inevitable muscle atrophy that occurs in chronic severe hypoxia, therefore, we are seeing a pattern of chronic deterioration rather than acclimatization. The same arguments may apply to the reduction in oxidative enzymes at extreme altitude. These may well be a reflection of the general muscle atrophy rather than a specific response of the oxygen transport system.

HIGH ALTITUDE ACCLIMATIZATION, ADAPTATION, AND DETERIORATION

It is useful to reserve the terms acclimatization and adaptation for two different responses to high altitude. *Acclimatization* is the process that occurs in lowlanders who spend weeks, months, or even years at high altitude. As indicated previously, if the altitude is over about 6000 m, acclimatization may give way to high altitude *deterioration*. *Adaptation* is best reserved for the changes that occur over many generations of residents at high altitude, and it presumably represents a true genetic selective response to the hostile environment. Many of the features of acclimatization and adaptation are similar and indeed in this discussion no distinction has been made between the two. There is some evidence, however, of differences between the two processes.

One example is in the ventilatory response to hypoxia. There is evidence that acclimatized lowlanders tolerate extreme altitude best when they have a high hypoxic ventilatory response (24, 25, 34). By contrast, both high Andean natives and Sherpas have been shown to have a blunted (reduced) hypoxic ventilatory response (20, 35). In spite of this apparent limitation, the exercise tolerance of high Andean natives and Sherpas at high altitude is superior to that of lowlanders, as judged by load carrying and stamina. This has been recognized ever since Barcroft et al. (3) remarked on the ability of high-altitude natives to play football in Cerro de Pasco. Presumably this means that what high-altitude natives lose in the level of ventilation and, therefore, arterial and alveolar Po_2, they more than gain in some tissue or metabolic changes, as yet unidentified.

Another difference between acclimatized lowlanders and some high-altitude natives is the occurrence of nocturnal periodic breathing in the former but not in the latter, for example, Sherpas. It has been suggested that this is related to the difference in hypoxic ventilatory response in that the lowlanders at high altitude have such a high drive to ventilation that the control system becomes unstable (21). Instability of a control system with a very high gain is well recognized in control theory. The fact that high-altitude natives have developed a blunted hypoxic ventilatory response is advantageous in this context because they avoid nocturnal periodic breathing with the inevitable troughs of arterial hypoxemia that follow the apneic periods.

There is some evidence that the blunted hypoxic ventilatory response seen at high altitude is not due to genetic selection. For example, Weil et al. (44) showed that lowlanders living for 3 to 39 years at an altitude of 3100 m developed gradual blunting of their hypoxic response. In addition, Lahiri et al. (19) reported that the children of Andean Indians had a normal hypoxic ventilatory response that only became blunted as they grew into adulthood at altitude. Finally, children born at sea level with cyanotic congenital heart disease have been shown to have a low hypoxic ventilatory response (11).

Another possible difference between acclimatization and adaptation is the degree of polycythemia as discussed by Winslow in Chapter 13. The hypothesis is that the Tibetan race, which has been at high altitude for a much longer period than the high Andean natives, has developed lower hemoglobin levels for a given altitude. As described earlier, the very high hematocrits of high altitude may be disadvantageous because abnormalities of capillary blood flow caused by the increased viscosity of the blood may interfere with oxygen unloading. Thus, adaptation in this setting would be a more modest increase in red blood cell concentration.

In summary, although a great deal is known about the more obvious features of acclimatization and adaptation to high altitude, such as the hyperventilation and polycythemia, our knowledge of the cellular and metabolic responses is in its infancy. This is an area where a great acceleration of knowledge can be expected over the next few years.

REFERENCES

1. ANTHONY, A., E. ACKERMAN, AND G. K. STROTHER. Effects of altitude acclimatization on rat myoglobin. Changes in myoglobin content of skeletal and cardiac muscle. *Am. J. Physiol. 196*:512–516, 1959.
2. APPELL, H. J. Capillary density and patterns in skeletal muscles. III. Changes of the capillary pattern after hypoxia. (Abstr) *Pflugers Arch. 377*:R–53, 1978.
3. BARCROFT, J., C. A. BINGER, A. V. BOCK, J. H. DOGGART, H. S. FORBES, G. HARROP, J. C. MEAKINS, AND A. C. REDFIELD. Observations upon the effect of high altitude on the physiological processes of the human body, carried out in the Peruvian Andes, chiefly at Cerro de Pasco. *Phil. Trans. Royal. Soc., Ser. B, 211*:351–480, 1923.
5. BANCHERO, N. Long-term adaptation of skeletal muscle capillarity. *Physiologist 25*:385–389, 1982.
6. BENCOWITZ, H. Z., P. D. WAGNER, AND J. B. WEST. Effect of change in P_{50} on exercise tolerance at high altitude: a theoretical study. *J. Appl. Physiol. 53*:1487–1495, 1982.
7. BERT, P. *La Pression Barométrique.* Paris: Masson, 1878. English translation by M. A. Hitchcock and F. A. Hitchcock. Columbus, OH: College Book Co., 1943, p. 1004.
8. CASSIN, S. R., D. GILBERT, C. F. BUNNELL, AND E. M. JOHNSON. Capillary development during exposure to chronic hypoxia. *Am. J. Physiol. 220*:448–451, 1971.
9. CASTELLINI, M. A., AND G. N. SOMERO. Buffering capacity of vertebrate muscle: correlations with potentials for anaerobic function. *J. Comp. Physiol. 143*:191–198, 1981.
10. CLARK, R. T., JR., D. CRISCUOLO, AND D. K. COULSON. Effects of 20,000 feet simulated altitude on myoglobin content of animals with and without exercise. *Federation Proc. 11*:25, 1952.
11. EDELMAN, N. H., S. LAHIRI, L. BRUADO, N. S. CHERNIACK, AND A. P. FISHMAN. The blunted ventilatory response to hypoxia in cyanotic congenital heart disease. *N. Engl. J. Med. 282*:405–411, 1970.

12. GREEN, H. J., J. R. SUTTON, A. CYMERMAN, AND C. S. HOUSTON. Enzyme levels measured on muscle biopsies during Operation Everest II. *J. Appl. Physiol.* 66:142–150, 1989.

13. HARRIS, P., Y. CASTILLO, K. GIBSON, D. HEATH, AND J. ARIAS-STELLA. Succinic and lactic dehydrogenase activity in myocardial homogenates from animals at high and low altitude. *J. Mol. Cell. Cardiol.* 1:189–193, 1970.

14. HOLLOSZY, J. O., AND E. F. COYLE. Adaptations of skeletal muscle to endurance exercise and their metabolic consequences. *J. Appl. Physiol.* 56:831–838, 1984.

15. HOPPELER, H., S. R. KAYAR, H. CLAASEN, E. UHLMANN, AND R. H. KARAS. Adaptive variation in the mammalian respiratory system in relation to energetic demand: III. Skeletal muscles: setting the demand for oxygen. *Respir. Physiol.* 69:27–46, 1987.

16. HURTADO, A., A. ROTTA, AND C. MERINO. Studies of myohemoglobin at high altitudes. *Am. J. Med. Sci.* 194:708–713, 1937.

17. JANSSON, E., C. SYLVEN, AND E. NORDEVANG. Myoglobin in the quadriceps femoris muscle of competitive cyclists and untrained men. *Acta Physiol. Scand.* 114:627–629, 1982.

18. KEARNEY, M. S. Ultrastructural changes in the heart at high altitude. *Pathologia et Microbiologia* 39:258–265, 1973.

19. LAHIRI, S., R. G. DELANEY, J. S. BRODY, M. SIMPSER, T. VELASQUEZ, E.K. MONTOYAMA, AND C. POLGAR. Relative role of environmental and genetic factors in respiratory adaptation to high altitude. *Nature (London)* 261: 133–135, 1976.

20. LAHIRI, S., F. F. KAO, T. VELASQUEZ, C. MARTINEZ, AND W. PEZZIA. Irreversible blunted sensitivity in high altitude natives. *Respir. Physiol.* 6:360–367, 1969.

21. LAHIRI, S., K. MARET, AND M. G. SHERPA. Dependence of high altitude sleep apnea on ventilatory sensitivity to hypoxia. *Respir. Physiol.* 52:281–301, 1983.

22. LAWRIE, R. A. Effect of enforced exercise on myoglobin concentration in muscle. *Nature (London)* 171:1069–1070, 1953.

23. MERCKER, H., AND M. SCHNEIDER. Über Capillarveranderungen des Gehirns bei Hohenanpassung. *Pflugers Arch.* 251:49–55, 1949.

24. MUSUYAMA, S., H. KIMURA, T. SUGITA, T. KURIYAMA, F. KUNITOMO, S. OKITA, H. TOJIMA, Y. YUGUCHI, S. WATANABE, AND Y. HONDA. Control of ventilation in extreme-altitude climbers. *J. Appl. Physiol.* 61:500–506, 1986.

25. OELZ, O., H. HOWALD, P. E. DIPRAMPERO, H. HOPPELER, H. CLASSEN, R. JENNI, A. BÜHLMANN, G. FERRETTI, J. C. BRÜCHNER, A. VEICSTEINAS, M. GUSSONI, AND P. CERRETELLI. Physiological profile of world-class high-altitude climbers. *J. Appl. Physiol.* 60:1734–1742, 1986.

26. OPITZ, E. Increased vascularization of the tissue due to acclimatization to high altitude and its significance for oxygen transport. *Exper. Med. Surg.* 9:389–403, 1951.

27. OU, L. C., AND S. M. TENNEY. Properties of mitochondria from hearts of cattle acclimatized to high altitude. *Respir. Physiol.* 8:151–159, 1970.

28. PATTENGALE, P. K., AND J. O. HOLLOSZY. Augmentation of skeletal muscle myoglobin by a program of treadmill running. *Am. J. Physiol.* 213:783–785, 1967.

29. PIIPER, J., AND P. SCHEID. Blood-gas equilibration in lungs. In: *Pulmonary Gas Exchange, Volume 1, Ventilation, Blood Flow, and Diffusion,* ed. J. B. West. New York: Academic Press, 1980, pp. 131–171.

30. POOLE, D. C., AND O. MATHIEU-COSTELLO. Skeletal muscle capillary geometry: adaptation to chronic hypoxia. *Respir. Physiol.* 77:21–30, 1989.

31. PUGH, L. G. C. E. Animals in high altitudes: Man above 5000 m—Mountain exploration. In: *Handbook of Physiology Section 4,* eds. D. B. Dill, E. F. Adolph, and C. G. Wilber. Washington, D.C.: American Physiological Society, 1964.

32. REYNAFARJE, B. Myoglobin content and enzymatic activity of muscle and altitude adaptation. *J. Appl. Physiol.* 17:301–305, 1962.

33. SARNQUIST, F. H., R. B. SCHOENE, P. H. HACKETT, AND B. D. TOWNES. Hemodilution of polycythemic mountaineers: effects on exercise and mental function. *Aviat. Space Environ. Med.* 57:313–317, 1986.

34. SCHOENE, R. B., S. LAHIRI, P. H. HACKETT, R. M. PETERS, JR., J. S. MILLEDGE, C. J. PIZZO, F. H. SARNQUIST, S. J. BOYER, D. J. GRABER, K. H. MARET, AND J. B. WEST. Relationship of hypoxic ventilatory response to exercise performance on Mount Everest. *J. Appl. Physiol.* 56:1478–1483, 1984.

35. SEVERINGHAUS, J. W., C. R. BAINTON, AND A. CARCELEN. Respiratory insensitivity to hypoxia in chronically hypoxic man. *Respir. Physiol.* 1:308–334, 1966.

36. SUTTON, J. R., J. T. REEVES, P. D. WAGNER, B. M. GROVES, A. CYMERMAN, M. K. MALCONIAN, P. B. ROCK, P. M. YOUNG, S. D. WALTER, AND C. S. HOUSTON. Operation Everest II: oxygen transport during exercise at extreme simulated altitude. *J. Appl. Physiol.* 64:1309–1321, 1988.

37. SVEDENHAG, J., J. HENRIKSSON, AND C. SYLVEN. Dissociation of training effects on skeletal

muscle mitochondrial enzymes and myoglobin in man. *Acta Physiol. Scand. 117*:213–218, 1983.

38. TAPPAN, D. V., AND B. D. REYNAFARJE. Tissue pigment manifestation of adaptation to high altitudes. *Am. J. Physiol. 190*:99–103, 1957.
39. TENNEY, S. M., AND L. C. OU. Physiological evidence for increased tissue capillarity in rats acclimatized to high altitude. *Respir. Physiol. 8*:137–150, 1970.
40. TILMAN, H. W. *Nepal—Himalaya.* Cambridge: Cambridge University Press, 1952, p. 79.
41. VALDIVIA, E. Total capillary bed in striated muscle of guinea pigs native to the Peruvian mountains. *Am. J. Physiol. 194*:585–589, 1958.
42. VAUGHAN, B. E., AND N. PACE. Changes in myoglobin content of the high altitude acclimatized rat. *Am. J. Physiol. 185*:549–556, 1956.
43. WARD, M. P., J. S. MILLEDGE, AND J. B. WEST. *High Altitude Medicine and Physiology.* London: Chapman and Hall Medical, 1989.
44. WEIL, J. V., E. BYRNE-QUINN, I. E. SODAL, G. F. FILLEY, AND R. F. GROVER. Acquired attenuation of chemoreceptor function in chronically hypoxic man at high altitude. *J. Clin. Invest. 50*:186–195, 1971.
45. WEST, J. B. Rate of ventilatory acclimatization to extreme altitude. *Respir. Physiol. 74*:323–333, 1988.
46. WEST, J. B., S. J. BOYER, D. J. GRABER, P. H. HACKETT, K. H. MARET, J. S. MILLEDGE, R. M. PETERS, JR., C. J. PIZZO, M. SAMAJA, F. H. SARNQUIST, R. B. SCHOENE, AND R. M. WINSLOW. Maximal exercise at extreme altitudes on Mount Everest. *J. Appl. Physiol. 55*:688–698, 1983.
47. WEST, J. B., P. H. HACKETT, K. H. MARET, J. S. MILLEDGE, R. M. PETERS, JR., C. J. PIZZO, AND R. M. WINSLOW. Pulmonary gas exchange on the summit of Mt. Everest. *J. Appl. Physiol. 55*:678–687, 1983.
48. WEST, J. B., S. LAHIRI, K. H. MARET, R. M. PETERS, JR., AND C. J. PIZZO. Barometric pressures at extreme altitudes on Mt. Everest: physiological significance. *J. Appl. Physiol. 54*:1188–1194, 1983.
49. WEST, J. B., AND P. D. WAGNER. Predicted gas exchange on the summit of Mt. Everest. *Respir. Physiol. 42*:1–16, 1980.
50. WINSLOW, R. M., AND C. C. MONGE. *Hypoxia, Polycythemia, and Chronic Mountain Sickness.* Baltimore: Johns Hopkins University Press, 1987, p. 184.
51. WINSLOW, R. M., MONGE, C. C., STATHAM, J. J., GIBSON, C. G., CHARACHE, S., WHITTEMBURY, J., MORAN, O., AND BERGER, R. L. Variability of oxygen affinity of blood: human subjects native to high altitude. *J. Appl. Physiol. 51*:1411–1416, 1981.
52. WINSLOW, R. M., M. SAMAJA, AND J. B. WEST. Red cell function at extreme altitude on Mount Everest. *J. Appl. Physiol. 56*:109–116, 1984.

17

Inborn Resistance to Hypoxia in High Altitude Adapted Humans

P. W. HOCHACHKA, G. O. MATHESON, W. S. PARKHOUSE,
J. SUMAR-KALINOWSKI, C. STANLEY, C. MONGE, D. C. MCKENZIE, J. MERKT,
S. F. P. MAN, R. JONES, and P. S. ALLEN

Whereas the theme of these chapters aims to unravel mechanisms of adaptation to the environment, most of our analyses to this point have focused more on the mechanisms and less on adaptation per se. At least a part of our assignment is to explore the connections between these two processes, as the latter sets limits and requirements on the former. That is why biologists have long recognized the intricate interplay between clock time and adaptational strategies or "options" available to organisms in specific hostile environments. Long-term adaptations are compensatory processes that are selectively advantageous and may be developmentally or genetically fixed and unchangeable. Acclimations (or acclimatizations) are less constrained, usually fully reversible adaptational processes that may be activated within a fraction of the organism's life cycle. Finally, acute adaptations are those that can be turned on as a practically instantaneous response to (change in) the environment (3,5). In this chapter we briefly review very recent evidence that we have accumulated, which bears on these three kinds of adaptations in high-altitude adapted Andean people.

Although we are not the first to have addressed these problems [for example, see reviews of this area in Winslow and Monge (9)], our program apparently is the first to have reversed the time-honored research strategy of taking the laboratory to the subjects under study. To maximize our chances of working out fundamental adaptational strategies in indigenous highlanders we reasoned that we should take our subjects to our home laboratories, rather than vice versa. To this end, six Quechua Indians, born and living essentially all of their lives in the La Raya area of Peru at altitudes ranging from 3600 to 4500 m, volunteered to fly to Vancouver, Canada, to participate in a 6-week deacclimation study. Several functional links in the transfer of oxygen from air to working mitochondria (8) were closely monitored, including the lung, the heart, the blood and circulation, and skeletal muscles; the path was examined invasively and noninvasively, when the subjects were at rest, and when they were exercising at varying intensities ultimately to fatigue.

As may well have been anticipated from animal studies (8), we found that some processes in gas exchange and metabolism showed evidence of long-term (developmental or genetic) adaptation, some showed acclimation capacities, and some showed acute adaptational capacities. For example, several functional features of the lung were measurably unique and dramatically different from homologous lung functions in lowlanders, yet showed no change on deacclimation. Our tentative interpretation is that these functions or links in the path of oxygen in high-altitude adapted Quechuas are long-term developmental or genetic adaptations, analogous to the interspecies scaling adaptations studied in detail by Taylor (7) and Weibel (8). A number of similar conclusions arose from functional studies of the heart at rest and during exercise and in the metabolic properties of skeletal muscle. The latter was particularly instructive and deserves special emphasis.

In the first place, we found that, as was previously reported by others (1, 2, 10), Andean natives display the lactate paradox: during incremental aerobic (bicycle ergometer) exercise tests to fatigue under hypoxic conditions they form less lactate and accumulate it to lower levels than in normoxic lowlanders. In lowlanders, this characteristic is an acclimation: it requires about 10 to 20 days at altitude to be expressed (6, 10) and it is lost along a similar time course on descent. Andean natives, in contrast, express the lactate paradox even 6 weeks after descent, and indeed after 6 weeks of reacclimation to high altitude. Thus, we conclude that it too is a fixed metabolic feature that we tentatively term the *perpetual lactate paradox*. Because it is an expression of oxidative metabolism, a part of the last link in the path of oxygen from atmosphere to mitochondria (7, 8) that seems fixed and does not deacclimate, we also assume at least for now that it is a developmental or genetic adaptation.

Although the adaptive significance of the lactate paradox at high altitude is well recognized (both the excessive production of lactate and its accumulation under these conditions are counterproductive), the metabolic or molecular mechanisms underlying this unique regulatory interaction between aerobic and anaerobic metabolism have remained a mystery for more than 50 years (2). 31P-NMR spectroscopy studies using a calf muscle ergometer arranged for function within a 1-m 1.5 T magnet allowed us to look for mechanisms underlying the lactate paradox. Earlier on, West (10) and Cerretelli (1) hypothesized that high-altitude adapted individuals may display a more labile intracellular muscle pH; they supposed that an inordinately large drop in muscle pH for a given level of work would serve to inhibit glycolysis (by phosphofructokinase inhibition). If real, this process could well account for the lactate paradox. Our NMRS measurements rule out that alternative: if anything, skeletal muscle in Quechuas displays more stable intracellular pH than in lowlanders, and this difference is retained during work while breathing hypoxic air. Instead of differences in muscle pH homeostasis, it appears that differences in energy coupling stabilization lie at the heart of the lactate paradox in Quechua muscle (4). We hypothesize that the difference between skeletal muscle metabolism in Quechuas and lowlanders is similar to the difference between cardiac and skeletal muscles, but that the difference is less extreme. In the cardiac muscle, energy demand and energy supply functions are so closely balanced that large changes in work rate are achieved with minimal or no changes in concentrations of high energy phosphate metabolites and with minimal or no lactate production at all. In contrast, in working skeletal muscle, change in work rate is usually accompanied by changes in high energy phosphate metabolites and particularly in the phosphorylation potential. The latter is usually considered to supply kinetic and thermodynamic drive for oxidative metabolism and to account for the large increase in oxygen consumption that skeletal muscle can sustain during work. What is often overlooked, or at least underemphasized, is that the same signals that are used to turn on oxidative metabolism serve (kinetically and thermodynamically) to activate glycolysis. That is why aerobically working skeletal muscle generates lactate in proportion to the work rate, in contrast to cardiac muscle that does not produce lactate under these conditions. Given this spectrum of metabolic organization (from the classic skeletal muscle situation as exemplified by the dog gracilis muscle to the situation in the cardiac muscle), we hypothesize that high-altitude acclimation in healthy lowlanders moves skeletal muscle metabolic regulation toward the cardiac end of the spectrum (4) and that in high-altitude adapted Quechuas, this requirement for close energy demand–supply coupling has improved even further. At this time we infer that the tighter energy coupling observed in muscles of Andean natives is a constrained or fixed metabolic characteristic: this regulatory component in the final link of the path of oxygen in vivo (8) is thus tentatively assumed to be a developmental or genetic adaptation.

In contrast to the fixed characteristics, change in hematocrit and hemoglobin content of the blood as a function of time at sea level is a classic example of an acclimation process; as far as we know, this process starts soon after descent and apparently is approaching a new steady state after 6 weeks at sea level, as often observed in the past (9). From data in the literature (9, 10), it is known that concomitant changes in hemoglobin modulators also occur over time courses of days to weeks; again we consider these to be standard acclimations (3, 5). Correlated with these compensatory adjustments, in our study we observed systematic changes in cardiac function that compensate for changes in oxygen-carrying capacity of the blood; as a result, oxygen delivery for a given intensity of work is the same as before, during, and after deacclimation at sea level for at least 6 weeks.

Finally, to complete the adaptational sequence, it is instructive to note that we also observed at least two examples of acute adaptational response to hypoxia: in both anaerobic and maximum aerobic metabolism tests, our Quechua subjects showed a high degree of resistance to hypoxia. With acute exposure to hypoxic air (equivalent in oxygen content to that found in their indigenous environment in the Andes), metabolic and physiological compensatory mechanisms were so effective that they allowed near (89 to 95%) normal performance despite reduced oxygen availability in the inspired air. Similarly, switching from normoxia to breathing hypoxic air did not significantly alter the 31P-NMR spectra of high energy phosphate metabolites in working skeletal muscles, implying that here too acute adjustments were able to fully compensate for the reduced oxygen availability in the inspired air.

Taken together, we consider that our data clearly demonstrate some adaptable and some constrained (largely unchangeable) components in the path of oxygen from air in the lungs to water in the mitochondria. Generally, however, we do not understand what constraints require some functions to behave in a seemingly fixed and unchangable way, whereas other functions can be adjusted through acute (very short-term) adaptations or through acclimatory (medium-term) compensations. The principle, however, that adaptive change in one component of the path of oxygen must be matched by appropriate tuning up of all other links in the overall pathway is strongly supported by these new data on adaptation in humans. This principle was first and most forcefully illustrated in scaling studies of animals varying greatly in body mass (7, 8); although cast as a universal principle, to date it has been missing the elements of time course and kinetics of adaptation. At least some of these missing elements are now clarified for humans during adaptation to the hypobaric hypoxia of the high Andes.

ACKNOWLEDGMENTS

These studies could not have been performed without the enthusiastic cooperation and assistance of numerous volunteers from La Raya, Peru. Especial thanks are due the Univ. of Cusco, the Univ. of San Marcos, and Cayetano Heredia University, all of Peru, for collaborative and cooperative efforts far beyond our wildest expectations. Financial support for the work was provided by NSERC and MRC (Ottawa, Canada) as well as by the Alberta Heritage Foundation for Medical Research. It is planned to have the work published in entirety in an upcoming issue of *Respiration Physiology*.

REFERENCES

1. CERRETELLI, P. Gas exchange at high altitude. In: *Pulmonary Gas Exchange*, Vol. II, ed. West, J. B. New York: Academic Press, 1980, pp. 97–147.
2. EDWARDS, H. T. Lactic acid in rest and work at high altitude. *Am. J. Physiol. 116*:367–375, 1936.
3. HOCHACHKA, P. W. Exercise limitations at high altitude: the metabolic problem and search for its solution. In: *Circulation, Respiration and Metabolism*, ed. Gilles, R. Berlin: Springer-Verlag, 1985, pp. 240–249.
4. HOCHACHKA, P. W. The lactate paradox: analysis of underying mechanisms. *Annals Sports Med. 4*(4), 1989.
5. HOCHACHKA, P. W., AND G. N. SOMERO. *Biochemical Adaptation*. Princeton: Princeton Univ. Press, 1984.
6. SUTTON J. R., J. T. REEVES, P. D. WAGNER, B. M. GROVES, A. CYMERMAN, M. K. MALCONIAN, P. B. ROCK, P. M. YOUNG, S. D. WALTER, AND C. S. HOUSTON. Operation Everest II: oxygen transport during exercise at extreme simulated altitude. *J. Appl. Physiol. 64*:1309–1321, 1988.
7. TAYLOR, C. R. Structural and functional limits to oxidative metabolism: insights from scaling. *Ann. Rev. Physiol. 49*:135–147, 1987.
8. WEIBEL, E. R. *The Pathway For Oxygen*. Cambridge, MA: Harvard Univ. Press, 1984.
9. WINSLOW, R. M., AND C. MONGE. *Hypoxia, Polycythemia, and Chronic Mountain Sickness*. Baltimore: Johns Hopkins Univ. Press, 1987.
10. WEST, J. B. Lactate during exercise at extreme altitude. *Fed. Proc. 45*:2953–2957, 1986.

18

Differences in Pulmonary and Systemic Arterial Endothelial Cell Adaptation to Chronic Hypoxia

HARRISON W. FARBER

In vivo, vascular beds often respond to changes in ambient oxygen in diverse ways. For example, a decrease in oxygen concentration causes pulmonary vascular beds to vasoconstrict, while causing systemic vascular beds to vasodilate. This differential response to the same stimulus suggests some inherent difference in the oxygen-sensing mechanism or the translation of this signal within the vascular bed. Because endothelial cells are positioned such that they should be the initial cell within the vascular wall to detect a change in blood oxygen concentration, studies on the effect of acute and chronic hypoxia on these cells might define the oxygen-sensing mechanisms and uncover the inherent differences between aortic and pulmonary arterial endothelial cells. Because whole animal preparations are composed of numerous cell types, use of cultured endothelial cells would seem to be an excellent alternative to investigate the differences between endothelial cells of the two vascular beds. Until now, however, most studies have examined the effects of hypoxia on endothelial cells from a single vascular bed. In addition, endothelial cells from several different species have been used. Optimally, to obviate potential species differences or variability of animals within the same species, it would be better to use endothelial cells from both the pulmonary and the systemic circulation from the same animal and compare the responses in the same study.

DEFINITION OF CHRONIC HYPOXIA

In vivo, most studies of the effects of chronic hypoxia have used hypoxic exposures of at least 1 week. What consitutes chronic hypoxia in an in vitro system, however, is not known. In most in vitro studies, the duration of hypoxia has been less than 24 hours and in no previous study has the endothelial cell exposure to hypoxia been greater than 96 hours. Whether this exposure to hypoxia is sufficient to be termed chronic hypoxia or whether it corresponds to an in vivo model is not yet known. But, for the purposes of this discussion, studies of endothelial cells exposed to hypoxia for 24 hours or more are examined.

CHARACTERIZATION OF ENDOTHELIAL CELLS MAINTAINED IN
CHRONIC HYPOXIA

In an attempt to avoid the problems noted previously, we have maintained
endothelial cells in an hypoxic environment from the time of harvesting for
periods of several months (6). Once we were able to maintain bovine aortic and
pulmonary artery endothelial cells in a chronic hypoxic environment (10% or
3% oxygen), we characterized the endothelial cells maintained under these
conditions to prove that they continued to function as endothelial cells.

Even after several months in 10% oxygen, endothelial cells retained a
characteristic "cobblestone appearance"; however, in 3% oxygen, the endothelial cells become somewhat elongated. In either hypoxic condition, the endothelial cells demonstrated immunofluorescence to Factor VIII and retained angiotensin converting enzyme (ACE) activity, although it was decreased in cells
maintained in 3% oxygen. In addition, chronically hypoxic endothelial cells
took up a specific marker, fluorescent acetylated-low density lipoprotein, in a
similar manner as endothelial cells maintained in standard culture conditions
(21% oxygen) for the same amount of time (15).

Once we had determined that chronically hypoxic endothelial cells retained markers associated with normal endothelial cell function, we then assessed their growth patterns and some of their metabolic functions and compared our results with those obtained in endothelial cells maintained in
hypoxia for shorter periods.

CELL GROWTH/CELLULAR PROTEIN

In studies of bovine pulmonary arterial endothelial cells grown initially in 20%
oxygen and then exposed to 3% oxygen during a 48-to-72 hour experimental
period, a downward, although not significant, trend in cell number was noted
at both 48 and 72 hours when compared with cell growth in 20% oxygen (11,
12). In these studies, cell viability in 3% oxygen, as assessed by phase contrast
microscopy, trypan blue exclusion, LDH release, or ATP content, was not com-
promised (11, 12). Our studies (6) of cell growth after exposure to hypoxia dif-
fered somewhat from those studies cited. We used bovine pulmonary arterial
and aortic endothelial cells from the same animal and compared the growth of
each type of cell with cells grown in 21% oxygen and cells from the other vascular bed. We investigated cell growth for periods up to 144 hours after seeding
and at different oxygen concentrations (10% or 3% oxygen). Finally, before
their utilization in these experiments, the cells had been maintained in the
same oxygen concentration since their harvesting. Under these conditions, we
have found that the growth of pulmonary arterial endothelial cells is much
less affected by long-term exposure to hypoxia than aortic endothelial cells. In
10% oxygen, pulmonary arterial endothelial cells grow as well as in 21% oxygen. In 3% oxygen, there is a downward trend in cell number as noted, that
becomes greater, and significant, the longer the hypoxic exposure. In contrast,
in 10% oxygen, aortic endothelial cells grow in a fashion similar to pulmonary
arterial cells grown in 3% oxygen. In 3% oxygen, the growth of aortic endothelial cells is markedly depressed.

TABLE 18.1. Effect of Chronic Hypoxia on Cultured Endothelial Cells
(Characterization of Cells)

		AEC	PAEC
LDL uptake	10% oxygen	+	+
	3% oxygen	+	+
Factor VIII	10% oxygen	+	+
	3% oxygen	+	+
Cell growth	10% oxygen	↓	0
	3% oxygen	↓ ↓	↓
Protein content	10% oxygen	↓	0/ ↓
	3% oxygen	↓ ↓	↓

AEC, aortic endothelial cells; PAEC, pulmonary arterial endothelial cells.
Data from Ref. 6.

   Associated with the decrease in cell growth is a reduction in cellular protein content. In other studies (11, 12), a trend toward decreased protein content/cell has been noted. We have found that, during the first few weeks in an hypoxic environment, the protein content of the cells slowly falls (Barnett, H.F. and Farber, H.W., unpublished data). After several weeks in hypoxia the protein content/cell stabilizes and remains constant for the duration of the culture period. Similar to what was found with growth rates, aortic endothelial cells are much more sensitive to chronic hypoxia than are pulmonary arterial endothelial cells. Protein content/cell in aortic endothelial cells grown long-term in 3% oxygen falls to about half of that seen in cells grown in standard culture conditions. The protein content/cell in pulmonary artery endothelial cells grown long-term in 3% oxygen also decreases, but to a much smaller extent (approximately 25%).
   In summary (Table 18.1), it appears that both aortic and pulmonary arterial endothelial cells can be grown chronically in a low oxygen environment, that they retain characteristics associated with cultured endothelial cells, and that pulmonary arterial endothelial cells are more tolerant of a low oxygen environment than aortic endothelial cells with respect to cell growth and protein content/cell.

METABOLIC FUNCTIONS

There is little information concerning the effect of chronic hypoxia on endothelial cell function and even less examining a difference between the response of aortic and pulmonary arterial endothelial cells. In this section, we review the currently available data on enzyme activity, cell surface integrity, and production of cytokines in chronically hypoxic endothelial cells.

Enzyme Activity

Study of bioenergetic enzyme activity in bovine aortic and pulmonary arterial endothelial cells exposed to 0% oxygen for 96 hours has demonstrated a pattern favoring glycolysis (2). In both cell types there was an increase in the activity of two glycolytic enzymes (pyruvate kinase and phosphofructokinase) and no significant change in the activity of cytochrome oxidase, an enzyme of oxidative phosphorylation. This pattern was the reverse of the pattern seen in both cell types in normoxic conditions; that is, a pattern favoring oxidative phosphorylation. Study of freshly isolated intimal strips from the aorta and pulmonary artery seemed to indicate that a similar pattern exists in vivo (2). Strips from the pulmonary artery had greater activity of the glycolytic enzyme, pyruvate kinase, than strips isolated from the aorta, apparently reflecting the difference in blood oxygen tension to which the two vascular beds are exposed in vivo.

In a study of ACE activity, bovine pulmonary arterial endothelial cells exposed to 3% oxygen for 24 to 48 hours demonstrated increased cellular ACE activity, without a concomitant increase in ACE activity released into the supernatant (11). Only pulmonary arterial endothelial cells, however, were studied. We find a decrease in ACE activity in both cell types maintained in chronic hypoxia (6), but this is not inconsistent with the above study. In our experiments, ACE activity was assessed at times in which the endothelial cells had been maintained in hypoxia for much longer periods than 48 hours. The ACE activity seemed to mirror the cellular protein content/synthesis of the cells at this time, which had decreased with the continued hypoxia.

Membrane and Cell Surface Integrity

Exposure to 3% oxygen for 72 hours significantly altered proteoglycan production of bovine pulmonary arterial endothelial cells (10). The amount of ^{35}S-proteoglycan released into the medium in the subsequent 5-hour labeling period was decreased to a greater extent than the amount of ^{35}S-proteoglycan that remained cell associated. The decrease was secondary to a reduction in heparan sulfate, as the amount of chondroitin sulfate did not change. In these experiments, proteoglycans produced after hypoxic exposure were of similar size as those produced by endothelial cells cultured in 20% oxygen; in addition, glycosaminoglycan sulfation did not appear to change. In these experiments, there was no evaluation of the effect of hypoxic exposure on proteoglycan production in aortic endothelial cells.

Another marker of cell membrane integrity is the uptake of serotonin by endothelial cells. Serotonin is avidly taken up by vascular endothelial cells both in vivo and in vitro and this uptake has been used as a marker of endothelial cell injury (8). In vitro, pulmonary arterial endothelial cells exposed to 3% oxygen for 24 to 48 hours demonstrated a twofold increase in the uptake of serotonin compared with control cells (12). This increase in serotonin uptake was not accompanied by evidence of cell injury and was similar in both pulmonary arterial and aortic cells. Further investigation of the mechanism of this increase in serotonin uptake has demonstrated an apparent association with enhanced glycolytic activity in the cell (13), but the direct connection between these two phenomena remains unclear.

Cytokine Production

By definition, cytokines are substances produced by one cell type that have a functional or activational effect on another cell type. In one study, bovine pulmonary arterial endothelial cells exposed to 0% oxygen for 24 hours released a peptide(s) that was mitogenic for pulmonary arterial smooth muscle cells (16). This factor did not appear after 24-hour exposure to 5% oxygen, was not apparent in cells maintained in 21% oxygen for a similar amount of time, and was not released by aortic endothelial cells exposed to 0% oxygen for 24 hours. Further study has demonstrated that this factor was not stored, but was apparently newly synthesized, by pulmonary arterial endothelial cells and had an approximate molecular weight of 30 to 65 kd (7). Other investigators, however, have not demonstrated release of a mitogen for smooth muscle cells from pulmonary arterial endothelial cells exposed to 3% oxygen for 48 hours; on the contrary, an inhibitor of smooth muscle growth with an apparent molecular weight of less than 10 kd has been found (9, 14). Although there were some differences in the methods of the two studies, the reason for the marked difference in results has not been clarified.

We have been interested in cytokine release by cultured endothelial cells (3, 4) and have been particularly intrigued by a differential release of a cytokine for neutrophils, neutrophil chemoattractant activity (NCA) by endothelial cells from different vascular beds maintained in 21% oxygen and exposed to 4 hours of acute hypoxia (5). We have found that bovine aortic endothelial cells release NCA when exposed acutely to either 10% or 3% oxygen, whereas pulmonary arterial endothelial cells release NCA only when exposed to 0% oxygen. When maintained long term in 10% or 3% oxygen, neither cell type releases this factor spontaneously (6). Aortic endothelial cells, however, maintained in long-term hypoxia release NCA when exposed acutely to an oxygen concentration below that in which they are maintained chronically. Once again, pulmonary arterial endothelial cells release NCA when exposed acutely to 0% oxygen if maintained long term in 10% oxygen, but this response is abolished when they are exposed to 0% oxygen after being maintained chronically in 3% oxygen. In all cases, these differences in NCA release are not associated with any evidence of cell injury.

In further experiments, we have examined the release of other mediators, such as prostacyclin and thromboxane, from endothelial cells (1). We have found that baseline prostacyclin production in both aortic and pulmonary arterial endothelial cells maintained long term in 3% oxygen is decreased by approximately 25% compared with production in cells maintained in 21% oxygen. Baseline thromboxane production under the same conditions is decreased by 50% in both cell types compared with production in cells maintained in 21% oxygen. Exposure of these chronically hypoxic endothelial cells to acute hypoxia (0% oxygen) causes a differential release of these cyclooxygenase metabolites. Acute exposure to 0% oxygen causes no change in release of prostacyclin from either cell type. In contrast, acute exposure to 0% oxygen causes a marked increase in thromboxane release from pulmonary arterial endothelial cells without any change in thromboxane release from aortic endothelial cells. This pattern of cyclooxygenase release is markedly different from the pattern seen after exposure of endothelial cells maintained in 21% oxygen and exposed to acute hypoxia. Under these conditions there is an increased release of both cylcooxygenase products from both cell types.

In summary (Tables 18.2 and 18.3), it appears that chronic hypoxia alters enzyme activity, proteoglycan synthesis, and serotonin uptake in bovine pulmonary arterial endothelial cells; the corresponding activity in chronically hy-

TABLE 18.2. Effect of Chronic Hypoxia on Cultured Endothelial Cells (Metabolic Functions)

		AEC	PAEC
Pyruvate kinase (2)	0% oxygen	↓	↓
Phosphofructokinase (2)	0% oxygen	↓	↓
Cytochrome oxidase (2)	0% oxygen	0	0
ACE activity	3% oxygen (<48 h) (11)		↑
	3% oxygen (>48 h) (6)	↓	↓
Proteoglycans (10)	3% oxygen		↓
Serotonin uptake (11)	3% oxygen	↑	↑
Smooth muscle mitogen	0% oxygen (7,16)	No	Yes
	3% oxygen (9,14)		No
NCA (6)	10% oxygen	0	0
	3% oxygen	0	0
Prostacyclin (1)	3% oxygen	↓	↓
Thromboxane (1)	3% oxygen	↓	↓

ACE, aortic endothelial cells; PAEC, pulmonary arterial endothelial cells; NCA, neutrophil chemoattractant activity.
Numbers in parentheses denote appropriate reference.

poxic aortic endothelial cells appears similar or has not been studied. With regard to cytokine release, there appears to be similar patterns of NCA and cyclooxygenase activity in chronically hypoxic aortic and pulmonary arterial endothelial cells in the unstimulated state; exposure of the cells to further hypoxia causes a differential pattern of release of these cytokines. The existence of a smooth muscle mitogen released from hypoxic pulmonary arterial endothelial cells requires further clarification.

CONCLUSION

In the in vivo situation differences in the response of the pulmonary and systemic vascular beds may be mediated in part by the endothelium. It is apparent from this review that elucidation of the effects of chronic hypoxia on cultured endothelial cells is in its infancy. In fact, it is not yet clear what the definition of chronic hypoxia, in vitro, actually is. What differences exist between aortic and pulmonary arterial endothelial cells in their response to chronic hypoxia is also not yet clear; but it is likely that some substantial differences will be found. It will then become crucial to understand the mechanisms of these differences.

TABLE 18.3. Effect of Chronic Hypoxia on Cultured Endothelial Cells (Acute Hypoxic Exposure, 0% Oxygen)

		AEC	PAEC
NCA (6)	10% oxygen	↑	↑
	3% oxygen	↑	0
Prostacyclin (1)	3% oxygen	0	0
Thromboxane (1)	3% oxygen	0	↑

AEC, aortic endothelial cells; PAEC, pulmonary arterial endothelial cells; NCA, neutrophil chemoattractant activity.
Numbers in parentheses denote appropriate reference.

ACKNOWLEDGMENTS

The author is grateful to Dr. Sharon Rounds, Emily Mar-Cain, and Hillary Barnett for their valuable input and assistance in performing the studies described.

REFERENCES

1. BARNETT, H. F., AND H. W. FARBER. Effect of decreased ambient oxygen on prostaglandin production in pulmonary arterial and aortic endothelial cells. *Am. Rev. Respir. Dis.* 137:A326, 1988.
2. CUMMISKEY, J. M., L. M. SIMON, T. THEODORE, U. S. RYAN, AND E. D. ROBIN. Bioenergetic alterations in cultivated pulmonary artery and aortic endothelial cells exposed to normoxia and hypoxia. *Exp. Lung. Res.* 2:155–163, 1981.
3. FARBER, H. W., D. M. CENTER, AND S. ROUNDS. Bovine and human endothelial cell production of neutrophil chemoattractant activity in response to components of the angiotensin system. *Circ. Res.* 57:898–902, 1985.
4. FARBER, H. W., P. F. WELLER, S. ROUNDS, D. J. BEER, AND D. M. CENTER. Generation of lipid neutrophil chemoattractant activity by histamine-stimulated cultured endothelial cells. *J. Immunol.* 137:2918–2924, 1986.
5. FARBER, H. W., D. M. CENTER, AND S. ROUNDS. Effect of ambient oxygen on cultured endothelial cells from different vascular beds. *Am. J. Physiol.* 253:H878–H883, 1987.
6. FARBER, H. W., AND S. ROUNDS. Effect of long-term hypoxia on cultured aortic and pulmonary arterial endothelial cells. (in press).
7. FRIEDMAN, M., AND D. R. CLEMMONS. Hypoxia stimulates the de novo synthesis and release of a pulmonary vascular smooth muscle mitogen in cultured pulmonary endothelial cells. *Am. Rev. Respir. Dis.* 137:A326, 1988.
8. HART, C. M., AND E. R. BLOCK. Lung serotonin metabolism. *Clin. Chest Med.* 10:59–70, 1989.
9. HASSOUN, P. M., S-L. LEE, AND B. L. FANBURG. Hypoxia, pulmonary endothelial cells and smooth muscle cell growth. *Am. Rev. Respir. Dis.* 137:A325, 1988.
10. HUMPHRIES, D. E., S-L. LEE, B. L. FANBURG, AND J. E. SILBERT. Effects of hypoxia and hyperoxia on proteoglycan production by bovine pulmonary artery endothelial cells. *J. Cell. Physiol.* 126:249–253, 1986.
11. KRULEWITZ, A. H., AND B. L. FANBURG. The effect of oxygen tension on the in vitro production and release of angiotensin-converting enzyme by bovine pulmonary artery endothelial cells. *Am. Rev. Respir. Dis.* 130:866–869, 1984.
12. LEE, S-L., AND B. L. FANBURG. Serotonin uptake by bovine pulmonary artery endothelial cells in culture II. Stimulation by hypoxia. *Am. J. Physiol.* 250:C766–C770, 1986.
13. LEE, S-L., AND B. L. FANBURG. Glycolytic activity and enhancement of serotonin uptake by endothelial cells exposed to hypoxia/anoxia. *Circ. Res.* 60:653–658, 1987.
14. PASHIRA, P. J., P. M. HASSOUN, E. TEUFEL, AND B. L. FANBURG. Hypoxic endothelial cells actively secrete an inhibitor for smooth muscle growth. *FASEB J.* 3:A1309, 1989.
15. STEIN, O., AND Y. STEIN. Bovine aortic endothelial cells display macrophage-like properties towards acetylated [I-125]-labeled low density lipoprotein. *Biochem. Biophys. Acta* 620:631–635, 1980.
16. VENDER, R. L., D. R. CLEMMONS, L. KWOCK, AND M. FRIEDMAN. Reduced oxygen tension induces pulmonary endothelium to release a pulmonary smooth muscle mitogen(s). *Am. Rev. Respir. Dis.* 135:622–627, 1987.

19

Pulmonary Hypoxic Vasoconstrictor Response: Modulation by the Peripheral Arterial Chemoreceptors

ROBERT S. FITZGERALD, GHOLAM ABBAS DEHGHANI, JAMES S. K. SHAM, AND MACHIKO SHIRAHATA

The focus of this chapter is on the role of the carotid and aortic bodies in controlling the pulmonary vasculature during hypoxia. It should be stated at the outset that control of the pulmonary vasculature is an extremely controversial area. On first survey it would appear that data presented by one distinguished investigator simply contradicts the data presented by a second equally distinguished investigator. Closer inspection of the fairly abundant literature in this area reveals that responses of the pulmonary vasculature to almost any challenge can vary, sometimes radically, among species, can be a function of the preexisting tone in the vessel, can be influenced by anesthesia, and can be difficult even to measure. Hence, making generalizations about the pulmonary vasculature can be a rather risky business.

There is substantial evidence, however, that both the sympathetic and parasympathetic nervous systems are present in the pulmonary vasculature. Hence, there is anatomical potential for some kind of reflex control either arising in the central nervous system spontaneously, or by a reflex arc involving peripheral receptors and afferent pathways, such as the peripheral chemoreceptor input into the autonomic nervous system. Some investigators tend to dismiss or greatly minimize any role for neural influence on the pulmonary vasculature during hypoxia because the hypoxic vasoconstrictor response can be observed in excised lungs ventilated with an hypoxic mixture (7). This, although true, seems to be a somewhat limited view of the determinants of pulmonary vascular control. For it would surely be significant if the hypoxic vasoconstrictor response, initiated in the vasculature, could be in any way modulated by extrapulmonary neurohumoral influences. The autonomic nervous system sends both myelinated and unmyelinated fibers to the pulmonary vasculature. Sympathetic innervation is more heavily represented on the precapillary vessels where the density of innervation coincides with vessel diameter. The smallest vessels are not innervated (<30 to 40 μm). Pulmonary veins are by comparison hardly innervated by the sympathetic system.

Parasympathetic neurons also innervate the pulmonary circulation. Again the concentration is greater on the arteriolar side with little to none on the pulmonary veins. Larger elastic arteries have a more dense innervation than smaller muscular arteries and as in the sympathetic innervation, branching points in the vasculature are more heavily innervated.

Activation of the sympathetic nerves by direct electrical stimulation or an infusion of norepinephrine provokes pulmonary vasoconstriction in a wide variety of species under most conditions. Alpha-adrenergic blockade abolishes both effects (4, 10, 17). Precisely where the vasconstriction in response to nerve stimulation takes place is not well understood. Interestingly, if alpha-adrenergic receptors are blocked, then sympathetic nerve stimulation or norepinephrine provokes a pulmonary vasodilation (9). And this is blocked by propranolol. Selective beta$_1$ antagonists do not block this response. Hence, on the basis of anatomical structures and pharmacological challenges the pulmonary vasculature appears capable of responding to alpha-activation with vasoconstriction and beta$_2$ stimulation with vasodilation. These responses are modified substantially by the preexisting tone of the vessels. And this may account for some of the differences in responses reported in the literature.

Parasympathetic activation produces a less clear picture. There appears to be a marked species difference. For example, cats (16) show a vasodilation, whereas dogs and rabbits show a vasoconstriction (2, 8). Again, tone plays a big part in the outcome of either vagal stimulation or the administration of acetylcholine. Blocked by atropine these effects are mediated by muscarinic receptors. In some of these responses the cyclooxygenase metabolites have a role. But again there is controversy over where the vasoconstriction occurs.

Finally, it should be stated that both vasoactive intestinal polypeptide and substance P have been identified in neurons supplying the pulmonary vasculature of some species. Both delivered exogenously produce a pulmonary vasodilation if the vascular tone is high. But how the substances are released endogenously is not well understood. Hence, there is both an anatomical substrate and a sensitivity to the respective neurotransmitters applied pharmacologically or released by artificially stimulating the nerve.

Selective stimulation of the carotid bodies produces both a bradycardia (vagally mediated) and a subsequent tachycardia. Indeed, sympathetic output to the heart from carotid body stimulation is lateralized, that is, stimulation of left carotid body activates the right cardiac sympathetic nerve and vice versa (11). It has also been reported (14) that carotid body stimulation in dogs provokes an increase in peripheral airways resistance that is abolished by vagotomy. Hence, carotid body stimulation activates sympathetic and parasympathetic input into the thorax. This suggests the possibility that the carotid body could control pulmonary vascular smooth muscle reflexly. The impact of aortic bodies stimulation on autonomic output has been less well studied.

Among the first to study the role of the carotid body in the control of the pulmonary vasculature was Aviado et al. (1). Calculating the pulmonary vascular resistance by dividing pulmonary arterial pressure by pulmonary venous outflow, they concluded from their study that anoxic stimulation of the aortic and carotid chemoreceptors produced reflex pulmonary vasoconstriction. Daly and Daly first reported (5) that stimulation of the carotid body chemoreceptors by venous blood usually caused a reflex decrease in pulmonary vascular resistance in lungs perfused at constant blood volume. But if they temporarily interrupted blood flow through the bronchial circulation they invariably saw an increase in pulmonary vascular resistance (6). Stern et al. (18) reported that selective stimulation of the aortic bodies by an injection of nicotine produced a pulmonary vasoconstriction.

Over the last several years, Levitsky and his colleagues have published a series of papers (3, 12, 13, 19) in which the basic technique was to measure total pulmonary blood flow and blood flow to the left lung while ventilating that lung with oxygen or nitrogen. The right lung was ventilated with oxygen or room air. They demonstrated a shift of the blood flow away from the hypoxic left lung when the right lung was ventilated with oxygen making the arterial blood gases normoxic. But when they subsequently ventilated the right lung with room air making the blood gases hypoxic, blood flow in the hypoxic lung increased. This increase did not take place in the sinoaortic denervated dog. They have recently identified the efferent limb of this apparent reflex vasodilation as being the result of parasympathetic mediation.

Although the studies presented do not identify the efferent limb of the carotid body–pulmonary vasculature interaction, they suggest that both the carotid bodies and the aortic bodies acting together or individually promote a decrease in the pulmonary vascular resistance, a vasodilation, both when tone is high (alveolar hypoxia) and when it is normal (alveolar normoxia).

STUDY 1

Methods

Fifteen anesthetized, paralyzed, artificially ventilated cats were prepared for recording right and left atrial, left ventricular, pulmonary artery pressure (catheters to pressure transducers) and aortic flow (electromagnetic flow probe at the base of the aorta). Aortic depressor nerves were prepared for transection. The experimental design took advantage of the fact that the aortic bodies increase their neural output when exposed to CO, whereas the carotid bodies do not; both, of course, increase neural output when exposed to a decreased PaO_2, hypoxic hypoxia (HH, Fig. 19.1). Therefore, after a 3-hour recovery period from surgery and a control period the cats were exposed to 8% O_2 in N_2 for 15 minutes lowering their SaO_2 to 42% (Table 19.1). Measurements were made throughout the exposure. The animals were returned to room air for an hour of recovery. After control measurements, the animals were then exposed to CO lowering SaO_2 to the same level (at a normal, or above PaO_2). This was called CO hypoxia (COH). The animals were then hyperventilated on 92% O_2/8% CO_2 to eliminate the CO for 1.5 hours. During this time the aortic nerves were transected. The protocol for exposing the aortic nerve-transected (abr) animals to HH and to COH was repeated. Cardiac output was calculated as aortic flow plus the coronary blood flow. Coronary blood flow (ml/min) was determined by labeled microspheres in a separate study ($n = 5$) using the identical preparation and protocol. Statistical significance (at the 0.05 level) was established with a three-way analysis of variance and a Duncan new multiple range test.

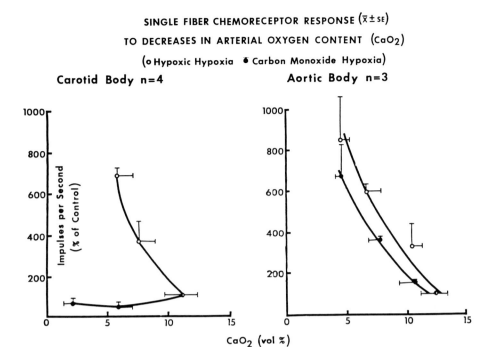

FIGURE 19.1. The response of carotid and aortic bodies to carbon monoxide hypoxia (COH) and to hypoxic hypoxia (HH). Insets show an individual experiment for each chemoreceptor. Letters signify points where blood samples were taken. Lowering contents by lowering PaO_2 stimulates both chemoreceptors, whereas lowering content by the use of carbon monoxide stimulates only the aortic body.

Results

In these experiments cardiac output increased to 161%, 142%, 150%, and 112% of the control in the intact HH, intact COH, abr HH, and abr COH conditions, respectively. In the first and third conditions (involving alveolar hypoxia) the rise to maximum pulmonary arterial pressure (Ppa) occurred rapidly (within 3 minutes) before half the maximum rise in cardiac output had occurred; hence, approximately 50% of the increase in cardiac output occurs at constant Ppa. This indicated a vasodilation, a decrease in pulmonary vascular resistance (PVR) (Fig. 19.2). The PVR in the HH-exposed intact cat (PVR = pulmonary arterial pressure [Ppa]-left atrial pressure [Pla]/cardiac output) rose rapidly to a maximum of 143% of its control value at 3 minutes. It then fell precipitously, and at 15 minutes of exposure was 117% of control, significantly lower than the maximum, as were the PVR values at 4,5,7,10, and 13 minutes. This suggested the possibility that an active vasodilation mediated by the aortic and carotid bodies followed an initial, locally mediated vasoconstriction.

In the aortic body-resected condition, the PVR in cats exposed to HH, where only the carotid body was operating, rose even more rapidly and higher, reaching a maximum of 150% of the control in 2 minutes. Again the fall from the maximum was precipitous; values from 5 minutes onward were significantly lower than the maximum, suggesting the possibility of carotid body-

TABLE 19.1. Blood Gas Values During HH and COH Challenges

	pH_a	Pa_{CO_2} (mm Hg)	Pa_{O_2} (mm Hg)	Sa_{O_2} (%)	Hb (g/dl)
Intact					
Control	7.439	33.8	117	99.0	8.4
	± 0.020	± 1.2	± 4	± 0.4	± 0.5
HH	7.361	36.5	28^a	43.7^a	9.7
	± 0.016	± 1.1	± 2	± 3.9	± 0.6
Control	7.420	35.8	121	100.0	8.5
	± 0.014	± 1.0	± 5	± 0.0	± 0.5
COH	7.409	34.3	130	44.8^a	9.0
	± 0.015	± 1.1	± 5	± 2.5	± 0.5
Aortic Body Resected					
Control	7.487	33.1	124	99.3	7.6
	± 0.012	± 0.9	± 4	± 0.3	± 0.5
HH	7.379	34.3	33^a	47.4^a	8.3
	± 0.024	± 1.1	± 3	± 4.0	± 0.6
Control	7.429	35.1	128	99.1	7.0
	± 0.020	± 0.8	± 5	± 0.4	± 0.5
COH	7.390	32.4	126	40.2^a	7.4
	± 0.023	± 1.7	± 4	± 3.7	+ 0.5

[a]Different from control at the 0.001 level.

$n = 15$ cats

HH, hypoxic hypoxia; lower Sa_{O_2} by lowering Pa_{O_2}.

COH, carbon monoxide hypoxia; lower Sa_{O_2} by increasing HbCO.

Hb, hemoglobin.

mediated vasodilation. The displacement of the abr HH curve (only carotid bodies acting) above the intact HH curve (both aortic bodies and carotid bodies acting), and the more rapid decline from the maximum of the intact HH PVR curve suggested again a vasodilatory role for the aortic body. Furthermore, support for this possibility was seen in the COH intact condition where there was a rise in cardiac output but not in Ppa or Pla. The PVR, thus, showed a significant decrease from 2 to 15 minutes, indicative of an active vasodilation.

STUDY 2

Methods

A second set of experiments was designed to determine in the normoxic cat the effect of stimulating the carotid bodies on the PVR. Four anesthetized, paralyzed, artificially ventilated cats were prepared for recording aortic flow, pulmonary artery, left atrial, and femoral artery blood pressures. Perfusion loops were placed bilaterally in the common carotid arteries. After interrupting blood flow, either a small volume of arterial blood or a small volume of venous blood with varying concentrations of NaCN was infused while recording Ppa, Pla, and aortic flow. Infusions lasted 3 to 6 seconds and contained 0.3 to 0.5 µg of NaCN. Statistical significance was determined either by Student's *t*-test (paired comparisons) or a two-way analysis of variance followed by a Duncan new multiple range test.

Results

Figures 19.3 and 19.4 present the results of infusions of arterial blood and of venous blood containing 0.3 to 0.5 µg of NaCN in a 1-ml infusion. There was no significant response to the infusion of arterial blood. But the response to venous blood containing NaCN was a reduction in PVR becoming significant 15 seconds after the initiation of the infusion and reaching a maximum of 17% below control at 25 seconds. We attempted to see if the effect was dose dependent by increasing the concentration of NaCN from 3 to 5 µg. Although this produced the maximum decrease more rapidly (20 seconds after start of infusion), PVR began to rise at 25 to 30 seconds. We interpreted this as the recirculation of the NaCN into the pulmonary vasculature stimulating locally a vasoconstriction. This decrease in PVR upon carotid body stimulation in the normoxic lung, suggestive of active vasodilation, received subsequent anecdotal support in three hypoxic animals. In these experiments we infused 10 ml of hyperoxic, hypocapnic blood into the common carotid arteries of these hypoxic cats. There was a clear increase in PVR. In view of the data already presented a reasonable interpretation of these last three observations is that carotid body output (vasodilatory) was silenced and locally generated vasoconstriction was allowed full expression.

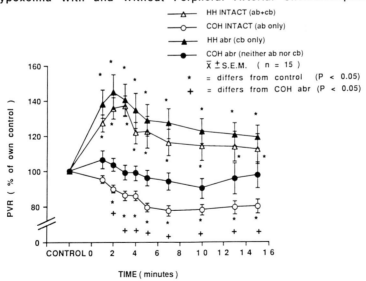

Pulmonary Vascular Resistance (PVR) - Response To Acute Hypoxemia With and Without Perpheral Arterial Chemoreceptors

FIGURE 19.2. Response of the pulmonary vascular resistance during hypoxia with four different conditions of chemoreceptor involvement. Intact, aortic depressor nerve is not transected; abr, aortic body resected; i.e., aortic nerve has been transected. In the intact COH condition (alveolar normoxia) there was no change in Ppa accompanying the 42% increase in cardiac output, again indicating a vasodilation, a decrease in PVR.

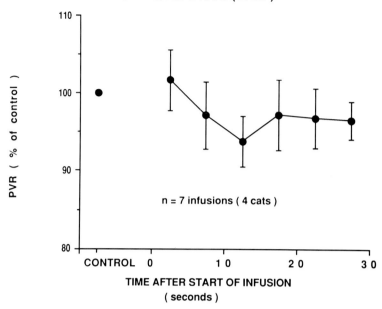

FIGURE 19.3. Response of the PVR to selective bilateral perfusion of the carotid bodies with arterial blood. One milliliter of arterial blood was infused (3 seconds). No significant change in PVR was observed.

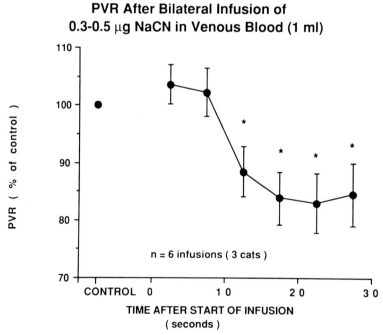

FIGURE 19.4. Response of the PVR to selective bilateral perfusion of the carotid bodies with venous blood containing sodium cyanide. Under conditions of alveolar normoxia, selective transient stimulation of the carotid bodies significantly reduced PVR. Whether the efferent limb is parasympathetic (vagal) or sympathetic (β_2) is controversial.

DISCUSSION

The interpretation of these results in the cat is limited because of the presence of anesthesia, the use of an open-chested animal (left lateral thoracotomy, fifth interspace), and the brevity of some of the procedures. The data, however, are consistent with those of Levitsky and his colleagues in the dog (3, 12, 13, 19) and, ideed, extend them somewhat. Their results clearly support a reflex modulation of the pulmonary vasculature in the hypoxic lung by activation of the arterial chemoreceptors during unilateral alveolar hypoxia. Our experiments have demonstrated that the peripheral chemoreceptors provoke a decrease in PVR during systemic hypoxia, presumably by active vasodilation in both lungs. To our knowledge, outside of the older study by Stern et al. (18), there are no other studies of a specific role for the aortic bodies in pulmonary vascular control. It is not clear why they observed vasoconstriction, whereas we saw the aortic body mediating a vasodilatory response in both the normoxic and hypoxic animal. Most recently, Naeije and his colleagues (15), using the technique of multipoint pulmonary artery pressure–cardiac index plots in dogs, concluded that stimulation of the peripheral chemoreceptors inhibits hypoxic pulmonary vasoconstriction.

In conclusion, whereas hypoxia clearly provokes pulmonary vasoconstriction primarily by local mechanisms, several recent studies support the hypothesis that stimulation of both carotid and aortic bodies modulate this response by provoking vasodilation.

REFERENCES

1. AVIADO, D. M. JR., J. S. LING, AND C. F. SCHMIDT. Effects of anoxia on pulmonary circulation: reflex pulmonary vasoconstriction. *Am. J. Physiol. 189:*253–262, 1957.
2. CATRAVAS, J. D., J. J. BUCCAFUSCO, AND H. A. EL-KASHEF. Effects of acetylcholine in the pulmonary circulation of rabbits. *J. Pharmacol. Exp. Ther. 231:*236–241, 1984.
3. CHAPLEAU, M. W., L. B. WILSON, T. J. GREGORY, AND M. G. LEVITSKY. Chemoreceptor stimulation interferes with regional hypoxic pulmonary vasoconstriction. *Respir. Physiol. 71:*185–200, 1988.
4. DALY, I. DEB., An analysis of active and passive effects on the pulmonary vascular bed in response to pulmonary nerve stimulation. *Q. J. Exp. Physiol. 46:*257–271, 1961.
5. DALY, I. DEB, AND M. DEB. DALY. The effects of stimulation of the carotid body chemoreceptors on pulmonary vascular resistance in the dog. *J. Physiol. (London) 137:*436–446, 1957.
6. DALY, I. DEB., AND M. DEB. DALY. The effects of stimulation of the carotid body chemoreceptors on the pulmonary vascular bed in the dog: the 'vasosensory controlled perfused living animal' preparation. *J. Physiol. (London) 148:*201–219, 1959.
7. GROVER, R. F., W. W. WAGNER, JR., I. F. MCMURTRY, AND J. T. REEVES. Pulmonary circulation. In: *Handbook of Physiology,* Section 2: *The Cardiovascular System, Volume. III: Peripheral Circulation and Organ Blood Flow, Part I,* eds. J. T. Shepherd and F. M. Abboud. Bethesda, MD: American Physiological Society, 1983, p. 122.
8. HYMAN, A. L. The direct effect of vasoactive agents on pulmonary veins. Studies of response to acetylcholine, serotonin, histamine, and isoproterenol in intact dogs. *J. Pharmacol. Exp. Ther. 168:*96–105, 1969.
9. HYMAN, A. L., P. NANDIWADA, D. S. KNIGHT, AND P. J. KADOWITZ. Pulmonary vasodilator responses to catecholamines and sympathetic nerve stimulation in the cat. *Circ. Res. 48:* 407–415, 1981.
10. KADOWITZ, P. J., AND A. L. HYMAN. Effect of sympathetic nerve stimulation on pulmonary vascular resistance in the dog. *Circ. Res. 32:*221–227, 1973.
11. KOLLAI, M., AND K. KOIZUMI. Differential responses in sympathetic outflow evoked by chemoreceptor activation. *Brain Res. 138:*159–165, 1977.

12. LEVITSKY, M. G. Chemoreceptor stimulation and hypoxic pulmonary vasoconstriction in conscious dogs. *Respir. Physiol. 37:*151–160, 1979.

13. LEVITSKY, M. G., J. C. NEWELL, J. A. KRASNEY, AND R. E. DUTTON. Chemoreceptor influence on pulmonary blood flow during unilateral hypoxia in dogs. *Respir. Physiol. 31:*345–356, 1977.

14. NADEL, J. A., AND J. G. WIDDICOMBE. Effect of changes in blood gas tensions and carotid sinus pressure on tracheal volume and total lung resistance to airflow. *J. Physiol. (London) 163:* 13–33, 1962.

15. NAEIJE, R., P. LEJEUNE, M. LEEMAN, C. MELOT, AND J. CLOSSET. Pulmonary vascular responses to surgical chemodenervation and chemical sympathectomy in dogs. *J. Appl. Physiol. 66:*42–50, 1989.

16. NANDIWADA, P. A., A. L. HYMAN, AND P. J. KADOWITZ. Pulmonary vasodilator responses to vagal stimulation and acetylcholine in the cat. *Circ. Res. 53:*86–95, 1983.

17. PORCELLI, R. J., AND E. H. BERGOFSKY. Adrenergic receptors in pulmonary vasoconstrictor responses to gaseous and humoral agents. *J. Appl. Physiol. 34:*483–488, 1973.

18. STERN, S., R. E. FERGUSON, AND E. RAPAPORT. Reflex pulmonary vasoconstriction due to stimulation of the aortic body by nicotine. *Am. J. Physiol. 206:*1189–1195, 1964.

19. WILSON, L. B., AND M. G. LEVITSKY. Chemoreflex blunting of hypoxic pulmonary vasoconstriction is vagally mediated. *J. Appl. Physiol. 66:*782–791, 1989.

20

The Renin–Angiotensin–Aldosterone System during Hypoxia

HERSHEL RAFF

The adaptation to hypoxia is an integrated response of the respiratory, cardiovascular, hematopoietic, renal, and endocrine systems. Disturbances of water and electrolyte balance during the adaptation to high altitude led investigators to analyze the renin–angiotensin–aldosterone system during a variety of hypoxic states.

The renin–angiotensin–aldosterone system is involved in the control of electrolyte metabolism, peripheral and pulmonary vascular resistance, and plasma volume. To understand the dynamics of this system during hypoxia, it is necessary to review briefly the normal control system. Extensive reviews have been published recently (8, 9, 13, 17, 28, 37, 50, 60).

Renin is an enzyme secreted by the kidney in response to an increase in sympathetic efferent tone, a decrease in sodium delivery to the macula densa, a decrease in renal perfusion pressure, and an increase in circulating catecholamines. Renin secretion is inhibited by the converse of these as well as increased atrial natriuretic peptide and circulating angiotensin II. Renin catalyzes the cleavage of angiotensin I from angiotensinogen, a hepatic $alpha_2$-globulin. Angiotensin I is a substrate for the generation of angiotensin II in vivo by converting enzyme (kininase II). Angiotensin II is a potent vasoconstrictor, a stimulator of aldosterone, and a mild dypsogen.

Aldosterone is a potent mineralocorticoid that increases potassium excretion and sodium reabsorption and is synthesized and secreted almost exclusively by the zona glomerulosa (outer zone) of the adrenal cortex. The magnitude of the aldosterone secretory rate at any one time is the result of a multifactorial interaction between stimulatory [angiotensin II, adrenocorticotropic hormone (ACTH), potassium] and inhibitory (atrial natriuretic peptide, sodium) inputs. For example, increased plasma potassium not only increases the secretion of aldosterone per se but increases the magnitude of the aldosterone response to angiotensin II (9).

Evaluation of the control of aldosterone during hypoxia requires consideration of these factors. This chapter takes a historic and mechanistic approach. It concentrates on the controllers of aldosterone secretion during acute and chronic hypoxia in healthy subjects rather than to review extensively disturbances in fluid and electrolyte balance.

211

DISSOCIATION OF RENIN AND ALDOSTERONE DURING HYPOXIA:
DISCOVERY AND DESCRIPTION OF THE PHENOMENON (1969–1977)

The advent of reliable assays for the measurement of plasma renin activity (angiotensin I generation in vitro) and aldosterone led to the investigation of the adaptation to high altitude. Although measurements of aldosterone during hypoxia had been made earlier (58, 59), Slater et al. (53, 54) were the first to describe the apparent dissociation of renin and aldosterone during hypobaric hypoxia. They studied healthy men (themselves) at altitude (4 to 5 days at 3500 m) under controlled conditions and showed a decrease in the rate of aldosterone excretion despite potassium retention and an increase in cortisol (reflecting an increase in ACTH). The dramatic decrease in aldosterone could not be explained by changes in plasma renin activity or other "known control mechanisms." The authors hypothesized that the decrease in aldosterone was a normal homeostatic mechanism by which the potassium balance could be maintained in the face of respiratory alkalosis induced by hyperventilation.

Hogan et al. (23) measured plasma renin activity and urinary aldosterone excretion in healthy men exposed to hypobaric hypoxia for 72 hours ($PET_{O_2} = 45$ to 55 mm Hg). Hypoxia resulted in a decrease in plasma renin activity and aldosterone excretion, a negative sodium and water balance, a positive potassium balance, and an increase in urinary 17-hydroxycorticosteroid excretion. It was concluded that plasma renin activity decreased due to increased renal blood flow and that the decrease in aldosterone excretion was due to diminished renin release.

Frayser et al. (21) studied healthy male volunteers during several expeditions to the St. Elias mountain range in the Canadian Rockies. There was a significant increase in plasma renin activity, aldosterone, and cortisol in subjects receiving acetazolamide, although the increase in aldosterone appeared to be less than one would expect from the magnitude of the increase in renin activity. In subjects not receiving acetazolamide, plasma renin activity, aldosterone and cortisol appeared to increase appropriately. The authors found no evidence for a dissociation of renin and aldosterone during hypoxia.

Maher et al. (30) studied subjects at Pike's Peak (PaO_2, 53 to 57 mm Hg) for 11 days. In general, a suppression of renin and aldosterone was found consistent with the study by Hogan et al. (23), but contrary to the one by Frayser et al. (21). Interestingly, angiotensin II concentration measured by radioimmunoassay remained elevated during exercise at altitude despite a persistent suppression of plasma renin activity. This would suggest either that the renin measurements were in error or that extrarenin production of angiotensin II was significant. This study discounts an inhibition of converting enzyme activity as an important factor in the decrease of aldosterone secretion during hypoxia. Unfortunately, these measurements of angiotensin II were largely ignored by subsequent proponents of the converting enzyme inhibition hypothesis.

Sutton et al. (57) studied four subjects during hypoxic decompression to a simulated altitude of 4760 m for 2 days. Plasma sodium, potassium, and renin activity did not change significantly, whereas plasma aldosterone decreased and cortisol increased consistent with the study by Slater et al. (53, 54). Urinary potassium and aldosterone excretion also decreased. The authors thought it unlikely that the decrease in aldosterone was due to a decrease in ACTH because cortisol increased.

In summary, investigators in the 1960s and 1970s evaluated renin, aldosterone, and cortisol with the hope that it would give some insight into the cause of changes in electrolyte balance observed at altitude. These studies concentrated on longer term hypoxic exposures. The studies generally agree (with exceptions) that aldosterone excretion and secretion are decreased during hypoxia and that this might be responsible for the decrease in potassium excretion. The studies disagreed as to whether the decrease in aldosterone was beneficial or detrimental to the control of fluid and electrolyte balance. A mechanism was not proposed, although decreases in plasma ACTH and angiotensin II were discounted. It was clear that the phenomenon was worth pursuing and that hypoxia would prove to have an unusual effect on aldosterone secretion.

ALDOSTERONE DYNAMICS DURING HYPOXIA: STIMULATION TESTS AND
POSSIBLE MECHANISMS (1980–1988)

To begin to analyze the mechanisms, subsequent studies were brought into the laboratory. The studies described are a mixture of acute and chronic hypoxia and of normobaric and hypobaric hypoxia in the laboratory or the field. This section is organized as follows: Studies on hypoxia per se are presented first. Then, studies using various stimulation tests (exercise, ACTH, etc.) are presented. Finally, evidence for and against endogenous inhibitors of aldosterone release are described.

Hypoxia per se

Martin and her co-workers (31, 32) investigated the renin and aldosterone adaptations to hypoxia in rats. In the first study (32), rats were exposed to 380 mm Hg barometric pressure (approximately 5500 m) in a hypobaric chamber for 7 months. Blood samples were obtained either by decapitation or by cardiac puncture under light ether anesthesia. Plasma renin activity was increased, whereas aldosterone did not increase and tended to decrease in female rats. This lack of increase in aldosterone is significant as, under normoxic conditions, ether anesthesia increases aldosterone by an increase in plasma ACTH (unpublished observations). An important variable, plasma potassium, was not measured. A subsequent study (31) evaluated rats exposed to 440 mm Hg barometric pressure (approximately 4400 m) in a hypobaric chamber for 10 weeks. Despite a lack of a significant change in plasma renin activity, aldosterone increased significantly in male but not in female rats. Interestingly, decreases in plasma angiotensinogen concentration were found in rats exposed to altitude. This paper was not in agreement with a previous study from the same group under similar conditions (32).

Heyes et al. (22) studied 11 healthy male subjects exposed to 1 hour of hypobaric (Pio_2, 74 mm Hg) or normobaric (Fio_2, 0.105) hypoxia. Plasma aldosterone concentration decreased in the four subjects with relatively constant urine flow despite no change in plasma renin activity. Interestingly, small but significant decreases in plasma potassium concentration were noted. The subjects also displayed an increase in sodium excretion that the authors thought might be due in part to the suppression of aldosterone.

Ashack et al. (2) exposed 10 healthy male volunteers to 60 minutes of normobaric hypoxia by a mask (FiO_2, 0.105 or 0.12). No significant changes were found in renin or aldosterone. It is interesting that plasma bradykinin levels were also unchanged by hypoxia as bradykinin metabolism is also controlled by angiotensin-converting enzyme activity. Raff and Roarty (47) could not demonstrate an inhibition of the aldosterone response to endogenous increases in ACTH induced by acute hypoxia in conscious rats (PaO_2, 45 mm Hg). This was attributed to the lack of hypokalemia due to the short-term exposure.

A recent study by Curran-Everett et al. (16) exposed conscious sheep to normobaric hypoxia (PaO_2, ~40 mm Hg) in a chamber for 96 hours with and without prevention of hypocapnia. Plasma sodium, potassium, and renin levels were unchanged during hypoxia. There were, however, significant decreases in urinary aldosterone and potassium excretion. A marked negative potassium balance was observed. The authors hypothesized that plasma potassium was preserved during hypoxia by potassium flux from the intracellular compartment and that this change in potassium distribution somehow resulted in a decrease in aldosterone secretion. Interestingly, plasma atrial natriuretic peptide, a known inhibitor of aldosterone secretion (14), was not elevated in two sheep in which measurements were made.

Stimulation Tests

Exercise

Milledge and his co-workers (35, 36) performed studies on healthy male subjects both at altitude (3100 m) and in the laboratory (FiO_2, 0.128). Hypoxic exercise for 1 hour led to significant increases in plasma renin activity but decreases in plasma aldosterone in the laboratory study. In the altitude study, more prolonged exercise was performed and plasma renin and aldosterone significantly increased. The increase in aldosterone was inappropriately low, however, for the increase in plasma renin activity (Fig. 20.1). Shigeoka et al. (52) and subsequently, Bouissou et al. (7) found a marked decrease in the aldosterone response to exercise during hypoxia in humans.

ACTH

Although plasma ACTH is clearly not inhibited during hypoxia, it was hypothesized that the sensitivity of the zona glomerulosa to ACTH is diminished. To evaluate this, several investigators injected physiological and pharmacological doses of ACTH. Keynes et al. (27) studied healthy male subjects; plasma renin activity and potassium concentration were unchanged at day 9 and 10 at 4350 m, whereas plasma aldosterone was undetectably low. Administration of ACTH resulted in a normal increase in urinary cortisol excretion at altitude. The absolute urinary aldosterone response to ACTH was decreased at altitude,

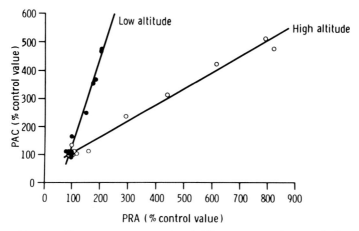

FIGURE 20.1. Plasma aldosterone concentration (PAC) response to increased plasma renin activity (PRA). Each point represents the mean result for 1 day from six subjects in the high-altitude study (*open circles*) and five subjects in the low-altitude study. High altitude significantly decreased the slope of the aldosterone versus renin relationship. From Milledge et al. (36).

although the percent increase from the lower baseline was unchanged. Colice and Ramirez (10) studied healthy subjects on a normal or low salt diet exposed to 1 hour of hypoxia (FiO$_2$, 0.15 to 0.16). Hypoxia decreased aldosterone significantly despite no change in plasma renin activity. The aldosterone and cortisol response to a large dose of ACTH (25 U) was normal under hypoxemic conditions.

Both of these previous experiments used pharmacological doses of ACTH. Raff and Chadwick (43) measured the plasma aldosterone response to physiological infusion of ACTH or a pharmacological injection in conscious male rats exposed to hypoxia for 42 hours (PaO$_2$, 44 mm Hg). Basal plasma aldosterone and potassium concentrations were suppressed despite no change in plasma renin activity. The aldosterone response to the physiological infusion rates of ACTH were significantly attenuated during hypoxia, whereas the response to a pharmacological dose was normal (Fig. 20.2). It was concluded that decreased adrenal sensitivity to ACTH is subtle and is either due to diminished potassium or a direct effect of hypoxia on the adrenal gland. Ramirez et al. (49) confirmed this in humans, finding that despite no change in plasma renin activity or potassium in high altitude acclimatized subjects (3000 m), the aldosterone response to increasing but relatively small doses of ACTH was inhibited.

Angiotensin II
Colice and Ramirez (11) performed a well-controlled study in which they infused angiotensin II at physiological rates (2 to 12 ng/kg per minute) and found no difference in the aldosterone response between normoxic and hypoxic human subjects. Interestingly, the hypoxic subjects did not appear to demonstrate a complete suppression of plasma renin activity during angiotensin II infusion.

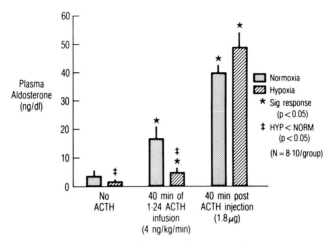

FIGURE 20.2. Rats exposed to 42 hours of hypoxia (FiO_2, 0.10) demonstrate suppressed aldosterone levels during time control (no ACTH) and at 40 minutes of a physiological ACTH infusion (4 ng/kg per minute). The aldosterone response to a pharmacological dose of ACTH (1.8 μg) was normal. *$P<0.05$, hypoxia<normoxia ($n = 8$ to 10/group). From Raff and Chadwick (43).

Furosemide
Colice and Ramirez (12) also studied the aldosterone response to furosemide infusion in healthy subjects and patients with chronic obstructive lung disease (COPD). It was concluded that "hypoxemia does not affect the plasma aldosterone concentration increase or urinary volume and sodium response to furosemide."

Hemorrhage and Tilt
Raff et al. (48) measured the response to hemorrhage (15 ml/kg) in rats exposed to hypoxia for 42 hours. Despite a significantly augmented ACTH and corticosterone response to hemorrhage under hypoxic conditions, the aldosterone response to hemorrhage was not increased. It was concluded that the aldosterone response to physiological increases in *endogenous* ACTH was inhibited during hypoxia, although the decreased plasma potassium concentrations during hypoxia confounded this interpretation. Keynes et al. (27) found a dissociation of the renin and aldosterone response to head-up tilt in human subjects at altitude.

Summary
The aldosterone response to exercise and physiological increases in ACTH may be inhibited during hypoxia. Studies in rats found hypokalemia and were concerned that this confounded interpretation of the data. The lack of hypokalemia in humans and sheep, however, suggest that this is not a unifying hypothesis. The studies involved acute or chronic normobaric or hypobaric hypoxia. Regardless of these factors, the results were fairly consistent and suggested that a factor (or factors) was selectively inhibiting aldosteronogenesis during hypoxia.

Inhibitors

What, in addition to hypokalemia, might inhibit the aldosterone response to exercise and ACTH at altitude? There are several possibilities.

Angiotensin Converting Enzyme Inhibition
Despite increased plasma angiotensin II concentration reported by Maher et al. (30) in 1975, it was proposed that aldosterone was decreased during hypoxia due to inhibition of pulmonary angiotensin II production. This controversial and troublesome hypothesis is not consistent with the known control of the system. First, as pointed out by Keynes et al. (27), inhibition of angiotensin converting enzyme (ACE) (e.g., with captopril) leads to large increases in plasma renin activity due to the loss of angiotensin II inhibition of renin secretion. Second, extrapulmonary ACE is sufficient to maintain normal angiotensin II production (8, 19). It is noteworthy that extrapulmonary ACE activity was known as early as 1974 (19), yet largely ignored by subsequent investigators. The effect of hypoxia on pulmonary and peripheral ACE appears to be a real phenomenon (41). Serum ACE has been reported to decrease (35, 36) or be unchanged (10) during hypoxia. The significance of serum ACE as an index of angiotensin II production in vivo, however, is suspect; it probably reflects loss of ACE from endothelial cells and can be used as a clinical marker of certain pulmonary diseases (see Ref. 39), rather than as an index of angiotensin II production in vivo. The inconsistency of the ACE inhibition hypothesis was confirmed when it was shown that acute hypoxia did *not* alter angiotensin II production in dogs (46) or in patients with COPD (45). Therefore, although hypoxia may have an effect on ACE, this does not result in an inhibition of arterial angiotensin II concentration nor is it responsible for a decrease in aldosterone during hypoxia. An interesting and as yet unstudied hypothesis is that hypoxia decreases intraadrenal converting enzyme, local concentrations of angiotensin II and, therefore, aldosterone secretion (38).

Atrial Natriuretic Peptide
Atrial natriuretic peptide (ANP) infusion at physiological doses decreases the aldosterone response to angiotensin II but not ACTH in normoxic humans (14). The ANP is increased during acute (4) and chronic hypoxia (48) possibly due to a direct cardiac effect (3), although McKenzie et al. (33) failed to find an increase early in hypoxia (3 days) before the development of severe pulmonary hypertension but when aldosterone levels are low. It is possible that increases in ANP are responsible for the dissociation of aldosterone and its controllers during hypoxia. There are inconsistencies in this hypothesis as hypoxia decreases the aldosterone response to ACTH but not angiotensin II (10, 49), whereas ANP decreases the aldosterone response to angiotensin II but not ACTH (14). Future studies should also examine a novel neuropeptide with homology to ANP, which is synthesized in the adrenal medulla and may inhibit aldosteronogenesis by a paracrine action (40).

Neural Input
Schmidt et al. (51) found a decrease in plasma aldosterone in cats with hypoxic–hypercapnic perfusion of isolated carotid bifurcations and systemic normoxia. Hypoxia activates carotid body afferents, which may lead to a suppres-

sion of aldosterone by an increase in efferent nerve activity to the adrenal cortex. This pathway may involve central dopamine (14) or serotonin (29) and/ or efferent vasoactive intestinal polypeptinergic nerves (15).

DOES HYPOXIA DIRECTLY INHIBIT ALDOSTERONE SECRETION BY
INHIBITING STEROID SYNTHESIS WITHIN THE ZONA GLOMERULOSA?

A recent study by McLean et al. (34) found a decrease in saliva aldosterone but not cortisol in six healthy young men at 4450 mm for 16 days. They suggested that hypobaric hypoxia might have a direct, inhibitory effect on the zona glomerulosa. The steroidogenic enzymes of the adrenal cortex use oxygen to hydroxylate sequentially cholesterol to aldosterone, cortisol, or adrenal androgens. It seemed possible that the limitation of oxygen delivery to these cytochrome P_{450} enzymes could result in decreased steroid synthesis. This was recently studied (42) using acutely dispersed bovine adrenocortical cells exposed to increasing levels of secretagogues under normoxic (P_{O_2}, ~150 mm Hg) or mildly hypoxic (P_{O_2} ~85 mm Hg) conditions (Fig. 20.3).

Decreased buffer P_{O_2} diminished the aldosterone response to angiotensin II, cyclic AMP (second messenger for ACTH action), and progesterone; hypoxic inhibition was reversed by returning the cells to normoxic conditions. Progesterone increased aldosterone production by entering after the first two steroidogenic steps. The inhibition of the aldosterone response to progesterone suggests a distal locus. At first glance, one might assume that this is a trivial effect merely due to O_2 limitation to the steroidogenic cytochrome P_{450} enzymes; however, cortisol secretion from fasciculata cells was not inhibited by hypoxia under similar conditions. Because the genes encoding the steroidogenic enzymes in the zona glomerulosa and fasciculata are remarkably similar if not the same (37), O_2 limitation is unlikely. Furthermore, P_{O_2} levels of 85 mm Hg are not close to the level required to inhibit other cytochromes studied (25), although hepatic cytochrome P_{450} have been shown to be affected by exposing rats to 7% O_2 in vivo (26). It may also be that low P_{O_2} alters intraadrenal paracrine regulation of aldosteronogenesis (38,40).

Does a direct effect make sense? Because adrenal blood flow is very high (2 to 4 ml/min per g), the adrenal cortex does not seem to require significant desaturation of hemoglobin to maintain O_2 delivery ($P_{V_{O_2}}$ >70 mm Hg) (5).

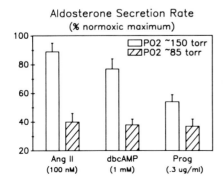

FIGURE 20.3. Normalized aldosterone response of dispersed bovine adrenocortical glomerulosa cells to angiotensin II (Ang II), dibutyryl cAMP (dbcAMP), and progesterone (Prog) in vitro. Low P_{O_2} significantly decreased aldosterone secretion ($P<0.05$). Replotted from Raff et al. (42).

Because the outer layer of the adrenal receives its blood first, the P_{O_2} in the zona glomerulosa is probably even higher and may even be in the 85 mm Hg range. It has been suggested that the dissociation of renin and aldosterone during critical illness may be due to ischemia of the zona glomerulosa (55) and that this effect is reversible (20). Therefore, the zona glomerulosa may be very sensitive to decreased oxygen delivery. Carbon monoxide poisoning, however, does not seem to adversely affect adrenocortical function (44).

Summary
Decreased aldosterone secretion during hypoxia may be due to (1) increased ANP, (2) a change in potassium balance across the zona glomerulosa cell, and/or (3) a direct effect of low O_2 on the adrenal.

TELEOLOGY

Curran-Everett et al. (16) summarized the teleogical reasons for reduced aldosterone as a normal homeostatic adaptation to hypoxia. Decreases in aldosterone may help maintain potassium balance in the face of respiratory alkalosis due to hypoxia-induced hyperventilation. Decreases in aldosterone might also help to maintain sodium excretion, thereby minimizing the formation of edema. Curran-Everett et al. proposed that the decreased aldosterone may help to maintain a normal systemic transmembrane potassium distribution, a concept supported by studies in anephric humans (56).

It is interesting that converting enzyme inhibitors may be beneficial for treating patients with advanced COPD (18) in whom the hypoxic inhibition of aldosterone has been overridden by the stimulatory effects of CO_2 retention. It is also of interest that captopril or ANP decreases normocapnic hypoxic pulmonary vasoconstriction (1, 6, 24). Future therapies for altitude-induced pulmonary hypertension or chronic lung disease should consider these treatments.

The suppression of aldosterone during hypoxia may be an important homeostatic component of an overall adaptation to hypoxia. A direct and specific inhibitory effect on the zona glomerulosa of the adrenal cortex may lead to a decrease in aldosterone secretion without a decrease in ACTH and cortisol, necessary for the adaptation to hypoxia. Furthermore, this would allow a decrease in aldosterone without a decrease in plasma angiotensin II concentration, which may be necessary for the maintenance of peripheral vascular resistance in hypoxic states.

ACKNOWLEDGMENTS

The author wishes to thank Dr. Gene Colice for his critical review of the manuscript.

REFERENCES

1. ADNOT, S., P. E. CHABRIER, C. BRUN-BUISSON, I. VIOSSAT, AND P. BRAQUET. Atrial natriuretic factor attenuates the pulmonary pressor response to hypoxia. *J. Appl. Physiol.* 65:1975–1983, 1988.

2. ASHACK, R., M. O. FARBER, M. H. WEINBERGER, G. L. ROBERTSON, N. S. FINEBERG, AND F. MANFREDI. Renal and hormonal responses to acute hypoxia in normal individuals. *J. Lab. Clin. Med.* 106:12–16, 1985.

3. BAERTSCHI, A. J., C. HAUSMANINGER, R. S. WALSH, R. M. MENTZER JR., D. A. WYATT, AND R. A. PENCE. Hypoxia-induced release of atrial natriuretic factor (ANF) from the isolated rat and rabbit heart. *Biochem. Biophys. Res. Comm.* 140:427–433, 1986.

4. BAERTSCHI, A. J., J. M. ADAMS, AND M. P. SULLIVAN. Acute hypoxemia stimulates atrial natriuretic factor secretion in vivo. *Am. J. Physiol.* 255:H295–H300, 1988.

5. BRESLOW, M. J., T. D. BALL, C. F. MILLER, H. RAFF, AND R. J. TRAYSTMAN. Adrenal blood flow and secretory relationships during hypoxia in anesthetized dogs. *Am. J. Physiol.* 257:H1458–H1465, 1989.

6. BOSCHETTI, E., C. TANTUCCI, M. COCCHIERI, G. FORNARI, V. GRASSI, AND C. A. SORBINI. Acute effects of captopril in hypoxic pulmonary hypertension. *Respiration* 48:296–302, 1985.

7. BOUISSOU, P., F. PERONNET, G. BRISSON, R. HELIE, AND M. LEDOUX. Fluid-electrolyte shift and renin-aldosterone responses to exercise under hypoxia. *Horm. Metabol. Res.* 19:331–332, 1987.

8. CAMPBELL, D. J. The site of angiotensin production. *J. Hypertension* 3:199–207, 1985.

9. COGHLAN, J. P., J. R. BLAIR-WEST, D. A. DENTON, D. T. FEI, R. T. FERNLEY, K. J. HARDY, J. G. MCDOUGALL, R. PUY, P. M. ROBINSON, B. A. SCOGGINS, AND R. D. WRIGHT. Control of aldosterone secretion. *J. Endocr.* 81:55P–67P, 1979.

10. COLICE, G. L., AND G. RAMIREZ. Effect of hypoxemia on the renin–angiotensin–aldosterone system in humans. *J. Appl. Physiol.* 58:724–730, 1985.

11. COLICE, G. L., AND G. RAMIREZ. Aldosterone response to angiotensin II during hypoxemia. *J. Appl. Physiol.* 61:150–154, 1986.

12. COLICE, G. L., AND G. RAMIREZ. The effect of furosemide during normoxemia and hypoxemia. *Am. Rev. Resp. Dis.* 133:279–285, 1986.

13. CUCHE, J. L. Dopaminergic control of aldosterone secretion. State-of-the-art review. *Fundam. Clin. Pharmacol.* 2:327–339, 1988.

14. CUNEO, R. C., E. A. ESPINER, M. G. NICHOLLS, T. G. YANDLE, AND J. H. LIVESEY. Effect of physiological levels of atrial natriuretic peptide on hormone secretion: inhibition of angiotensin-induced aldosterone secretion and renin release in normal man. *J. Clin. Endocrinol. Metab.* 65:765–772, 1987.

15. CUNNINGHAM, L. A., AND M. A. HOLZWARTH. Vasoactive intestinal peptide stimulates adrenal aldosterone and corticosterone secretion. *Endocrinology* 122:2090–2097, 1988.

16. CURRAN-EVERETT, D. C., J. R. CLAYBAUGH, K. MIKI, S. K. HONG, AND J. A. KRASNEY. Hormonal and electrolyte responses of conscious sheep to 96 h of hypoxia. *Am. J. Physiol.* 255:R274–R283, 1988.

17. DZAU, V. J., D. W. BURT, AND R. E. PRATT. Molecular biology of the renin-angiotensin system. *Am. J. Physiol.* 255:F563–F573, 1988.

18. FARBER, M. O., M. H. WEINBERGER, G. L. ROBERTSON, AND N. S. FINEBERG. The effects of angiotensin-converting enzyme inhibition on sodium handling in patients with advanced chronic obstructive pulmonary disease. *Am. Rev. Resp. Dis.* 136:862–866, 1987.

19. FAVRE, L., M. B. VALLOTON, AND A. F. MULLER. Relationship between plasma concentrations of angiotensin I, angiotensin II, and plasma renin activity during cardio-pulmonary bypass in man. *Europ. J. Clin. Invest.* 4:135–140, 1974.

20. FINDLING, J. W., V. O. WATERS, AND H. RAFF. Dissociation of renin and aldosterone during critical illness. *J. Clin. Endocrin. Metab.* 64:592–595, 1987.

21. FRAYSER, R., I. D. RENNIE, G. W. GRAY, AND C. S. HOUSTON. Hormonal and electrolyte response to exposure to 17,500 ft. *J. Appl. Physiol.* 38:636–642, 1975.

22. HEYES, M. P., M. O. FARBER, F. MANFREDI, D. ROBERTSHAW, M. WEINBERGER, N. FINEBERG, AND G. ROBERTSON. Acute effects of hypoxia on renal and endocrine function in normal humans. *Am. J. Physiol.* 243:R265–R270, 1982.

23. HOGAN, R. P. III, T. A. KOTCHEN, A. E. BOYD III, AND L. H. HARTLEY. Effect of altitude on renin-aldosterone system and metabolism of water and electrolytes. *J. Appl. Physiol.* 35:385–390, 1973.

24. JIN, H., R-H. YANG, R. M. THORNTON, Y-F CHEN, R. JACKSON, AND S. OPARIL. Atrial natriuretic peptide lowers pulmonary artery pressure in hypoxia-adapted rats. *J. Appl. Physiol.* 65:1729–1735, 1988.

25. JONES, D. P., AND F. G. KENNEDY. Intracellular oxygen supply during hypoxia. *Am. J. Physiol.* 243:C247–C253, 1982.

26. JORDI-RACINE, A. L., E. ALVAREZ, AND J. REICHEN. The effect of hypoxia on hepatic cytochromes and heme turnover in rats in vivo. *Experientia* 44:343–345, 1988.

27. KEYNES, R. J., G. W. SMITH, J. D. H. SLATER, M. M. BROWN, S. E. BROWN, N. N. PAYNE, T. P. JOWETT, AND C. C. MONGE. Renin and aldosterone at high altitude in man. *J. Endocr.* 92:131–140, 1982.

28. KURTZ, A. Intracellular control of renin release—an overview. *Klin. Wochenschr.* 64:838–846, 1986.

29. MAESTRI, E., L. CAMELLINI, G. ROSSI, M. DOTTI, M. MARCHESI, AND A. GNUDI. Serotonin regulation of aldosterone secretion. *Horm. Metab. Res.* 20:457–459, 1988.

30. MAHER, J. T., L. G. JONES, L. H. HARTLEY, G. H. WILLIAMS, AND L. I. ROSE. Aldosterone dynamics during graded exercise at sea level and high altitude. *J. Appl. Physiol.* 39:18–22, 1975.

31. MARTIN, I. H., N. BASSO, M. I. SARCHI, AND A. C. TAQUINI. Changes in the renin–angiotensin–aldosterone system in rats of both sexes submitted to chronic hypobaric hypoxia. *Arch. Int. Physiol. Bioch.* 95:255–262, 1987.

32. MARTIN, I. H., D. BAULAN, N. BASSO, AND A. C. TAQUINI. The renin–angiotensin–aldosterone system in rats of both sexes subjected to chronic hypobaric hypoxia. *Arch. Int. Physiol. Bioch.* 90:129–133, 1982.

33. McKENZIE, J. C., I. TANAKA, T. INAGAMI, K. S. MISONI, AND R. M. KLEIN. Alterations in atrial and plasma atrial natriuretic factor (ANF) content during development of hypoxia-induced pulmonary hypertension in rat. *Proc. Soc. Exp. Biol. Med.* 181:459–463, 1986.

34. McLEAN, C. J., C. W. BOOTH, T. TATTERSALL, AND J. D. FEW. The effect of high altitude on saliva aldosterone and glucocorticoid concentrations. *Eur. J. Appl. Physiol.* 58:341–347, 1989.

35. MILLEDGE, J. S., AND D. M. CATLEY. Renin, aldosterone, and converting enzyme during exercise and acute hypoxia in humans. *J. Appl. Physiol.* 52:320–323, 1982.

36. MILLEDGE, J. S., D. M. CATLEY, E. S. WILLIAMS, W. R. WITHEY, AND B. D. MINTY. Effect of prolonged exercise at altitude on the renin-aldosterone system. *J. Appl. Physiol.* 55:413–418, 1983.

37. MILLER, W. L. Molecular biology of steroid hormone synthesis. *Endocrine Rev.* 9:295–318, 1988.

38. MULROW, P. J., E. KUSANO, K. BABA, D. SCHIER, Y. DOI, R. FRANCO-SAENZ, G. STONER, AND J. RAPP. Adrenal renin: a possible local hormonal regulator of aldosterone production. *Cardiovasc. Drugs Ther.* 2:463–471, 1988.

39. NEILLY, J. B., C. J. CLARK, A. TWEDDEL, A. P. RAE, D. M. HUGHES, I. HUTTON, J. J. MORTON, AND R. D. STEVENSON. Transpulmonary angiotensin II formation in patients with chronic stable cor pulmonale. *Am. Rev. Respir. Dis.* 135:891–895, 1987.

40. NGUYEN, T. T., C. LAZURE, K. BABINSKI, M. CHRETIEN, H. ONG, AND A. DE LEAN. Aldosterone secretion inhibitory factor: a novel neuropeptide in bovine chromaffin cells. *Endocrinology* 124:1591–1593, 1989.

41. OPARIL, S., A. J. NARKATES, R. M. JACKSON, AND H. S. ANN. Altered angiotensin-converting enzyme in lungs and extrapulmonary tissues of hypoxia-adapted rats. *J. Appl. Physiol.* 65:218–227, 1988.

42. RAFF, H., D. L. BALL, AND T. L. GOODFRIEND. Low oxygen selectively inhibits aldosterone secretion from bovine adrenocortical cells in vitro. *Am. J. Physiol.* 256:E640–E644, 1989.

43. RAFF H., AND K. J. CHADWICK. Aldosterone responses to ACTH during hypoxia in conscious rats. *Clin. Exp. Pharm. Physiol.* 13:827–830, 1986.

44. RAFF H., R. W. GOLDMANN, AND E. P. KINDWALL. Adrenocortical function after acute carbon monoxide exposure in humans. *Arch. Env. Hlth.* 40:88–90, 1985.

45. RAFF H., AND S. A. LEVY. Renin-angiotensin-aldosterone and ACTH-cortisol control during acute hypoxemia and exercise in patients with chronic obstructive lung disease. *Am. Rev. Respir. Dis.* 133:396–399, 1986.

46. RAFF H., J. MASELLI, AND I. A. REID. Correlation of plasma angiotensin II concentration and plasma renin activity during acute hypoxia in dogs. *Clin. Exper. Pharm. Physiol.* 12:91–94, 1985.

47. RAFF H., AND T. P. ROARTY. Renin, ACTH, and aldosterone during acute hypercapnia and hypoxia in conscious rats. *Am. J. Physiol.* 254:R431–R435, 1988.

48. RAFF H., R. B. SANDRI, AND T. P. SEGERSON. Renin, ACTH, and adrenocortical function during hypoxia and hemorrhage in conscious rats. *Am. J. Physiol.* 250:R240–R244, 1986.

49. RAMIREZ, G., P. A. BITTLE, M. HAMMON, C. W. AYERS, J. R. DIETZ, AND G. L. COLICE. Regulation of aldosterone secretion during hypoxemia at sea level and moderately high altitude. *J. Clin. Endocrin. Metab.* 67:1162–1165, 1988.

50. REID, I. A. The renin-angiotensin system and body function. *Arch. Intern. Med.* 145:1475–1479, 1985.

51. SCHMIDT, M., B. WEDLER, C. ZINGLER, C. LEDDERHOS, AND A. HONIG. Kidney function during arterial chemoreceptor stimulation. II. Suppression of plasma aldosterone concentration due to hypoxic-hypercapnic perfusion of the carotid bodies in anesthetized cats. *Biomed. Biochim. Acta* 44:711–722, 1985.

52. SHIGEOKA, J. W., G. L. COLICE, AND G. RAMIREZ. Effect of normoxemic and hypoxemic exercise on renin and aldosterone. *J. Appl. Physiol.* 59:142–148, 1985.
53. SLATER, J. D. H., R. E. TUFFLEY, E. S. WILLIAMS, C. H. BERESFORD, P. H. SONKSEN, R. H. T. EDWARDS, R. P. EKINS, AND M. MCLAUGHLIN. Control of aldosterone secretion during acclimatization to hypoxia in man. *Clin. Sci.* 37:327–341, 1969.
54. SLATER, J. D. H., E. S. WILLIAMS, R. H. T. EDWARDS, R. P. EKINS, P. H. SONKSEN, C. H. BERESFORD, AND M. MCLAUGHLIN. Potassium retention during the respiratory alkalosis of mild hypoxia in man: its relationship to aldosterone secretion and other metabolic changes. *Clin. Sci.* 37:311–326, 1969.
55. STERN, N., F. W. J. BECK, J. R. SOWERS, M. TUCK, W. A. HSUEH, AND R. D. ZIPSER. Plasma corticosteroids in hyperreninemic hypoaldosteronism: evidence for diffuse impairment of the zona glomerulosa. *J. Clin. Endocrinol. Metab.* 57:217–220, 1983.
56. SUGARMAN, A., AND R. S. BROWN. The role of aldosterone in potassium tolerance: studies in anephric humans. *Kidney Int.* 34:397–403, 1988.
57. SUTTON, J. R., G. W. VIOL, G. W. GRAY, M. MCFADDEN, AND P. KEANE. Renin, aldosterone, electrolyte, and cortisol responses to hypoxic decompression. *J. Appl. Physiol.* 43:421–424, 1977.
58. WILLIAMS, E. S. Salivary electrolyte composition at high altitude. *Clin. Sci.* 21:37–42, 1961.
59. WILLIAMS, E. S. Electrolyte regulation during the adaptation of humans to life at high altitude. *Proc. Roy. Soc. B.* 165:266–280, 1966.
60. YOUNG, D. B. Quantitative analysis of aldosterone's role in potassium regulation. *Am. J. Physiol.* 255:F811–F822, 1988.

21

Hypoxic Birds: Temperature and Respiration

MARVIN H. BERNSTEIN

The extreme cold at high altitudes compounds the hypoxic challenge that resident animals must meet. A bird called the alpine chough (*Pyrrhocorax graculus*), for example, lives and reproduces at 6500 m (53) where the Po_2 is 69 mm Hg and the temperature averages $-27°C$ (43). Despite increased solar radiation and efficient insulation, this and similar species undoubtedly increase their O_2 utilization in defending homeothermy while at rest. Montane birds, like lowland birds, use flight as a primary mode of locomotion. Moreover, some sea-level residents climb to high altitudes where they may migrate great distances. Increased exposure, as birds spread the wings, along with increased convection to subfreezing air, unavoidably increase heat loss. The saving factor, perhaps, is that flight, the most metabolically demanding form of vertebrate exercise, is accompanied by huge quantities of heat production in the pectoral muscles. Thus, the source of power for the activity that causes the loss of heat also produces its replacement.

Thermoregulation has been studied in inactive birds exposed to hypoxia or to extreme cold, but not to both together, and few data exist for hypoxic birds in flight. In this chapter I attempt to summarize the sparse information available and to speculate about avian respiratory adaptations to hypoxic cold.

HYPOXIC BIRDS AT REST

Temperatures

Body Core
The diurnal oscillations of core body temperature (T_c) in birds and mammals have amplitudes of 1 to 3°C and represent small changes in thermostatic set point (32). In addition, heat production sometimes leads heat loss (e.g., exercise) or lags it (e.g., cold exposure), and this causes T_c fluctuations that can span 4°C. Because T_c in unstressed birds is already higher than that in similar-sized mammals, body heating associated with avian exercise frequently raises T_c above the upper lethal temperature for mammals. Hyperthermia is probably rare in hypoxic birds. In fact, hypoxia depresses avian T_c, often causing a 1 to 2°C fall, even at thermoneutral ambient temperature (T_a). In contrast, T_c remains unchanged in normoxic birds, even when they are exposed to cold air (25, 51, 56). The energy and O_2 saved by slight cooling can be substantial: a 1-kg bird at rest, for example, produces 3.8 W under basal conditions (calculated

from Ref. 42). If specific tissue–heat capacity is 3.47 J/(g°C), such a bird would use an additional 6.9 kJ and 344 ml O_2 to raise T_c by 2°C, and would have to double the basal O_2 uptake and heat production for 15 minutes to do so (assuming no additional heat loss). Because a rise in T_c increases the gradient for heat loss, the bird would also have to improve its insulation or sustain an above-basal metabolic rate.

Extremities and Skin
During heat stress birds, like mammals, engorge the rich vasculature of their extremities to void heat nonevaporatively, requiring just seconds for onset or reversal (1, 3, 8, 34, 38, 44, 52). In cold air body surface temperatures approximate air temperature (T_a), thereby reducing the thermal gradient and conserving heat in unfeathered regions (bill, legs, feet, and in some species the bare head and neck). During cold exposure many birds also take advantage of tibiotarsal and humeral vasculature that cools arterial blood by countercurrent heat exchange (1, 24). At high altitudes, resting birds in subfreezing air probably take maximum advantage of such blood coolers, and probably perfuse bare areas just enough to prevent tissue freezing. Still, heat loss from skin at perhaps 1°C to air at, say, -30°C must rapidly drain body heat, and it would be valuable to determine the importance of this to thermoregulation.

Brain
Bird brains are almost always cooler than the body core (19, 40). Brain cooling depends on the cooling of blood at the evaporative surfaces in the oral and nasal cavities and in the orbital cavities. This blood then flows to paired ophthalmic retia (OR) in the skull's temporal regions, where it acts as a heat sink, cooling cephalic arterial blood that then flows to the brain (45). The OR are supplied by branches of the carotid artery that ramify and intertwine with multiply branching veins, such that arterial and venous blood flow are countercurrent, improving heat-transfer efficiency. Bypass arteries in the OR of some species apparently allow proportioning of total flow through or around heat-exchanging vessels, finely regulating brain temperature (T_b) (47). The system also controls eye temperature (46, 49), and appears to protect the retina from overheating by sunlight and from becoming cold at altitude.

   During heat stress, independent T_b control allows an increase in the amount of heat stored in the more heat-tolerant body core. This decreases the amount of water needed for cooling and increases the thermal gradient for heat loss. Brain cooling occurs in cold air as well. For example, pigeons at -6°C kept T_b between 39 and 40°C, whereas T_c remained between 41 and 42°C (Fig. 21.1). The advantage of brain cooling during cold stress is not obvious. Perhaps the OR simply slows cranial heat loss to the cold environment, like heat exchangers in other extremities (28). Or maybe brain cooling keeps T_b close to a temperature optimum that may be lower than that in the core. Birds exposed to hypoxia, as well as to cold, sacrifice whatever advantage may be afforded by reduced T_b. At 7 km, for example, T_c in inactive pigeons fell, becoming indistinguishable from T_b. As T_a was reduced, both T_b and T_c fell further. At 9 km, the pigeons underwent further controlled hypothermia, but reached a stable T_c provided that T_a remained above freezing (Fig. 21.1). At lower T_a their

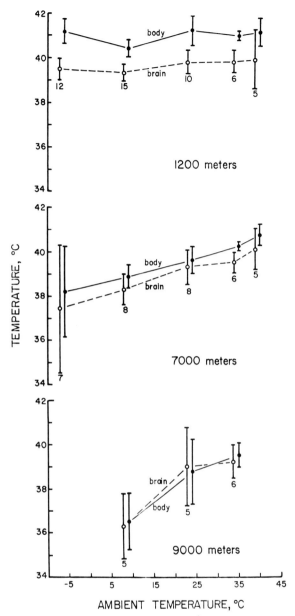

FIGURE 21.1. Body (colonic) and brain (hypothalamic) temperatures in pigeons exposed to air temperatures from −6 to 40°C and to hypobaric hypoxia corresponding to altitudes of 1.2, 7, or 9 km. Points are means for numbers of measurements indicated by small numerals. (Where they overlap at each ambient temperature, points are slightly offset for clarity.) Error bars span 95% confidence intervals. At 1.2 km brain temperature was 1 to 2°C below body temperature over the range of air temperatures used. At high altitudes, colonic temperature decreased to the level of brain temperature, indicating a cessation of brain cooling, and both temperatures decreased with ambient temperature. Pigeons exposed to −6°C at 9 km became irreversibly hypothermic, whereas those exposed to 40°C underwent explosive heat rise. Data from Ref. 14.

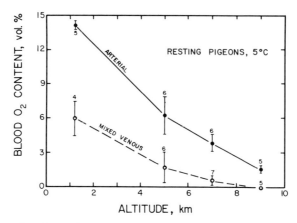

FIGURE 21.2. Arterial and mixed venous O_2 content in pigeons at rest, in air at 5°C, during exposure to hypobaric hypoxia corresponding to the altitudes indicated. Values are means for the numbers of measurements, as indicated by small numerals. Vertical bars span ±2 SD. No O_2 was detected in mixed venous blood at 9 km, indicating 100% tissue O_2 extraction. Data from Ref. 60.

hypothermia became uncontrolled and T_c never stabilized, in spite of increases in both pulmonary and tissue O_2 extraction to nearly 100% (60) (Fig. 21.2). Despite this, it is possible that brain cooling is restored in hypoxic birds when they fly (discussed later).

Heat

Metabolism

Birds at rest shiver when their heat loss exceeds the heat gain from basal metabolism, but at high altitude shivering appears to be inhibited. When pigeons with a PiO_2 of 76 mm Hg were exposed to 5°C air, pectoral electromyogram (EMG) intensity decreased along with T_c and the EMG was eliminated completely at 53 mm Hg (29). The same results were obtained in vagotomized pigeons (30), and as vagotomy in birds prevents pulmonary and arterial chemoreceptor input, the hypothalamus itself must have inhibited shivering when it became hypoxic. If muscle hypoxia had instead been responsible for suppressing shivering, EMG activity would still have been observed in vagotomized birds, although it would have been uncoupled from contraction (30).

The inhibition of shivering in pigeons occurred at PiO_2 corresponding to 4.5, 5.8, and 8.4 km, altitudes at which mean T_a is *not* 5°C, the temperature used in the above experiments, but -14, -23, and -40°C, respectively (43). As already noted, pigeons did not tolerate subfreezing T_a at 9 km, and became severely hypothermic at 5°C. It is curious that lowland birds should have evolved pulmonary and tissue O_2 extractions that approach 100% and that permit tolerance to extreme hypoxia in moderate cold, but not in the extreme cold characteristic of corresponding altitudes. Perhaps, as suggested previously (60), this situation is really just a coincidental manifestation of physiological adaptations to the intensive exercise of flight, rather than to high altitude per se.

Respiration

Birds exposed to cold and to either isobaric or hypobaric hypoxia increased both breathing rate and parabronchial ventilation (15–17, 20, 23, 51). To avoid a simultaneous increase in evaporative heat loss, they appear to lower their exhaled air temperature (T_E) during hypoxic hyperventilation (22), as do birds exposed to cold alone (see Refs. 6, 18, 50). The contribution of respiratory evaporation to heat balance is, therefore, probably negligible in hypoxic birds (22). Even though T_E may approach 1°C at high altitude, it is many degrees warmer than inspired air temperature. The low heat capacity of the air, however, makes the energy cost of "warming" the exhalant negligibly low.

BIRDS FLYING AT HIGH ALTITUDE

Temperature

Body Core

For several minutes after the onset of low-altitude flight, birds store the majority of their metabolic heat (2, 35, 37). Starlings (*Sturnus vulgaris*), for example, raise T_c to 43 or 44°C in 2 minutes of flight (54), and maintain their high T_c during long flights, even at 3°C T_a (54). White-necked ravens (*Corvus cryptoleucus*) that increase T_c from 42.2 to 45.0°C during 5 minutes of flight at 36 km/hour store 64% of their metabolic heat (37). Flying through still air at that speed, a bird could travel 3 km in 5 minutes, far enough perhaps to reach food or water. Hyperthermia during short flights saves water and aids heat loss, as in resting birds. During long flights, however, birds must accelerate evaporation to prevent T_c from rising excessively.

   That birds fly hot in cold air suggests other advantages: A high T_c may increase the efficiency of muscular contraction, and thus the amount of work performed by a unit mass of muscle (54). It may also increase the rate of isotonic shortening (5). Birds, thus, appear to develop the power for flight with smaller muscles, lighter body mass, and lower energy cost, and to cover more distance on a unit of fuel, than if they did not become hyperthermic (54). Rapid heat production and the advantages of a high T_c strongly suggest that high-flying birds have high body temperatures. Although no information is available about T_c during high-altitude flight, hypoxic Pekin ducks running on a treadmill did raise their T_c (39).

Extremities and Integument

Spreading the wings and extending the feet may dissipate much of the heat produced by flying birds (27, 36, 37, 54, 57). In flying gulls (*Larus argentatus*), for example, 46% of heat loss occurs from the feet (3). High blood flow rates and nonevaporative heat loss from the bill characterize heat-stressed pigeons (36), ducks (34), and ravens (59). Temperature of skin overlying the pectoral muscles is higher than T_a in flying starlings (54) and pigeons (35), aiding heat loss as well. All of these responses offset the need to evaporate water in flight. During flight in cold air, however, particularly at high altitude, one might expect birds to minimize heat loss. Some species may thus use countercurrent heat exchangers in the wings and legs to conserve body heat. Further study is needed to determine the patterns of thermoregulation in birds flying at high altitude.

Brain

Brain temperature has been measured during flight in only one bird species, the American kestrel (*Falco sparverius*) (10). At T_a of 23°C, T_c increased by 2°C, but T_b increased by only 1°C. This means the bird confined much of its heat storage to noncranial tissue. Similar results were observed in quail that ran on a treadmill (41). The surface temperature of the eyes in flying birds is near T_c (59); therefore, rapid air flow probably increases corneal heat loss, and this probably cools some of the blood that flows to the OR, as in resting birds (12, 49). This in turn would cool the venous blood supply of the OR, and thereby increase brain cooling. If T_c is as high during hypoxic as during normoxic flight, as suggested earlier, it seems likely that brain cooling during hypoxic flight might be restored or even enhanced, despite its abolition in hypoxic pigeons at rest. Further study is required to confirm this.

Heat

Metabolism

Birds flying at low altitude do the work of producing lift and thrust using only about 20% of their metabolic energy; the balance appears as body heat (13). Soaring birds use metabolic energy only twice as fast as at rest (4, 31), whereas the fly to rest ratio in flapping fliers may be 10 or greater (9). For example, pigeons in flight consume 79 ml O_2 STPD more each minute than at rest (21). If their pectoral muscles were to account for, say, 80% of this increase, then their heat output would be 17 W, a 20-fold increase over basal heat production. If this heat increment were then stored, T_c would rise by 0.66°C/minute, or 2°C in 3 minutes of flight. This is in the range of observed T_c increases noted for flying birds, but is only an estimate, as the pigeons probably lose some of the heat they produce and as these estimates of muscle efficiency and of the muscular contribution to total O_2 uptake are speculative.

Pectoral muscle perfusion, calculated from muscle O_2 uptake estimated above and from the whole body arteriovenous (AV) difference in O_2 content during flight (21), would be about 765 ml/minute or 72% of measured cardiac output. If pectoral AV difference were in fact twice that of the body, representing nearly complete tissue O_2 extraction, then pectoral perfusion would be only 36% of cardiac output. In this range of perfusion rates blood would warm by between 0.4 and 0.7°C while traversing the pectoral muscles. These values would be lower if heat loss from ventral skin were taken into account. Thus, a reasonable estimate of pectoral blood warming is about 0.5°C in flying pigeons, and this would cause T_c to rise initially at a rate of about 0.5°C/minute.

To ascend requires more work than to fly horizontally or to descend at the same speed (57). Birds climbing to high altitude can achieve the necessary work performance either by increasing their total energy expenditure, or by increasing their energy-use efficiency. In fact, flight efficiency has been shown to increase during ascent, compared with level flight, and the amount is evidently just enough to provide the required increase in energy cost (57); therefore, ascent to altitude probably requires no increase in total energy use compared with level flight. Using a larger share of its total energy to ascend also means that a bird produces less heat than when flying horizontally, and this undoubtedly affects thermoregulation.

Once having reached high altitude, a flying bird encounters lower air densities and viscosities, reducing lift and requiring more muscular effort. Thus, the metabolic cost of flying high is greater than at sea level (58). When this is taken into account in calculations for pigeon pectoral muscles during flight at 4 km, the increase in heat production is 33 W. Assuming no body heat is lost, T_c would rise at the rate of 1.3°C/minute, more than twice that calculated for low-altitude flight. The low T_a would assure significant body heat loss, however, even in the earliest stages of a flight; therefore, the actual rate of heating is probably slower. The rise in T_c would also be slower if muscle efficiency were greater, if the pectorals contributed less to total metabolism, or if pectoral perfusion rate were lower. Still, compensation for the physical properties of high-altitude air probably requires greater metabolic and respiratory performance during flight, leading to faster muscular heat production than at low elevations. This lends additional weight to the suggestion that birds flying at high altitude may be hyperthermic, despite their hypothermia at rest. Therefore, rather than the thermoregulatory limitations of resting hypoxic birds, the greatest constraint on the height at which birds fly may be O_2 delivery to flight muscle (26).

Respiration

Skin evaporation in many birds, despite the absence of demonstrable sweat glands, contributes as much as half of evaporative cooling, while at rest, even during heat stress (7). In flying ravens, however, cutaneous evaporation dissipated only 10% of the metabolic heat. The same rate of evaporation would have eliminated 42% of the resting metabolic heat production (37); therefore, cutaneous evaporation apparently did not increase during flight, despite greater convection. Respiratory evaporation is higher during normoxic flight because of increased respiratory ventilation, but even in warm air this pathway dispels half or less of metabolic heat (37, 55, 57). Indeed, it is likely that, during flight in cool air, respiratory evaporation dissipates only about 17% of metabolically produced heat, leaving the majority of heat for convective dissipation from skin. If during high-altitude flight T_E is reduced in proportion to T_a, as it is in resting birds, skin convection would dissipate an even higher percentage of the metabolic heat.

TEMPERATURE AND OXYGEN TRANSPORT

Body

The fall of T_c in hypoxic, inactive birds is not likely to affect blood O_2 affinity except at the highest altitudes. For example, based on model calculations illustrated in Fig. 21.3, SaO_2 in pigeons at 9 km would be 46% in hypothermic and alkalotic blood, but only 34% in blood that is alkalotic but not hypothermic, at the same PaO_2. At 7 km, however, the change in T_c (1.9°C decrease) would be too small to modify the effect of alkalosis. The significance of lowered T_c in hypoxic birds at rest, thus, seems primarily to be that it reduces O_2 de-

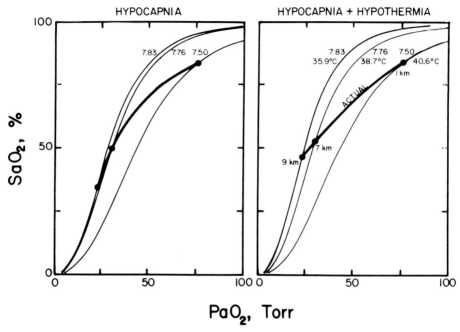

FIGURE 21.3. Oxygen equilibrium curves for pigeon blood calculated from Ref. 48 at pHa of 7.50, 7.76, or 7.83. These correspond to steady-state data for anaerobic samples obtained during acute exposure to 5°C T_a and to hypobaric hypoxia simulating 1.2, 7, or 9 km, respectively (60). *Thick lines* connect points corresponding to Po_2 measured in the same samples. **Left panel.** Curves for hypothetical birds that undergo hypocapnic alkalosis but remain isothermic (40.6°C) with increasing altitude. **Right panel.** Curves for birds that become both alkalotic and hypothermic with increasing altitude. Temperatures and pH indicated, corresponding to actual steady-state data at the altitudes shown, were used to calculate curves. Results indicate that hypothermia provides a significant advantage in blood O_2 loading only at the highest altitude. Modified from Ref. 14.

mand, except at the extremes of high altitude where it may be great enough to contribute to O_2 loading.

If, as suggested earlier, T_c rises in birds flying at high altitude, the increase is not likely to be great enough to affect blood O_2 affinity, compared with the effects of hyperventilation (which may only offset metabolic acid production). In any case, higher T_c in flying birds may have importance in improving muscle performance. Further study will be necessary to ascertain its role in blood gas transport.

An important factor in O_2 transport during flight may be an increase in Pao_2, which in normoxic pigeons was found to be higher during flight than at rest (21). If Pao_2 also increases in birds flying at high altitude, O_2 saturation could rise significantly, as hypoxia would place the blood in the steep segment of the O_2 equilibrium curve, and this could result in greater tissue O_2 delivery.

Brain

Indirect evidence from experiments on normoxic, inactive pigeons suggests that blood may give up CO_2 and take up O_2 as it perfuses the moist mucosa of the head exposed to air (11). Its Po_2, thus, rises, and the cooling and reduction of P_{CO_2} simultaneously decrease the blood's P_{50}. Because O_2 saturation is normally incomplete in resting birds, this combination of factors could also raise S_{O_2}. In the OR, blood takes up heat from the arteries, as described previously; if its P_{CO_2} were sufficiently low, due to losses at mucosal surfaces, it might also take up arterial CO_2. Either or both of these events would enhance O_2 unloading from the OR veins, and thereby increase Pa_{O_2}, perhaps compensating for the reduction that would otherwise accompany cooling. It is even possible that due to countercurrent gas exchange the P_{O_2} in arterial blood leaving the OR approaches that in the venous blood entering it, raising Sa_{O_2} and aiding brain oxygenation (11,48). This possibility gains credence from observations of cerebrospinal fluid P_{O_2} amounting to 115 mm Hg in pigeons, compared with a simultaneous Pa_{O_2} of 83 mm Hg (Fig. 21.4).

Can such a mechanism aid brain oxygenation at high altitude? As noted earlier, the difference between T_b and T_c disappears in resting pigeons during exposure to extreme hypoxia, indicating a shutdown of retial heat exchange that would preclude operation of the proposed O_2-enhancing system. As suggested previously, however, birds flying at high altitudes may resume brain cooling, allowing cooled mucosal blood with a high P_{O_2} to return to the OR. Only additional investigation will tell whether or not high fliers cool their brains and whether they supplement their brain's O_2 supply. If so, the effect

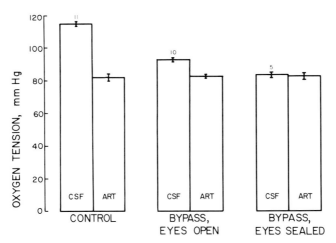

FIGURE 21.4. Oxygen tension measured in cerebrospinal fluid (CSF) sampled anaerobically from the dorsal ventricle, and in arterial blood (ART) sampled anaerobically from the brachial artery of pigeons. Bar heights represent means for the number of individual measurements indicated; error lines span ± 2 SD. Controls (*left*) were undisturbed and at rest at 25°C. Experimental animals breathed through a tracheostomy (BYPASS) with the eyes open (*middle*), or breathed through a tracheostomy while the eyes were sealed (*right*). Results show that P_{O_2} was greater in CSF than in arterial blood in controls, but that the CSF–arterial difference was diminished in bypassed birds, presumably because contact between air and the mucous membranes of oral, pharyngeal, or nasal cavities was prevented. The difference between CSF and arterial blood is fully abolished if contact between air and eyes is also prevented. The experimental data preclude the possibility that the results in the control group are due to acidification of blood in the choroid plexus. They are consistent, however, with the hypothesis that P_{O_2} in cephalic arterial blood is enhanced by countercurrent gas exchange with O_2-enriched venous blood in the ophthalmic retia, and that the moist surfaces of the head in contact with the air are the O_2 source. Data from Ref. 11.

may be only to compensate the Po_2 reduction associated with cooling; this could improve tissue diffusion by raising brain–capillary Po_2. On the other hand, if So_2 also increases in cerebral arteries, a hypoxic bird might not require as large an increase in cerebral blood flow during flight as at rest (25, 33).

CONCLUSIONS

Birds resting at high altitude regulate body temperature lower than during normoxia, reducing energy and O_2 demands. They probably cool their expirate to nearly freezing, saving almost all the water vapor and losing little convective heat, despite hyperventilation. Homeothermic lowland birds normally cool the brain and eyes below T_c, even in cold air, whereas birds resting at high altitude apparently do not. The overall T_c reduction, however, combined with hypocapnic alkalosis, can increase blood O_2 saturation during extreme hypoxia well above levels ascribable to alkalosis alone.

Tolerance of hypoxia by resting lowland birds is related to nearly 100% pulmonary and tissue O_2 extraction, as well as to the effects of hyperventilation and hypothermia on O_2 transport, but it is uncoupled from cold-stress tolerance. This is apparently because hypoxia inhibits the central nervous drive for shivering heat production, and this may be a primary factor limiting the altitude that birds can invade. Extreme hypoxia tolerance in resting lowland birds is correlated with moderate T_a only and, thus, may not reflect the evolution of high-altitude tolerance. Rather, it may be a secondary effect of physiological adaptations to the extreme metabolic requirements of flight.

Unlike resting birds, birds that fly at high altitude probably raise T_c due to heat production in the working pectoral muscles. They may simultaneously minimize heat loss from exposed extremities; cool expired air to minimize respiratory heat loss; and cool the brain as in resting, lowland birds. They probably compensate for the effects of temperature on hemoglobin by hyperventilating, driving Pao_2, pHa, and blood O_2 affinity up. A rise in muscle temperature would improve muscle performance, and this would be an advantage at the reduced air density and viscosity found at high altitudes, where more work is needed to remain airborne, but may not affect O_2 delivery significantly. Brain cooling entails loss of heat by blood perfusing the mucosal surfaces of the head, and this may be accompanied by gas exchange between blood and air at these sites. Countercurrent arteriovenous gas exchange in the OR of the head may also occur. If so, this could enhance the O_2 supply in the brain, with potential advantages during high-altitude flight.

ACKNOWLEDGMENTS

Preparation of this contribution supported in part by NSF grant BSR-8806604.

REFERENCES

1. ARAD, Z., U. MIDTGÅRD, AND M. H. BERNSTEIN. Thermoregulation in turkey vultures: vascular anatomy, arteriovenous heat exchange, and behavior. The Condor 91:505–514, 1989.

2. AULIE, A. Body temperatures in pigeons and budgerigars during sustained flight. *Comp. Biochem. Physiol. 39*:173–176, 1971.
3. BAUDINETTE, R. V., J. P. LOVERIDGE, K. J. WILSON, AND K. SCHMIDT-NIELSEN. Heat loss from feet of herring gulls at rest and during flight. *Am. J. Physiol. 230*:920–924, 1976.
4. BAUDINETTE, R. V., AND K. SCHMIDT-NIELSEN. Energy cost of gliding flight in herring gulls. *Nature 248*:83–84, 1974.
5. BENNETT, A. F. Thermal dependence of muscle function. *Am. J. Physiol. 247*:R217–R229, 1984.
6. BERGER, M., J. S. HART, AND O. Z. ROY. Respiratory water and heat loss of the black duck during flight at different ambient temperatures. *Can. J. Zool. 49*:767–774, 1971.
7. BERNSTEIN, M. H. Cutaneous water loss in small birds. *Condor 73*:468–469, 1971.
8. BERNSTEIN, M. H. Vascular responses and foot temperature in pigeons. *Am. J. Physiol. 226*:1350 1355, 1974.
9. BERNSTEIN, M. H. Respiration in flying birds. In: *Bird Respiration,* ed. T. J. Sellers. Boca Raton: CRC Press, II: 1987, pp. 43–74.
10. BERNSTEIN, M. H., M.B. CURTIS, AND D. M. HUDSON. Independence of brain and body temperatures in flying American kestrels, *Falco sparverius. Am. J. Physiol. 237*:R58–R62, 1979.
11. BERNSTEIN, M. H., H. L. DURAN, AND B. PINSHOW. Extrapulmonary gas exchange enhances brain oxygen in pigeons. *Science 226*:564–566, 1984.
12. BERNSTEIN, M. H., I. SANDOVAL, M. B. CURTIS, AND D. M. HUDSON. Brain temperature in pigeons: effects of anterior respiratory bypass. *J. Comp. Physiol. 129*:115–118, 1979.
13. BERNSTEIN, M. H., S. P. THOMAS, AND K. SCHMIDT-NIELSEN. Power input during flight of the fish crow, *Corvus ossifragus. J. Exper. Biol. 58*:401–410, 1973.
14. BERNSTEIN, M. H., C. TIQUI, K. M. RAMIREZ, AND J. MANZANARES. Brain and body temperatures in pigeons at simulated high altitudes. (submitted).
15. BLACK, C. P., AND S. M. TENNEY. Oxygen transport during progressive hypoxia in high-altitude and sea-level waterfowl. *Respir. Physiol. 39*:217–239, 1980.
16. BLACK, C. P., S. M. TENNEY, AND M. VAN KROONENBURG. Oxygen transport during progressive hypoxia in bar-headed geese (*Anser indicus*) acclimated to sea level and 5600 m. In: *Respiratory Function in Birds, Adult and Embryonic,* ed. J. Piiper, New York: Springer-Verlag, 1978.
17. BOUVEROT, P., G. HILDWEIN, AND P. OULHEN. Ventilatory and circulatory O_2 convection at 4000 m in pigeon at neutral or cold temperature. *Respir. Physiol. 28*:371–385, 1976.
18. BRENT, R., P. F. PEDERSEN, C. BECH, AND K. JOHANSEN. Lung ventilation and temperature regulation in the European coot (*Fulica atra*). *Physiol. Zool. 57*:19–25, 1984.
19. BURGOON, D. A., D. L. KILGORE, JR., AND P. J. MOTTA. Brain temperature in the calliope hummingbird (*Stellula calliope*): a species lacking a *rete mirabile ophthalmicum. J. Comp. Physiol. B 157*:583–588, 1987.
20. BUTLER, P. J. The effect of progressive hypoxia on the respiratory and cardiovascular systems of the pigeon and duck. *J. Physiol. 201*:527–538, 1970.
21. BUTLER, P. J., N. H. WEST, AND D. R. JONES. Respiratory and cardiovascular responses of the pigeon to sustained, level flight in a wind-tunnel. *J. Exp. Biol. 71*:7–26, 1977.
22. CHAPPELL, M. A., AND T. L. BUCHER. Effects of temperature and altitude on ventilation and gas exchange in chukars (*Alectoris chukar*). *J. Comp. Physiol. B 157*:129–136, 1987.
23. COLACINO, J. M., D. H. HECTOR, AND K. SCHMIDT-NIELSEN. Respiratory responses of ducks to simulated altitude. *Respir. Physiol. 29*:265–281, 1977.
24. EDERSTROM, H. E., AND S. J. BRUMLEVE. Temperature gradients in the legs of cold-acclimatized pheasants. *Am. J. Physiol. 207*:457–459, 1964.
25. FARACI, F. M., D. L. KILGORE, JR., AND M. R. FEDDE. Oxygen delivery to the heart and brain during hypoxia: pekin duck vs. bar-headed goose. *Am. J. Physiol. 247*:R69–R75, 1984.
26. FEDDE, M. R., F. M. FARACI, D. L. KILGORE, JR., G. H. CARDINET, III, AND A. CHATTERJEE. Cardiopulmonary adaptations in birds for exercise at high altitude. In: *Circulation, Respiration, and Metabolism,* ed. R. Gilles. New York: Springer-Verlag, 1985.
27. FROST, P. G. H., AND W. R. SIEGFRIED. Use of legs as dissipators of heat in flying passerines. *Zool. Afr. 10*:101–102, 1975.
28. FROST, P. G. H., W. R. SIEGFRIED, AND P. J. GREENWOOD. Arteriovenous heat exchange systems in the jackass penguin, *Spheniscus demersus. J. Zool. 175*:231–241, 1975.
29. GLEESON, M., G. M. BARNAS, AND W. RAUTENBERG. The effects of hypoxia on the metabolic and cardiorespiratory responses to shivering produced by external and central cooling in the pigeon. *Pflügers Archiv 407*:312–319, 1986.
30. GLEESON, M., G. M. BARNAS, AND W. RAUTENBERG. Cardiorespiratory responses to shivering in vagotomized pigeons during normoxia and hypoxia. *Pflügers Archiv 407*:664–669, 1986.
31. GOLDSPINK, G., C. MILLS, AND K. SCHMIDT-NIELSEN. Electrical activity of the pectoral mus-

cles during gliding and flapping flight in the herring gull (*Larus argentatus*). *Experientia 34*:862–865, 1978.

32. GRAF, R. Diurnal cycles of thermoregulation and hypothermia. *International Ornithological Congress (17th), Berlin, Germany, Acta* 1:331–335, 1978.

33. GRUBB, B., J. M. COLACINO, AND K. SCHMIDT-NIELSEN. Cerebral blood flow in birds: effect of hypoxia. *Am. J. Physiol. 234*:H230–H234, 1978.

34. HAGAN, A. A., AND J. E. HEATH. Regulation of heat loss in the duck by vasomotion in the bill. *J. Thermal Biol. 5*:95–101, 1980.

35. HART, J. S., AND O. Z. ROY. Temperature regulation during flight in pigeons. *Am. J. Physiol. 213*:1311–1316, 1967.

36. HIRTH, K.-D., W. BIESEL, AND W. NACHTIGALL. Pigeon flight in a wind tunnel. *J. Comp. Physiol. B. 157*:111–116, 1987.

37. HUDSON, D. M., AND M. H. BERNSTEIN. Temperature regulation and heat balance in flying white-necked ravens, *Corvus cryptoleucus. J. Exp. Biol. 90*:267–281, 1981.

38. JOHANSEN, K., AND R. W. MILLARD. Vascular responses to temperature in the foot of the giant fulmar, *Macronectes giganteus. J. Comp. Physiol. 85*:47–64, 1973.

39. KILEY, J. P., F. M. FARACI, AND M. R. FEDDE. Gas exchange during exercise in hypoxic ducks. *Respir. Physiol. 59*:105–115, 1985.

40. KILGORE, D. L., JR., M. H. BERNSTEIN, AND D. M. HUDSON. Brain temperatures in birds. *J. Comp. Physiol. 110*:209–215, 1976.

41. KILGORE, D. L., JR., G. F. BIRCHARD, AND D. F. BOGGS. Brain temperatures in running quail. *J. Appl. Physiol. 50*:1277–1281, 1981.

42. LASIEWSKI, R. C., AND W. R. DAWSON. A re-examination of the relation between standard metabolic rate and body weight in birds. *Condor 69*:13–23, 1967.

43. LENTNER, C. Geigy Scientific Tables. *Ciba-Geigy Limited, Basle, Switzerland,* Vol. 3, 1984.

44. MIDTGÅRD, U. Heat loss from the feet of mallards, *Anas platyrhynchos,* and arterio-venous heat exchange in the *rete tibiotarsale. Ibis 122*:354–359, 1980.

45. MIDTGÅRD, U. The blood vascular system in the head of the herring gull (*Larus argentatus*). *J. Morphology 179*:135–152, 1984.

46. MIDTGÅRD, U. Eye temperatures in birds and the significance of the *rete ophthalmicum. Vidensk. Meddr dansk naturh. Foren. 145*:173–181, 1984.

47. MIDTGÅRD, U. Innervation of the avian ophthalmic rete. *Fortschritte der Zoologie 30*:401–404, 1985.

48. PINSHOW, B., M. H. BERNSTEIN, AND Z. ARAD. Effects of temperature and P_{CO_2} on O_2 affinity of pigeon blood: implications for brain O_2 supply. *Am. J. Physiol. 249*:R758–R764, 1985.

49. PINSHOW, B., M. H. BERNSTEIN, G. E. LOPEZ, AND S. KLEINHAUS. Regulation of brain temperature in pigeons: effects of corneal convection. *Am. J. Physiol. 242*:R577–R581, 1982.

50. SCHMIDT-NIELSEN, K., F. R. HAINSWORTH, AND D. E. MURRISH. Countercurrent heat exchange in the respiratory passages: effect on water and heat balance. *Respir. Physiol. 9*:263–276, 1970.

51. SHAMS, H., AND P. SCHEID. Respiration and blood gases in the duck exposed to normocapnic and hypercapnic hypoxia. *Respir. Physiol. 67*:1–12, 1987.

52. STEEN, I., AND J. B. STEEN. The importance of the legs in the thermoregulation of birds. *Acta Physiol. Scand. 63*:285–291, 1965.

53. SWAN, L. W. The ecology of the high Himalayas. *Sci. Am. 205*:68–78, 1961.

54. TORRE-BUENO, J. R. Temperature regulation and heat dissipation during flight in birds. *J. Exp. Biol. 65*:471–482, 1976.

55. TORRE-BUENO, J. R. Evaporative cooling and water balance during flight in birds. *J. Exp. Biol. 75*:231–236, 1978.

56. TUCKER, V. A. Respiratory physiology of house sparrows in relation to high-altitude flight. *J. Exp. Biol. 48*:55–66, 1968.

57. TUCKER, V. A. Respiratory exchange and evaporative water loss in the flying budgerigar. *J. Exp. Biol. 48*:67–87, 1968.

58. TUCKER, V. A. Energetics of natural avian flight. In: *Avian Energetics,* ed. R. A. Paynter. Cambridge: Nuttall Ornithological Club, 1974.

59. VEGHTE, J. H. Thermal exchange between the raven, *Corvus corax,* and its environment. *Ph.D. Thesis, University of Michigan* 1976.

60. WEINSTEIN, Y., M. H. BERNSTEIN, P. E. BICKLER, D. V. GONZALES, F. C. SAMANIEGO, AND M. A. ESCOBEDO. Blood respiratory properties in pigeons at high altitudes: effects of acclimation. *Am. J. Physiol. 249*:R765–R775, 1985.

22

Central Adaptation to Hypoxia

NORMAN H. EDELMAN, JOSEPH E. MELTON,
AND JUDITH A. NEUBAUER

It is well established that in anesthetized animals, in the absence of peripheral chemoreceptor stimulation, hypoxia produces a depression of breathing. Recently, there has been considerable interest in discerning the mechanisms responsible for the central depression of respiration during hypoxia. A basic issue that arises when considering the mechanisms responsible for hypoxic modulation of central respiratory output is whether respiratory neuronal activity is simply limited by substrate availability within the brain, or whether this depression represents an active inhibition of neuronal activity. Such inhibition could serve to minimize energy use during hypoxia by limiting motor activity as well as conserving high energy substrates that would be used normally to reestablish transmembrane ionic gradients dissipated during neuronal activity. Thus, neuronal inhibition might subserve a protective function by affording tolerance to hypoxic environments. This ability to "down-regulate" metabolic activity during hypoxia is a well-characterized phenomenon in many lower vertebrates, for example, the diving turtle (46), but may also be physiologically relevant in both unanesthetized neonatal and adult mammals.

In the newborn of many species, the respiratory response to hypoxia consists of an initial increase in ventilation that is followed within a few minutes by a dramatic decline to levels that can actually be lower than normoxic values (1, 19, 28). It has been suggested that this secondary depression results from a failure of peripheral chemoreceptors (4). This seems unlikely, however, as other studies that have simultaneously recorded carotid sinus nerve activity and respiratory output have shown a sustained stimulation of the carotid chemoreceptors while the initial increase in respiratory output is not sustained (1, 28, 41). Thus, in the newborn, the central hypoxic depression of respiration appears to overcome the peripheral response to hypoxia within minutes, giving the response a biphasic character.

A biphasic response to hypoxia has also been identified in adult animals, although it is not as pronounced and has slower dynamics than that observed in the neonate (11, 26, 49). In unanesthetized humans (11), exposure to a constant level of isocapnic hypoxia results in an abrupt increase in ventilation that peaks in 3 to 5 minutes. If the hypoxia is maintained, ventilation declines over the next 15 to 30 minutes before achieving a new steady-state value that is above normoxic ventilatory levels, but 25% to 40% lower than the maximum. A similar response can be observed in goats with a secondary decline in ventilation occurring after an hour of relatively severe hypoxia (15). Evidence that the decline in respiration during hypoxia in the adult is also a central phenomenon and not a peripheral response comes from two observations: (1) an abrupt return to euoxia or hyperoxia results in a residual depression of ventilation (12, 23) that requires a substantial period of time (up to an hour) to resolve; and (2) blocking the hypoxic stimulation of the peripheral chemoreceptors with somatostatin eliminates the initial stimulation of ventilation by hypoxia and unmasks a pure respiratory depression with a time course consistent with a central phenomenon (14). The slow onset and recovery of central respiratory depression during hypoxia suggest that the mechanism responsible for this response requires an alteration in the release and/or accumulation of some neuroeffector.

The depressant action of brain hypoxia is probably best demonstrated in anesthetized, peripherally chemodenervated animals. Progressive isocapnic hypoxia in cats prepared in this manner, with blood pressure also controlled, results in a depression of the phrenic neurogram that is correlated with the degree of reduction in arterial oxygen content (30, 37, 53). This depression of respiration is characterized by an initial decline in the peak amplitude of the phrenic neurogram followed by a reduction in phrenic firing frequency after phrenic amplitude is reduced by approximately 50% (53). After arterial oxygen content is reduced by 50 to 60%, there is a complete silencing of the phrenic neurogram followed by gasping if the hypoxemia is made more severe (arterial oxygen content less than 20 vol %) (33).

Although depression appears to be a generalized response of respiratory efferent outputs to central hypoxia, there does appear to be differences in their vulnerability to this stress. Inspiratory activity measured in the hypoglossal nerve declines progressively with hypoxia but is silenced after less reduction in arterial oxygen content than is required to silence the phrenic nerve (48). Although depression of expiratory activity of the triangularis sterni appears to parallel the depression of the phrenic nerve (39), expiratory abdominal muscle and iliohypogastric nerve activities appear to be more vulnerable with depression of these respiratory outputs even manifested during hypoxia in unanesthetized animals (16). In contrast with other respiratory outputs, central hypoxia does not produce a generalized depression of central sympathetic activity (47). The sympathetic neurogram consists of two components: a tonic component and a phasic component, which is synchronous with respiratory (inspiratory) activity. The differential effect of hypoxia on both the tonic and inspiratory–synchronous activity of the preganglionic cervical sympathetic neurogram is shown in Fig. 22.1. Hypoxia produces a progressive decline in the phasic component in parallel with the depression of activity of the phrenic nerve. Tonic sympathetic nerve activity, however, is substantially increased at levels of hypoxia associated with silencing of respiratory activity. Thus, although the majority of central neurons are probably depressed by hypoxia, there is at least one central output that appears to be excited by hypoxia. It remains to be determined whether this increase in activity is due to a direct stimulation of the sympathetic neurons of the ventrolateral medulla or to an indirect excitation from disinhibition because of selective vulnerability within the central sympathetic neuronal network.

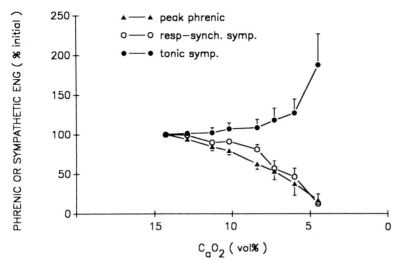

FIGURE 22.1. Mean phrenic and cervical sympathetic neurogram responses to brain hypoxia measured in anesthetized, peripherally chemodenervated, vagotomized cats. Cervical sympathetic activity is divided into inspiratory–synchronous and tonic components. Neurogram activities were measured at eight decreasing levels of arterial oxygen content (Ca_{O_2}). Values are means ± SEM.

We have characterized the mechanisms responsible for the central depression of respiratory output by hypoxia (36). This has led us to propose three categories of hypoxic respiratory depression based on both severity and presumed mechanism of action. Type I hypoxic depression occurs with mild or transient hypoxemia and is associated with a transient ventral medullary alkalosis secondary to sudden increases in brain blood flow. It presumably reflects decreased stimulation of the central chemoreceptor due to a "washout" of tissue CO_2 and is probably important mainly in specific non-steady-state circumstances such as during REM sleep (43). Type II hypoxic depression is associated with substantial medullary acidosis and progressive respiratory depression to complete apnea. We believe that this form of depression is due to an active inhibition because of an alteration in the balance of inhibitory and excitatory neuroeffectors toward greater inhibition. Finally, when hypoxia becomes very severe, there is a failure of membrane ionic pumps and an impairment of the respiratory neuron response that we have termed type III hypoxic depression.

It is the mechanisms responsible for type II hypoxic depression on which we have focused most of our recent attention. We have characterized type II depression by directly demonstrating that the respiratory depression observed during this phase is not due to a metabolic impairment of the respiratory neurons. We have shown this by determining that even moderate to severe respiratory depression (apnea) is not associated with a diminution of respiratory responsiveness to CO_2 and carotid sinus nerve stimulation (30, 40). The left panel of Fig. 22.2 illustrates the phrenic nerve response to a CO_2 rebreathing test before and after hypoxic depression of the phrenic neurogram to apnea in an anesthetized, peripherally chemodenervated cat. As can be seen from these responses, even after phrenic nerve activity is depressed to apnea with CO

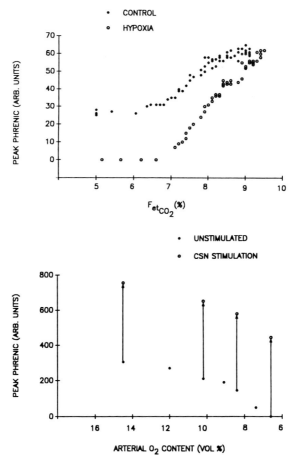

FIGURE 22.2. Intact afferent responses of the phrenic neurogram during hypoxic respiratory depression. The **left panel** shows the response of the phrenic neurogram of an anesthetized, peripherally chemodenervated, vagotomized cat to CO_2 rebreathing before and after hypoxic respiratory depression induced by inhalation of carbon monoxide (CO). Arterial oxygen content was maintained constant during the rebreathing. The slope of the response was unchanged despite hypoxic respiratory depression to the point of phrenic apnea. The **right panel** shows the effect of carotid sinus nerve (CSN) stimulation on the amplitude of the phrenic neurogram in the same cat preparation before and during CO inhalation. CSN stimulation resulted in the same increase in phrenic amplitude during hypoxic depression despite reduced prestimulation levels of phrenic amplitude.

hypoxia, the response to CO_2 during hypoxia was brisk and complete, reaching the same level of phrenic activation as seen without hypoxia. An intact CO_2 response during the secondary decline in ventilation with hypoxia has also recently been demonstrated in adult unanesthetized humans (17). Additionally, the right panel of Fig. 22.2 shows that the stimulatory effect of carotid sinus nerve stimulation on the phrenic neurogram is also unaffected by brain hypoxia. Phrenic nerve activity increases by the same amount at various points in the progressive depression caused by lowering the arterial oxygen content. These data indicate to us that the depression of respiratory neurons in this model is specific for brain hypoxia and does not prevent the neuronal circuitry from responding to other stimuli.

Further evidence that type II hypoxic depression is associated with maintenance of full integrity of respiratory neurons up to the point of gasping comes from studies that have examined the neuronal microenvironment for loss of membrane integrity as evidenced by a change in extracellular potassium concentration ($[K^+]ec$) (32). Using ion-specific microelectrodes, we have measured medullary $[K^+]ec$ during progressive hypoxic depression of phrenic nerve activity. Medullary $[K^+]ec$ was maintained constant up to and beyond the point of phrenic apnea (Fig. 22.3) and only began to rise when arterial oxygen content was reduced to a level low enough to initiate gasping. Thus, hypoxic depression of the sort we term type II is associated with intact transmembrane ionic gradients, at least as manifest by $[K^+]ec$ homeostasis, and hypoxia-induced gasping seems to mark a point when the capacity to maintain ionic gradients is beginning to fail.

The specific mechanisms responsible for hypoxic depression have not been clearly delineated. If we postulate that central hypoxic depression is a protective mechanism, then it is reasonable to suspect that it may be a conserved function whose general mechanisms are used more prominently by lower animals that have evolved a tolerance for hypoxic environments. In this regard, the turtle is an excellent example of a very hypoxia-tolerant animal, having the ability to sustain complete apnea in anoxic water for months (46). In addition to this sustained apneic response, Hitzig and Nattie (21) have shown that the ventilatory response of the turtle to hypoxia exhibits an increase in ventilation followed by a secondary decline with time, much like that seen in adult mammals.

The ability of the turtle to withstand hypoxic environments for such a prolonged time suggests that it has special strategies for maintaining the integrity of its cell membranes, and more specifically an ability to maintain the continued functioning of ionic pumps. That the turtle is better able to maintain

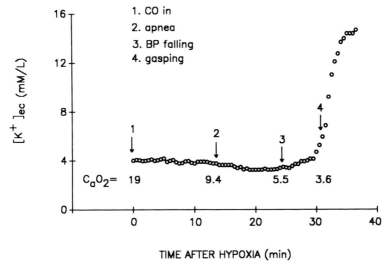

FIGURE 22.3. Medullary extracellular potassium concentration ($[K^+]ec$) as a function of time after initiation of inhalation of carbon monoxide in an anesthetized, peripherally chemodenervated, vagotomized cat. Values of arterial O_2 content (CaO_2) are also shown. $[K^+]ec$ was relatively unchanged until CaO_2 was reduced by 80%.

ionic gradients during anoxia than the rat is evidenced by measurements of brain extracellular K^+ concentrations (45). The specific strategies that assist in maintaining cellular integrity when oxygen becomes limited have been enumerated in a review by Hochachka (22). In brief, animals that can be classified as hypoxia tolerant generally are able to prevent accumulation of lactic acidosis with a reverse Pasteur effect, their membranes tend to be less permeable to ions, they decrease their metabolism so that ATP utilization is regulated to synthesis, and they are better able to maintain stable membranes with stable ion gradients. Of these strategies in hypoxia-tolerant animals, the most effective one has been found to be the ability to decrease their metabolism.

Although mammals appear to lack the special qualities that endow turtles with their extraordinary tolerance to hypoxia, there are mechanisms available to the mammalian nervous system that can minimize the effect of hypoxia at the cellular level. Because neuronal firing stresses the ionic pumps, reducing discharge rate could provide a means for delaying the loss of cellular integrity. An effective way of reducing neuronal activity would be through hyperpolarization of neuronal membranes. This could be accomplished by altering the balance between inhibitory and excitatory neuromodulators. The result would be a reduction of basal activity without necessarily impairing the response to intense stimuli such as hypercapnia or carotid sinus nerve stimulation.

There are several neuromodulator candidates that have been shown directly or indirectly to change with hypoxia. The synthesis and release of several excitatory neurotransmitters decrease during hypoxia (e.g., acetylcholine, adrenergic amines, glutamate, and aspartate (3, 7, 9, 13, 18), whereas there is a general increase in the concentrations of the neuronal depressants (e.g., adenosine, opioids, GABA, alanine, taurine, and lactic acid) (5, 9, 13, 20, 24, 37, 50, 51).

In an effort to identify which inhibitory neuromodulators are responsible for hypoxic depression of respiratory output, we have determined the effect of a number of selective antagonists in our cat model of progressive hypoxic depression using inhalation of carbon monoxide. Although antagonizing adenosine and opioids attentuates the amount of hypoxic depression, they seem to mediate only a minor portion of the respiratory depression during hypoxia (35, 38). Opioids may have a greater role in the secondary decline of ventilation in the biphasic response to the neonate (8), but not in the adult human biphasic response to hypoxia (26). The role of adenosine is somewhat more confusing as the use of adenosine antagonists appears to attenuate the secondary decline in ventilation in both the newborn (6) and the adult (10); however, use of these agents uncovers a rise in frequency with hypoxia rather than attenuating the decline in the amplitude of the breath.

The most dramatic effects that we have observed have been obtained by blocking the effects of hypoxia-induced brain acidosis or gamma-aminobutyric acid (GABA) (31, 37). Although we generally think of acidosis as a respiratory stimulant, this stimulation is a unique characteristic of a small population of chemosensitive cells located near the surface of the ventral medulla. In contrast to this stimulatory effect, most CNS neurons respond to acidosis with a hyperpolarization and diminished activity (25, 27, 29, 34). Because the acidosis of brain hypoxia is primarily the result of an early Pasteur shift with production of lactate, we determined the role of lactic acid in hypoxic depression by preventing the production of lactate with sodium dichloroacetate (DCA:37). Prevention of lactic acidosis with DCA prevented both the ventral medullary acidosis and the depression of phrenic nerve activity until the hypoxemia became very severe. Thus, the progressive and graded acidosis that is associated with brain hypoxia may provide a mechanism for progressive decreases in respiratory output. This effect of acidosis could be a direct effect on neuronal membrane potential or it could be an indirect effect mediated by another inhibitory neuromodulator such as GABA.

The synthetic rate of GABA is sensitive to both the effects of reductions in oxygen availability and to the intracellular acidity such that the production of GABA is favored when acidosis is present and degradation is significantly diminished (52). In addition, hypoxia significantly slows the reuptake mechanisms for GABA (20). Thus, the net effect is to increase both total brain concentration (13, 24, 51), as well as extracellular concentrations (20). The contribution of GABA to hypoxic depression of respiration was assessed in our cat model of brain hypoxia by determining the effect of hypoxia on the dose response of phrenic nerve activity to the GABA antagonist bicuculline (31). The dose responses before and during hypoxic depression are illustrated in Fig. 22.4. In the absence of hypoxia, only small doses of bicuculline are necessary to stimulate phrenic output maximally. In the presence of brain hypoxia, and significant respiratory depression, the dose-response curve is shifted toward higher doses. But most interesting is that the maximum level of response is the same with and without brain hypoxia, suggesting true competitive inhibition. These results suggest that GABA may be the principal inhibitory neurotransmitter mediating respiratory depression during brain hypoxia and that the levels of GABA may be regulated by the cellular acidosis.

Finally, it is necessary to speculate on the role of hypoxic depression in the integrated respiratory response to hypoxia. Initially, respiratory depression in the face of hypoxia may appear to be counterproductive as only an increase in ventilation can offset a reduction in inspired oxygen. Increases in ventilation during hypoxic exposure, however, do not maintain brain tissue oxygenation constant; thus, cellular mechanisms that are aimed at maintaining cellular integrity of the CNS are of adaptive value. Reducing cellular activity is a very important hypoxia-adaptive mechanism. In excitable cells, such as neurons, preventing neuronal activity is an effective means of preventing cell death (42). Thus, the observation that GABA levels increase during hypoxia and depress the neuronal activity responsible for respiratory output is consistent with a protective function for this inhibitory neurotransmitter. In addition, the protective value of lactic acidosis may be more than its indirect ability to enhance the production of GABA. Bonventre and Cheung (2) have demonstrated that during anoxia cells survive much better if they are more acidic. This protective effect of acidosis may in fact be specific for lactic acid, as Schurr and associates (44) have found that recovery of the synaptic function of hippocampal neurons made anoxic is improved when the concentration of lactic acid was increased.

In summary, we believe that the depression of respiratory neuronal activity during hypoxia is a potentially adaptive response mediated principally by the effects of acidosis and increased GABA levels. Its value in adult animals

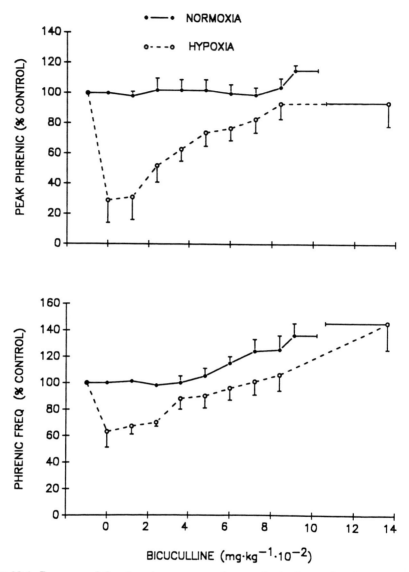

FIGURE 22.4. Response of the phrenic neurogram in anesthetized, peripherally chemodener-vated, vagotomized cats to intraveous infusion of the GABA antagonist bicuculline. Infusions were performed while cats were breathing 40% O_2 in N_2 (*closed circles*; $n = 5$) or after hypoxia (0.5% CO inhalation) sufficient to reduce phrenic amplitude to zero (*open circles*; $n = 5$). All values are mean $\pm$ SEM. Bicuculline reversed the depression of both phrenic amplitude and phrenic burst frequency characteristic of hypoxia.

may be limited but a very clear value may be recognized in the fetus. A fetal ventilatory response to hypoxia would certainly be counterproductive as the increased muscular activity would deplete O_2 stores without increasing O_2 supply, whereas lack of a response would conserve energy supplies for maintenance of ionic gradients. In addition, neonatal mammals can withstand considerably longer periods of anoxia with no loss of cellular integrity compared with adult mammals. Both considerations argue for a greater ability to reduce brain oxidative metabolism in response to hypoxia as compared with the adult. Thus, in regard to the respiratory response to hypoxia, the biphasic response of the neonate may represent a remnant adaption to life in utero.

REFERENCES

1. BLANCO, C. E., M.A. HANSON, P. JOHNSON, AND H. RIGATTO. Breathing pattern of kittens during hypoxia. *J. Appl. Physiol.* 56:12–17, 1984.
2. BONVENTRE, J. V., AND J. Y. CHEUNG. Effects of metabolic acidosis on viability of cells exposed to anoxia. *Am. J. Physiol.* 249:C149–C159, 1985.
3. BROWN, R. M., S. R. SNIDER, AND A. CARLSSON. Changes in biogenic amine synthesis and turnover induced by hypoxia and/or foot shock stress. II. The central nervous system. *J. Neurol. Trans.* 35:293–305, 1974.
4. BUREAU, M. A., J. LAMARCHE, P. FOULON, AND D. DALLE. The ventilatory response to hypoxia in the newborn lamb after carotid body denervation. *Respir. Physiol.* 60:109–119, 1985.
5. CHERNICK, V., AND R. J. CRAIG. Naloxone reverses neonatal depression caused by fetal asphyxia. *Science* 216:1252–1253, 1982.
6. DARNALL, R. A. Aminophylline reduces hypoxic ventilatory depression: possible role of adenosine. *Ped. Res.* 19:706–710, 1985.
7. DAVIS, J. N., AND A. CARLSSON. Effect of hypoxia on monoamine synthesis, levels and metabolism in rat brain. *J. Neurochem.* 21:783–790, 1973.
8. DEBOECK, C., P. VAN RAEMPTS, H. RIGATTO, AND V. CHERNICK. Naloxone reduces decrease in ventilation induced by hypoxia in newborn infants. *J. Appl. Physiol.* 56:1507–1511, 1984.
9. DUFFY, T. E., S. R. NELSON, AND O. H. LOWRY. Cerebral carbohydrate metabolism during acute hypoxia and recovery. *J. Neurochem.* 19:959–977, 1972.
10. EASTON, P. A., AND N. R. ANTHONISEN. Ventilatory response to sustained hypoxia after pretreatment with aminophylline. *J. Appl. Physiol.* 64:1445–1450, 1988.
11. EASTON, P. A., L. J. SLYKERMAN, AND N. R. ANTHONISEN. Ventilatory response to sustained hypoxia in normal adults. *J. Appl. Physiol.* 61:906–911, 1986.
12. EASTON, P. A., L. J. SLYKERMAN, AND N. R. ANTHONISEN. Recovery of the ventilatory response to hypoxia in normal adults. *J. Appl. Physiol.* 64:521–528, 1988.
13. ERECINSKA, M., D. NELSON, D. F. WILSON, AND I. A. SILVER. Neurotransmitter amino acids in the CNS. I. Regional changes in amino acid levels in rat brain during ischemia and reperfusion. *Brain Res.* 304:9–22, 1984.
14. FILUK, R. B., D. J. BEREZANSKI, AND N. R. ANTHONISEN. Depression of hypoxic ventilatory response in humans by somatostatin. *J. Appl. Physiol.* 65:1050–1054, 1988.
15. FREEDMAN, A., A. T. SCARDELLA, N. H. EDELMAN, AND T. V. SANTIAGO. Hypoxia does not increase CSF or plasma beta-endorphin activity. *J. Appl. Physiol.* 64:966–971, 1988.
16. FREGOSI, R. F., S. L. KNUTH, D. K. WARD, AND D. BARTLETT, JR. Hypoxia inhibits abdominal expiratory nerve activity. *J. Appl. Physiol.* 63:211–220, 1987.
17. GEORGOPOULOS, D., D. BEREZANSKI, AND N. R. ANTHONISEN. Effects of CO_2 breathing on ventilatory response to sustained hypoxia in normal adults. *J. Appl. Physiol.* 66:1071–1078, 1989.
18. GIBSON, G. E., M. SHIMADA, AND J. P. BLASS. Alterations in acetylcholine synthesis and in cyclic nucleotides in mild cerebral hypoxia. *J. Neurochem.* 31:757–760, 1978.
19. HADDAD, G. G., AND R. B. MELLINS. Hypoxia and respiratory control in early life. *Ann. Rev. Physiol.* 46:629–643, 1984.
20. HAGBERG, H., A. LEHMANN, M. SANDBERG, B. NYSTROM, I. JACOBSON, AND A. HAMBERGER. Ischemia-induced shift of inhibitory and excitatory amino acids from intra- to extracellular compartments. *J. Cereb. Blood Flow Metab.* 5:413–419, 1985.
21. HITZIG, B. M., AND E. E. NATTIE. Acid-base stress and central chemical control of ventilation in turtles. *J. Appl. Physiol.* 53:1365–1370, 1982.
22. HOCHACHKA, P. W. Defense strategies against hypoxia and hypothermia. *Science* 231:234–241, 1986.
23. HOLTBY, S. G., D. J. BEREZANSKI, AND N. R. ANTHONISEN. Effect of 100% O_2 on hypoxic eucapnic ventilation. *J. Appl. Physiol.* 65:1157–1162, 1988.
24. IVERSEN, K., T. HEDNER, AND P. LUNDBORG. GABA concentrations and turnover in neonatal rat brain during asphyxia and recovery. *Acta Physiol. Scand.* 118:91–94, 1983.
25. JODKOWSKI, J. S., AND J. LIPSKI. Decreased excitability of respiratory motoneurons during hypercapnia in the acute spinal cat. *Brain Res.* 386:296–304, 1986.
26. KAGAWA, S., M. J. STAFFORD, T. B. WAGGENER, AND J. W. SEVERINGHAUS. No effect of nalox-

one on hypoxia-induced ventilatory depression in adults. *J. Appl. Physiol. 52*:1030–1034, 1982.

27. KRYNJEVIC, K., M. RANDIC, AND B. K. SIESJO. Cortical CO_2 tension and neuronal excitability. *J. Physiol. (London) 176*:105–122, 1965.

28. LAWSON, E. E., AND W. W. LONG. Central origin of biphasic breathing pattern during hypoxia in newborns. *J. Appl. Physiol. 55*:483–488, 1983.

29. MARSHALL, K. C., AND I. ENGBERG. The effects of hydrogen ion on spinal neurons. *Can. J. Physiol. Pharmacol. 58*:650–655, 1980.

30. MELTON, J. E., J. A. NEUBAUER, AND N. H. EDELMAN. CO_2 sensitivity of cat phrenic neurogram during hypoxic respiratory depression. *J. Appl. Physiol. 65*:736–743, 1988.

31. MELTON, J. E., J. A. NEUBAUER, AND N. H. EDELMAN. GABA antagonism reverses hypoxic respiratory depression in the cat. *J. Appl. Physiol.* (provisionally accepted)

32. MELTON, J. E., L. M. OYER, J. A. NEUBAUER, AND N. H. EDELMAN. Brain extracellular [K^+] homeostasis during hypoxic respiratory depression (Abstr). *FASEB J. 3*(3):A251, 1989.

33. MELTON, J. E., M. J. WASICKO, J. A. NEUBAUER, AND N. H. EDELMAN. Patterns of phrenic depression during progressive brain hypoxia (Abstr). *FASEB J. 2*(4):A510, 1988.

34. MITCHELL, R. A., AND D. A. HERBERT. The effect of carbon dioxide on the membrane potential of medullary respiratory neurons. *Brain Res. 75*:345–349, 1974.

35. NEUBAUER, J. A., M. A. POSNER, T. V. SANTIAGO, AND N. H. EDELMAN. Naloxone reduces ventilatory depression of brain hypoxia. *J. Appl. Physiol. 63*:699–706, 1987.

36. NEUBAUER, J. A., T. V. SANTIAGO, M. A. POSNER, AND N. H. EDELMAN. Ventral medullary pH and ventilatory responses to hyperperfusion and hypoxia. *J. Appl. Physiol. 58*:1659–1668, 1985.

37. NEUBAUER, J. A., A. SIMONE, AND N. H. EDELMAN. Role of brain lactic acidosis in hypoxic depression of respiration. *J. Appl. Physiol. 65*:1324–1331, 1988.

38. NISSLEY, F. P., J. E. MELTON, J. A. NEUBAUER, AND N. H. EDELMAN. Effect of adenosine antagonism on phrenic nerve output during brain hypoxia. *Fed. Proc. 45*:1046, 1986.

39. OYER, L. M., J. E. MELTON, J. A. NEUBAUER, AND N. H. EDELMAN. Enhancement of expiratory triangularis sterni nerve (TSN) activity following severe hypoxia. *FASEB J. 3*(4):A1159, 1989.

40. PARISI, R. A., J. E. MELTON, M. J. WASICKO, J. A. NEUBAUER, Q. P. YU, AND N.H. EDELMAN. Phrenic responsiveness to carotid sinus nerve stimulation during progressive brain hypoxia. *FASEB J. 2*:1507, 1988.

41. RIGATTO, H. Control of ventilation in the newborn. *Ann. Rev. Physiol. 46*:661–674, 1984.

42. ROTHMAN, S. M. Synaptic activity mediates death of hypoxic neurons. *Science 220*:536–537, 1983.

43. SANTIAGO, T. V., J. A. NEUBAUER, AND N. H. EDELMAN. Correlation between ventilation and brain blood flow during hypoxic sleep. *J. Appl. Physiol. 60*:295–298, 1986.

44. SCHURR, A., W-Q. DONG, K. H. REID, C. A. WEST, AND B. M. RIGOR. Lactic acidosis and recovery of neuronal function following cerebral hypoxia *in vitro*. *Brain Res. 438*:311–314, 1988.

45. SICK, T. J., M. ROSENTHAL, J. C. LaMANNA, AND P. L. LUTZ. Brain potassium ion homeostasis, anoxia, and metabolic inhibition in turtles and rats. *Am. J. Physiol. 243*:R281–R288, 1982.

46. ULTSCH, G. R., AND D. C. JACKSON. Long-term submergence at 3°C of the turtle, *Chrysemys picta belli*, in normoxic and severely hypoxic water. I. Survival, gas exchange, and acid-base status. *J. Exp. Biol. 96*:11–28, 1982.

47. WASICKO, M. J., J. E. MELTON, J. A. NEUBAUER, N. KRAWCIW, AND N. H. EDELMAN. Cervical sympathetic and phrenic nerve responses to progressive brain hypoxia. *J. Appl. Physiol., 68*:53–58, 1990.

48. WASICKO, M. J., J. A. NEUBAUER, J. E. MELTON, A. M. HARANGOZO, AND N. H. EDELMAN. The effect of progressive brain hypoxia on the respiratory activity of the hypoglossal nerve (Abstr). *Fed. Proc. 46*:1418, 1987.

49. WEIL, J. V., AND C. W. ZWILLICH. Assessment of ventilatory response to hypoxia: methods and interpretation. *Chest 70*(Suppl):124–128, 1976.

50. WINN, H. R., R. RUBIO, AND R. M. BERNE. Brain adenosine concentration during hypoxia in rats. *Am. J. Physiol. 241*:H235–H242, 1981.

51. WOOD, J. D., W. J. WATSON, AND A. J. DRUCKER. The effect of hypoxia on brain gamma-aminobutyric acid levels. *J. Neurochem. 15*:603–608, 1968.

52. WU, J-Y. Purification, characterization, and kinetic studies of GAD and GABA-T from mouse brain. In: *GABA in Nervous System Function*, ed. E. Roberts, T. Chase and D. Tower. New York: Raven Press, 1976, pp. 7–55.

53. YU, Q. P., J. A. NEUBAUER, J. E. MELTON, M. J. WASICKO, J. K-J. LI, N. KRAWCIW, AND N.H. EDELMAN. Effect of brain hypoxia on the dynamic characteristics of the peak and frequency of phrenic nerve (Abstr). *FASEB J. 2*(5):A1508, 1988.

Index